Neurostereology

Unbiased Stereology of Neural Systems

Neurostereology
Unbiased Stereology of Neural Systems

Edited by
PETER R. MOUTON, PhD

WILEY Blackwell

Library of Congress Cataloging-in-Publication Data

Neurostereology : unbiased stereology of neural systems / edited by Peter R. Mouton.
    p. ; cm.
  Includes bibliographical references and index.
  ISBN 978-1-118-44421-4 (cloth : alk. paper) – ISBN 978-1-118-44413-9 (epdf) –
ISBN 978-1-118-44417-7 – ISBN 978-1-118-44418-4 (epub) – ISBN 978-1-118-44420-7 (emobi)
  I. Mouton, Peter R., editor of compilation.
  [DNLM: 1. Brain–anatomy & histology. 2. Brain–pathology. 3. Image Processing, Computer-Assisted.
4. Neuroimaging. 5. Stereotaxic Techniques. WL 300]
  QP360.5
  612.8'2–dc23
                                                                    2013029211

A catalogue record for this book is available from the British Library.

Set in 10.5/12 pt Times by Toppan Best-set Premedia Limited
Printed and bound in Malaysia by Vivar Printing Sdn Bhd

1 2014

Contents

Contributors

Niyazi Acer

Department of Anatomy
Erciyes Univesity School of Medicine
Kayseri, Turkey

Sandra A. Acosta

Center of Excellence for Aging and Brain Repair
Department of Neurosurgery and Brain Repair
University of South Florida College of Medicine
Tampa, FL, USA

S. Omar Ahmad

Doisy College of Health Sciences
St. Louis University
St. Louis, MO, USA

Clelia Ahrens-Barbeau

Department of Neuroscience
NIH-UCSD Autism Center of Excellence
University of California San Diego
La Jolla, CA, USA

Luis Alarcon-Martinez

Barrow Neurological Institute
Phoenix, AZ, USA

Phalguni Anand Alladi

Department of Neurophysiology
National Institute of Mental Health and Neurosciences
Bangalore, India

Hassan Azari

Department of Anatomical Sciences
School of Medicine
Shiraz University of Medical Sciences
Shiraz, Iran

Cynthia Carter Barnes

Department of Neuroscience
NIH-UCSD Autism Center of Excellence
University of California San Diego
La Jolla, CA, USA

Paula C. Bickford

Center of Excellence for Aging and Brain Repair
Department of Neurosurgery and Brain Repair
University of South Florida College of Medicine
Tampa, FL, USA
James A. Haley Veterans Affairs Hospital
Tampa, FL, USA

Cesar V. Borlongan   Center of Excellence for Aging and Brain Repair
                              Department of Neurosurgery and Brain Repair
                              University of South Florida College of Medicine
                              Tampa, FL, USA

Mark W. Burke   Department of Physiology and Biophysics
                              College of Medicine
                              Howard University School of Medicine
                              Washington, DC, USA

Mark T. Butt   Tox Path Specialists, LLC
                              Frederick, MD, USA

Michael E. Calhoun   Department of Neuroscience
                              NIH-UCSD Autism Center of Excellence
                              University of California San Diego
                              La Jolla, CA, USA

Eric Courchesne   Department of Neuroscience
                              NIH-UCSD Autism Center of Excellence
                              University of California San Diego
                              La Jolla, CA, USA

Peter Dockery   Anatomy School of Medicine
                              National University of Ireland
                              Galway, Ireland

Nina Eriksen   Research Laboratory for Stereology and Neuroscience
                              Bispebjerg Hospital
                              University Hospital of Copenhagen
                              Copenhagen, Denmark

Melodie J. Hallet   Department of Neuroscience
                              NIH-UCSD Autism Center of Excellence
                              University of California San Diego
                              La Jolla, CA, USA

Patrick R. Hof   Fishberg Department of Neuroscience
                              Seaver Autism Center
                              Mount Sinai School of Medicine
                              New York, NY, USA
                              Friedman Brain Institute
                              New York, NY, USA

Zahra Vojdani Jahromi   Department of Anatomical Sciences
                              School of Medicine
                              Shiraz University of Medical Sciences
                              Shiraz, Iran

Shozo Jinno   Department of Developmental Molecular Anatomy
                              Graduate School of Medical Sciences
                              Kyushu University
                              Fukuoka, Japan

Ahmad A. Khundakar   Institute for Ageing and Health
                           Newcastle University Campus for Ageing and Vitality
                           Newcastle upon Tyne, UK

Rocio Leal-Campanario Barrow Neurological Institute
                           Phoenix, AZ, USA

Zerina Lokmic   Department of Plastic and Maxillofacial Surgery
                           Department of Nursing Research
                           Murdoch Children's Research Institute
                           The Royal Children's Hospital
                           Parkville, Victoria, Australia

Stephen Macknik   Barrow Neurological Institute
                           Phoenix, AZ, USA

Kebreten F. Manaye   Department of Physiology and Biophysics
                           College of Medicine
                           Howard University
                           Washington, DC, USA

Susana Martinez-Conde Barrow Neurological Institute
                           Phoenix, AZ, USA

William L. Maxwell   Department of Anatomy
                           School of Biological Sciences
                           University of Glasgow
                           Glasgow, UK

Peter R. Mouton   Department of Pathology and Cell Biology
                           Byrd Alzheimer's Disease Institute
                           University of South Florida
                           Tampa, FL, USA

Mohammad Reza Namavar Histomorphometry and Stereology Research Center
                           Shiraz University of Medical Sciences
                           Department of Anatomical Sciences
                           School of Medicine
                           Shiraz, Iran

Bente Pakkenberg   Research Laboratory for Stereology and Neuroscience
                           Bispebjerg Hospital
                           University Hospital of Copenhagen
                           Copenhagen, Denmark

JiHyuk Park   Yonsei University
                           Seoul, South Korea

Karen Pierce   Department of Neuroscience
                           NIH-UCSD Autism Center of Excellence
                           University of California San Diego
                           La Jolla, CA, USA

Samira Raminfard
Department of Anatomical Sciences
School of Medicine
Shiraz University of Medical Sciences
Shiraz, Iran

Katarina Semendeferi
Department of Anthropology
University of California San Diego
San Diego, CA, USA

Naoki Tajiri
Center of Excellence for Aging and Brain Repair
Department of Neurosurgery and Brain Repair
University of South Florida College of Medicine
Tampa, Florida, USA

Alan J. Thomas
Institute for Ageing and Health
Newcastle University Campus for Ageing and Vitality
Newcastle upon Tyne, UK

Mehmet Turgut
Department of Neurosurgery
Adnan Menderes University School of Medicine
Aydın, Turkey

Neha Uppal
Fishberg Department of Neuroscience
Seaver Autism Center
Mount Sinai School of Medicine
New York, NY, USA
Friedman Brain Institute
New York, NY, USA

Preface

An interviewer once asked Woody Allen whether you could see the human soul with a microscope. "Yes, you can," he said, "but you need one of those good ones with two eyepieces."

Beyond seeing the microstructures that comprise the nervous system, one possible location for the human soul, neuroscientists often face the task of quantifying what we see. We also share the responsibility to do our best to accurately convey our results to each other, which led to the idea for this book.

After he finished his first stereology study a few years ago, a postdoctoral student in my lab sent his coauthors a manuscript to review, along with a statement that read, to the effect, "like most stereology papers, the discussion section is short."

When I asked him to elaborate, he said his reading of the literature showed that stereology papers generally have shorter discussion sections than nonstereology papers. With systematic-random sampling and unbiased estimators, the methodology avoids a wide range of potential pitfalls, problems, and assumptions associated with quantifying microstructures.

"When writing a paper," he said, "the author simply includes the details of their stereology approach in the methodology. There is little to no need for further justification in the discussion."

The situation is different for some areas of neuroscience, he explained, such as his field of experimental psychology, where the goal is to quantify animal behavior. Reviewers expect authors to detail all the possible confounds in the design and placement of the testing apparatus, motivational features of the task, and demands placed on the animal's abilities, along with a full statistical analysis of variables and covariables.

For stereology, he concluded, "you just discuss whether changes such as fewer neurons were revealed by the study and the implications of those findings for the hypothesis in question."

I reviewed his paper with this idea in mind. Well organized and written in the usual manner, the materials and methods section included descriptions of the procedures with correct citations for the stereological approaches such as the Cavalieri-point counting technique, disector principle, and the optical fractionator. As expected from a post doc in experimental psychology, the draft included a thorough statistical analysis of the findings with the total observed variability in the results partitioned into biological sources and method error. The concise discussion reviewed his findings relative to the original hypothesis and ended with a short conclusion. The study was submitted to a prominent peer-reviewed journal and was accepted with only minor revisions.

In the years since, my informal survey of stereology and nonstereology papers reveals that perhaps he was right. Because unbiased stereology has been carefully vetted for accuracy, with empirical comparisons to gold standards and rigorous reviews by theoretical experts, authors do not spend much effort justifying, rationalizing, or analyzing the approaches, other than to explain any caveats that apply. Provided the investigators clearly state and properly apply the methods, the results should be reliable.

Yet Luis M. Cruz-Orive, the esteemed stereologist from Spain, reminds us that the situation is not always that simple.

"Stereology," according to Professor Cruz-Orive, "is a committed task." That is, generating reliable stereology results requires a commitment by each investigator to thoroughly identify and eliminate all known sources of systematic error (bias) from his or her study design.

Neurostereology: Unbiased Stereology of Neural Systems brings together theory and research from neuroscientists who explore the issues, pitfalls, and potential confounds associated with the applications of design-based stereology to their research. Contributions from neuroscientists in Turkey, Iran, Denmark, India, Japan, Australia, the United Kingdom, and the United States use unbiased stereology to quantify a diverse range of neural structures, from macroscopic studies of brain volumes on MRI images to detailed microstructures of unmyelinated nerve fibers. Because the authors were encouraged to explore the practical issues in their work, readers will find the length of discussion sections perhaps a bit longer, and hopefully with more valuable insights, than those found in the majority of published stereology papers. For neuroscientists with previous experience, as well as those just starting to ease into stereology, these papers exemplify applications to a wide range of tissues, from human brains to marine mammals and genetic, toxicological, and chemical models in rodents. In each case, the authors identify and address a number of important pitfalls, such as the reference trap, recognition bias from inadequate staining, profile versus object counting, and poorly defined reference spaces.

Readers will note that despite the major differences in these studies with regard to the types of tissues analyzed, wide range of hypotheses tested, and different microstructures analyzed, each study applies similar principles and practices of unbiased stereology. In each case, the investigators identify an anatomical reference space of interest, apply systematic random sampling, use unbiased estimators, and sample with sufficient stringency to generate reliable results. In some cases, particularly those involving autopsied human brains or less common species of animals, unavoidable conditions complicate a fully unbiased study design, that is, one free of all methodological bias. In those cases, the authors point out to the readers if and how these issues might influence their findings.

My hope is that you find this book not only illuminating but helpful in your efforts to apply the methods of design-based stereology in an effective manner. Professor Cruz-Orive reminds us that stereology depends on a tacit agreement from each investigator to identify and eliminate all known sources of systematic error (bias) to the greatest extent possible. In line with this adage, *Neurostereology: Unbiased Stereology of Neural Systems* offers a multidisciplinary range of studies from an international group of neuroscientists who did their collective best to get it right.

Peter R. Mouton
Department of Pathology and Cell Biology
Byrd Alzheimer's Disease Institute
University of South Florida
Tampa, Florida, USA

Neurostereology

Unbiased Stereology of Neural Systems

1 Stereological Estimation of Brain Volume and Surface Area from MR Images

Niyazi Acer[1] and Mehmet Turgut[2]

[1] *Department of Anatomy, Erciyes University School of Medicine, Kayseri, Turkey*
[2] *Department of Neurosurgery, Adnan Menderes University School of Medicine, Aydın, Turkey*

Background

Stereology combines mathematical and statistical approaches to estimate three-dimensional (3D) parameters of biological objects based on two-dimensional (2D) observations obtained from sections through arbitrary-shaped objects (for reviews of design-based stereology, see Howard and Reed, 1998; Mouton, 2002, 2011; Evans et al., 2004). Among the first-order parameters quantified using unbiased stereology are *length* using plane or sphere probes, *surface area* using lines, *volume* using points, and *number* using the 3D disector probe. These approaches estimate stereology parameters with known precision for any object regardless of its shape.

These criteria for stereological estimation of volume and surface area are met by standard magnetic resonance imaging (MRI) and computed tomography (CT) scans, as well as tissue sections separated by a known distance with systematic random sampling, that is, taking a random first section followed by systematic sampling through the entire reference space (Gundersen and Jensen, 1987; Regeur and Pakkenberg, 1989; Roberts et al., 2000; Mouton, 2002, 2011; García-Fiñana et al., 2003; Acer et al., 2008, 2010). Numerous studies have been reported using MRI to estimate brain and related volumes by stereologic and segmentation methods in adults (Gur et al., 2002; Allen et al., 2003; Acer et al., 2007, 2008; Jovicich et al., 2009), children (Knickmeyer et al., 2008), and newborns (Anbeek et al., 2008; Weisenfeld and Warfield, 2009; Nisari et al., 2012).

The Cavalieri Principle

Named after the Italian mathematician Bonaventura Cavalieri (1598–1647), the Cavalieri principle estimates the first-order parameter volume (V) from an equidistant and parallel set of 2D slices through the 3D object. As detailed later, the approach uses the area on the cut surfaces of sections through the reference space (region of interest) to estimate size (volume) of whole organs and subregions of interest. The point counting technique for area estimation uses a point-grid system superimposed with random placement onto each section through the reference space (Gundersen and Jensen, 1987). The number of points falling within the reference area is counted for each section (Figure 1.1). Total *V* of a 3D object, *x*, is estimated by Equation 1.1:

Neurosterology: Unbiased Stereology of Neural Systems, First Edition. Edited by Peter R. Mouton.
© 2014 John Wiley & Sons, Inc. Published 2014 by John Wiley & Sons, Inc.

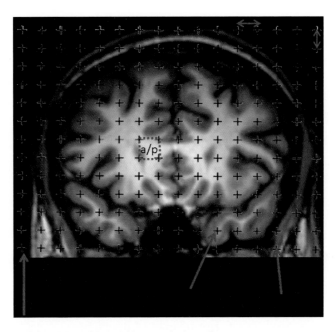

Figure 1.1   Illustration of point counting grid overlaid on one brain section.

$$V = \int_a^b A(x)dx, \tag{1.1}$$

where $A(x)$ is the area of the section of the object passing through the point $x \, \varepsilon \, (a, b)$, and b is the caliper diameter of the object perpendicular to section planes. The function $A(x)$ is bounded and integratable in a bounded domain (a, b), which represents the orthogonal linear projection of the object on the sampling axis (García-Fiñana et al., 2003; Kubínová et al., 2005).

The Cavalieri estimator of volume is constructed from a sample of equidistant observations of f, with a distance T apart, as follows (Eq. 1.2):

$$V = T\sum_{k \in Z} f(x_0 + kT) = T(f_1 + f_2 + f_3 + \cdots + f_n), \tag{1.2}$$

where x_0 is a uniform random variable in the interval $(0,T)$ and $\{f_1, f_2, \ldots, f_n\}$ is the set of equidistant observations of f at the sampling points which lie in (a, b). In many applications, Q represents the volume of a structure, and $f(x)$ is the area of the intersection between the structure and a plane that is perpendicular to a given sampling axis at the point of abscissa x (García-Fiñana et al., 2003; García-Fiñana, 2006; García-Fiñana et al., 2009).

Cavalieri Principle with Point Counting

Unbiased and efficient volume estimates with known precision (Roberts et al., 2000; García-Fiñana et al., 2003) can be obtained from a set of parallel slices separated by a known distance (T), and sampled in a systematic random manner. These criteria are easily obtained from standard sets of MRI and CT scans (Roberts et al., 2000; Acer et al., 2008, 2010).

To apply the point-counting method, a square grid system is superimposed with random placement onto each Cavalieri section or slice and the number of points falling within the reference area (area of interest) counted on each section (Figure 1.1). Finally, an unbiased estimate of volume is calculated from Equation 1.3:

$$V = T \times (a/p) \times (P_1 + P_2 + P_3 + \cdots + P_n), \qquad (1.3)$$

where n is the number of sections, P_1, P_2, . . . , P_n show point counts, a/p represents the area associated with each test point, and T is the sectioning interval.

We used software that allowed the user to automatically sum the area of each slice and determine brain volumes by the Cavalieri principle. An unbiased estimate of volume was obtained as the sum of the estimated areas of the structure transects on consecutive systematic sections multiplied by the distance between sections, that is, $V = \Sigma A \cdot T$. The program allowed the user to determine contrast, select true threshold value to estimate the point count automatically (Denby et al., 2009).

Coefficient of Error (CE) and Confidence Interval (CI) for Volume Estimation

The precision of volume estimation by the Cavalieri method was estimated by CE. Based on the original work of Matheron, the CE was adapted to the Cavalieri volume estimator by Gundersen and Jensen (1987) and more recently simplied by a number of stereologists (Gundersen et al., 1999; García-Fiñana et al., 2003; Cruz-Orive, 2006; Ertekin et al., 2010; Hall and Ziegel, 2011). The CE is useful for estimating the contribution of sampling error to the overall (total) variation for stereological estimates. A pilot study of the mean CE estimate allows the user to optimize sampling parameters, for example, mean CE less than one-half of total variation; to select the appropriate number of MRI sections through the reference space; and to set the optimal density of the point or cycloid grid.

García-Fiñana (2006) pointed out that the asymptotic distribution of the parameter volume as its variance is strongly connected with the smoothness properties of the measurement function. Using the Cavalieri method, we constructed both CE and a CI value for estimation of brain volumes. The first calculation involved the estimation of volume, variance of the volume estimate, and bounded intervals for the volume by Eq. (1.3).

Second, Var ($\mathbf{Q_T}$) was estimated via Eq. (1.4) according to Kiêu (1997), which first requires calculation of $\alpha(\mathbf{q})$, C_0, C_1, C_2, and C_4 (Table 1.1):

$$Var(\hat{Q}_T) = \alpha(q) \times (3C_0 - 4C_1 + C_2)T^2, \quad q \in [0, 1]. \qquad (1.4)$$

Eq. (1.5) leads to

$$C_k = \sum_{i=1}^{n-k} f_i f_{i+k}, \quad k = 1, 2, \ldots n - 1. \qquad (1.5)$$

The quantities C_0, C_1, and C_2 can be computed from the systematic data sample (García-Fiñana et al., 2003).

The smoothness constant (q) is then estimated from Eq. (1.6) as given in the following:

$$q = \max \left\{ 0, \frac{1}{2 \log 2} \log \left[\frac{(3C_0 - 4C_2 + C_4)}{(3C_0 - 4C_1 + C_2)} \right] - \frac{1}{2} \right\}. \qquad (1.6)$$

Table 1.1   Calculation of the constants C_0, C_1, C_2, and C_4 for brain volume

Section(i)	P_i	P_i^2	$P_i.P_{i+1}$	$P_i.P_{i+2}$	$P_i.P_{i+4}$
1	26	676	6468	2548	3432
2	66	4356	12,936	8712	10,296
3	98	9604	20,592	15,288	15,974
4	132	17,424	25,428	21,516	20,856
5	156	24,336	25,754	24,648	23,400
6	163	26,569	23,700	24,450	18,745
7	158	24,964	17,250	18,170	13,430
8	150	22,500	9775	12,750	3300
9	115	13,225	1870	2530	0
10	85	7225	0	0	0
11	22	484	0	0	0
		C_0	C_1	C_2	C_4
	1171	**151,363**	**143,773**	**130,612**	**109,433**

The coefficient $\alpha(q)$ has the following expression:

$$\alpha(q) = \frac{\Gamma(2q+2)\zeta(2q+2)\cos(\tau q)}{2\tau^{2q+2}(1 - 2^{2q-1})}, \quad q \in [0, 1], \tag{1.7}$$

where Γ and ζ denote the gamma function and the Riemann zeta function, respectively. For fairly regular, quasi-ellipsoidal objects, q approaches 1, and for irregular objects, q approaches 0. Under these circumstances, $\alpha(0) = 0.83$ and $\alpha(1) = 0.0041$ (García-Fiñana et al., 2003).

The bounded interval for the cerebral volume was obtained by Eq. (1.8):

$$\hat{Q}_T mT\lambda_q \sqrt{\alpha(q)(3C_0 - 4C_1 + C_2}. \tag{1.8}$$

Note that Eq. (1.8) gives the approximate lower and upper bounds for $V_2 - V_1$.

Example for Cerebral Volume, CE, and CI

Examples are provided for estimation of cerebral volume with upper and lower CI values and CE. To estimate brain volume, we used the total data set of 158 images with slice thickness 1 mm split into 15 Cavalieri planes, that is, every 10th magnetic resonance (MR) image with a different random starting point. Thus, each Cavalieri sample represents the area of cerebral cortex of a set of MR images at distance $T = 10 \cdot 1\,\text{mm} = 10\,\text{mm}$ apart (Table 1.1).

We illustrate the calculation steps involved in the estimation of a lower and upper bound for the true cerebral cortex volume by applying Eq. (1.8) to one set of Cavalieri planes (i.e., 26, 66, 98, 132, 156, 163, 158, 150, 115, 85, 22). This data sample represents the area of cerebral cortex in square centimeters on $n = 11$ MR sections a distance $T = 1\,\text{cm}$ apart. The Cavalieri volume for cerebrum was obtained using Eq. (1.3) as follows:

$$V = 1 \times 1^2 \times (26 + 66 + \cdots + 85 + 22) = 1171.0\,\text{cm}^3. \tag{1.9}$$

$$C_0 = (676^2 + 4356^2 + \cdots + 484^2) = 151363$$
$$C_1 = (26 \times 66 + 66 \times 98 + \cdots + 85 \times 22) = 145489$$
$$C_2 = (26 \times 98 + 66 \times 132 + \cdots + 115 \times 22) = 130612$$
$$C_4 = (26 \times 132 + 66 \times 156 + \cdots + 158 \times 22) = 109433.$$

(1.10)

The smoothness constant (q) is estimated from Eq. (1.6) as follows:

$$q = \left\{0, \frac{1}{2\log 2}\log\left[\frac{3 \times 151363 - 4 \times 130612 + 109433}{3 \times 151363 - 4 \times 145489 + 130612}\right] - \frac{1}{2}\right\} = 0.815.$$

(1.11)

Applying Eq. (1.7) with $q = 0.815$ leads to $\alpha(q)$ as follows:

$$\alpha(0.815) = \frac{\Gamma(2 \times 0.815 + 2)\zeta(2 \times 0.815 + 2)\cos(3.14 \times 0.815)}{(2\tau)^{2 \times 0.815 + 2}(1 - 2^{2 \times 0.815 - 1})} = 0.008.$$

(1.12)

Therefore, the estimate of $\mathrm{Var}\left(\hat{Q}_T\right)$ obtained via Eq. (1.4) is

$$\mathrm{Var}\left(\hat{Q}_T\right) = \alpha(q)(3C_0 - 4C_1 + C_2) \times T2$$
$$\mathrm{Var}\left(\hat{Q}_T\right) = 0.008 \times (3 \times 151363 - 4 \times 145489 + 130612) \times (1)^2$$
$$\mathrm{Var}\left(\hat{Q}_T\right) = 22.65.$$

The CE for this estimate is calculated as shown in Eq. (1.13):

$$CE(Q_T) = \sqrt{22.65/1171} = 4\%.$$

(1.13)

Values for CI were calculated using Eq. (1.8):

$$\left(1171 - 3.38 \times \sqrt{22.65}, 1171 + 3.38 \times \sqrt{22.65},\right) = (1154 - 1187)\,\mathrm{cm}^3$$
$$V_2 - V_1 = 1154\,\mathrm{cm}^3 - 1187\,\mathrm{cm}^3.$$

(1.14)

This example allowed us to identify the λ value as 3.38 according to García-Fiñana (2006). Predictive CE values were calculated using the R program using developed R codes to calculate the contribution to the predictive CE. After the initial setup and preparation of the formula, the point counts and other data were entered for each scan, and the final data were obtained automatically using the R program (Appendix A).

Volume Estimation Using Spatial Grid of Points

The method of volume estimation using a spatial grid of points (Gundersen and Jensen, 1987; Cruz-Orive, 1997; Kubínová and Janáček, 2001) is an efficient modification of the Cavalieri principle. If a cubic spatial grid of points is applied, the object volume can be estimated by the formula (Eq. 1.15):

$$V = u^3 \times P,$$

(1.15)

where u is the grid constant (distance between two neighboring points of the grid), and P is the number of grid points falling into the object.

Using slice thickness and distance between two test points of the grid for the same value such as 1 cm leads to simple estimates of brain volume. A 1 cm × 1 cm × 1 cm grid was chosen, indicating a grid point spacing of 1 cm^3 in the plane of the image and through the depth of the volume.

Surface Area Estimation

Surface area can be estimated on vertical uniform random (VUR) and isotropic uniform random (IUR) tissue sections (Baddeley et al., 1986). Estimations of surfaces require randomness of slice direction, also known as isotropy, as well as slice position (Henery and Mayhew, 1989; Mayhew et al., 1996; Roberts et al., 2000).

Estimation of Surface Area Using Vertical Sections

With this approach, surface area is sampled at systematic random positions in 3D and combines the Cavalieri principle with vertical sectioning (Baddeley et al., 1986), thus offering major advantages over earlier methods for estimation of surface area (Mayhew et al., 1990, 1996).

The vertical section technique for surface area estimation uses cycloid test probes (Baddeley et al., 1986). A cycloid probe is a line for which the length of arc oriented in a particular direction is proportional to the *sine* of the angle to vertical. The bias produced by taking VUR as opposed to IUR sections is exactly canceled by the inherent sine weighting of the orientation of the cycloid test lines; thus, IUR and VUR sections with cycloids are equivalent (Baddeley et al., 1986; Gual-Arnau and Cruz-Orive, 1998; Gokhale et al., 2004).

Vertical sections are planar sections longitudinal to either a fixed (but arbitrary) axial direction or perpendicular to a given horizontal plane. After rotating the object of interest by ø, the user cuts sections with uniform random position perpendicular to the vertical axis, thereby generating planes of fixed distance (T) apart, all vertical with respect to the horizontal reference plane (Baddeley et al., 1986; Howard and Reed, 2005). For example, if the horizontal plane is an axial section, coronal and sagittal sections will be vertical sections (Michel and Cruz-Orive, 1988; Pache et al., 1993). The 3D of objects is divided with uniform random position along each generating orientation to form n Cavalieri series of vertical sections (Figure 1.2a,b).

Both CT and MRI allow for sampling 3D objects into an exhaustive series of vertical sections in several systematic random orientations, each randomly offset with respect to a fixed vertical axis (Roberts et al., 2000). Thus, these data sets meet the requirement for isotropic and thus random orientations may be obtained for estimation of surface area as described previously (Roberts et al., 2000; Kubínová and Janácek, 2001).

A random direction of the uniform random line in the first orientation was selected as a random angle a from the interval (0°, 180°), then VUR sections generated a fixed distance T apart, $T = 1$ cm. Starting with a 5° random angle, the direction of vertical sections in the jth segment is given by the angle $aj = a_1 + (j - 1) \times (180°/m)$ ($j = 1, \ldots, m$) (Figure 1.3a–c). For example, if $m = 4$ and $a_1 = 5°$, then $a_2 = 5° + 1 \times (180°/4) = 50°$, $a_3 = 95°$, $a_4 = 140°$ (see Figure 1.3).

The relevant formula for estimating surface area from an exhaustive series of vertical sections was calculated from Equation 1.16 (Roberts et al., 2000; Ronan et al., 2006; Acer et al., 2010):

$$S = 2 \times T \times a / l \times I. \tag{1.16}$$

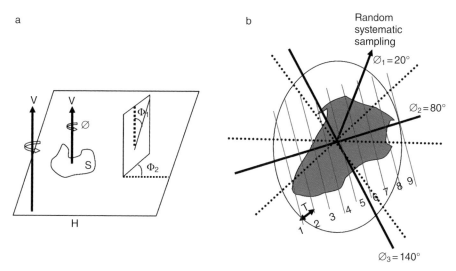

Figure 1.2 (a) The object is fixed horizontal plane (H), and is given isotropic rotation on the horizontal plane. (b) The object is divided with uniform random position along each generating orientation ($n = 3$) to form nine Cavalieri sections of vertical section. $\emptyset_1$ = random angle (obtained in the interural π/n, n = number of orientations, T is the interval of the sections. For example, if $n = 3$ and $\emptyset_1 = 20°$, then $\emptyset_2 = 20° + 1 \times (180°/3) = 80°$, $\emptyset_3 = 140°$.

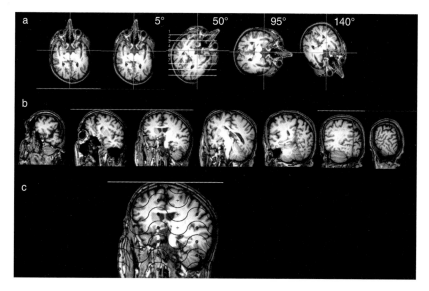

Figure 1.3 (a) An example of four systematic orientations (if $n = 4$ and $a_1 = 5°$, then $a_2 = 5° + 1 \times (180°/4) = 50°$, $a_3 = 95°$, $a_4 = 140°$. (b) A total of seven Cavalieri sections with slice separation (T) of 2 cm. (c) Illustration of cycloid probe overlaid on one subject all brain sections.

We modified the formula for surface area estimations of radiological images as shown in Equation 1.17:

$$S = \frac{2}{n} \times T \times \left(\frac{a/l \times SU}{SL} \right) \times I, \qquad (1.17)$$

where n is the number of random systematic orientation, a/l is the ratio of the test area to the cycloid length, T is the distance between serial sections, "SU" is the scale unit of the printed film, "SL" is the measured length of the scale printed on the film, and I is the number of intersections on all sections.

Eqs. (1.18, 1.19) that were used to estimate the surface area of an object by vertical sections are given in the following two formulas:

$$\tilde{S}_{n1} = \frac{\pi}{n}\left(\hat{f}_1 + \hat{f}_2 + \ldots + \hat{f}_n\right) \tag{1.18}$$

$$\hat{f}_i = \frac{2}{\pi} \cdot \frac{a}{l} \cdot T \cdot \sum_{j=1}^{k_i} I_{ij}, \quad i = 1, 2, \ldots, n \tag{1.19}$$

$$\hat{f}_1 = \frac{2}{\pi} \times 1 \times 1 \times 457 = 291.109$$

$$\hat{f}_2 = \frac{2}{\pi} \times 1 \times 1 \times 426 = 271.362$$

$$\hat{f}_3 = \frac{2}{\pi} \times 1 \times 1 \times 389 = 247.793 \tag{1.20}$$

$$\hat{f}_4 = \frac{2}{\pi} \times 1 \times 1 \times 382 = 243.334$$

$$\tilde{S}_{n1} = \frac{\pi}{4}(291.109 + 271.362 + 247.793 + 243.334) = 827.0749 \text{ cm}^2,$$

where n represents the number of random systematic orientation about a central vertical axis through the object, a/l represents the ratio of test area to cycloid test length, T represents distance between Cavalieri vertical sections, I_{ij} represent the number of intersections between cycloids and the jth vertical trace of the ith series; k_i is the number of nonempty vertical sections in that series ($n = 4$, $T = 1$ cm, $a/l = 1$ cm, $\sum_{i=1}^{n} I_i = 1654$):

$$\hat{S}_{n2} = \frac{2}{n} \cdot T \cdot \frac{a}{l} \cdot \sum_{i=1}^{n} I_i \quad I_i = \sum_{i=1}^{ki} I_{ij} \tag{1.19}$$

$$\hat{S}_{n2} = \frac{2 \times 1 \times 1 \times 1654}{4} \tag{1.21}$$

$$\hat{S}_{n2} = 827.074 \text{ cm}^2.$$

Four orientations were used to calculate the a/l using $d = 0.637$ cm. In our experiment, cycloid test lines had a 1-cm ratio of area associated with each cycloid for a/l according to Eq. 1.22 (Figure 1.4). In each orientation, the number of intersections on each of the MRI sections was counted on Cavalieri slices:

$$a/l = \pi \times d / 2 \tag{1.22}$$

$$a/l = 3.14 \times 0.637 / 2 = 1 \text{ cm}. \tag{1.23}$$

After transferring MR images to a personal computer, surface area estimation was done using different softwares. The first approach required conversion of the images to analyze format using

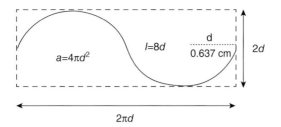

Figure 1.4 Cycloid test probe. Area per length (a/l) = 1 cm.

ImageJ, which is available free from the NIH (http://rsb.info.nih.gov/ij). After formatting, hdr or img file was opened using MRIcro (http://www.mccauslandcenter.sc.edu/mricro/mricro/index .html). MRIcro allows for rotation of each image for selection of random angles (Figure 1.3). Finally, the stereological parameters were estimated using EasyMeasure software.

Error Prediction for Surface Area for Vertical Section Method

Error prediction was divided into three processes: systematic orientations; systematic parallel sections for each orientation; and intersection counting with a cycloid test system on each section (Cruz-Orive and Gual-Arnau, 2002):

(1) $Var_\theta(\tilde{S}_n)$, the variance due to n systematic orientations
(2) $Var_{cav}(\tilde{S}_n)$, the variance due to Cavalieri vertical sections
(3) $Var_{cyc}(\tilde{S}_n)$, the variance due to application of cyloid probe,

where n represents the number of orientations.
    The CE is directly related to the variance of the surface area estimator:

$$CE(\tilde{S}_n) = \frac{\sqrt{Var(\tilde{S}_n)}}{S_n} \times 100 \qquad (1.24)$$

$$CE^2(\tilde{S}_n) = CE_\theta^2(\tilde{S}_n) + CE_{cav}^2(\tilde{S}_n) + CE_{cyc}^2(\tilde{S}_n) \qquad (1.25)$$

$$ce(\tilde{S}_n) = \sqrt{ce_\theta^2(\tilde{S}) + ce_{cav}^2(\tilde{S}) + ce_{cyc}^2(\tilde{S})}, \qquad (1.26)$$

where CE_θ, CE_{cav} and CE_{cyc} are orientation, Cavalieri, and cycloid CE values, respectively.
    Although error prediction for surface area on systematic sampled images has not been previously reported in the literature, Cruz-Orive and Gual-Arnau (2002) examined precision of circular sytematic sampling and discussed error prediction formulae for the surface area estimator on vertical sections. For this approach based on Cruz-Orive and Gual-Arnau (2002), the variance from each level sampling in vertical section provides useful information for optimization of sample size to design at different stages for estimation of cerebral surface. The error variance $\widehat{var}_m(\tilde{S}_n)$ based on a global model was calculated from systematic sampling using a semicircle:

$$\widehat{var}_m(\tilde{S}_n) = \frac{r^2 B_{2m+2}(\hat{C}_0 - \hat{C}_1 - \hat{v}_n)}{(B_{2m+2} - B_{2m+2}(1/n)) \cdot n^{2m+3}} + T^2\hat{v}_n, \quad n \geq 2, m = 0, 1, \ldots \qquad (1.27)$$

The right side of Eq. (1.27) $T^2\hat{v}_n$ estimates the local error. The constants $\hat{C}_0$ and $\hat{C}_1$ (Table 1.3) are determined by

$$C_k = \sum_{i=1}^{n-k} f_i f_{i+k}, \quad i = 1, 2, \ldots, n. \tag{1.28}$$

$B_{2j}(x)$ and $B_{2j}(0) \equiv B_{2j}$ are a Bernoulli polynomal and number, respectively, as shown in Eq. (1.29):

$$B_2(x) = x^2 - x + 1/6, \, B_4(x) = x^4 - 2x^3 + x^2 - 1/30. \tag{1.29}$$

Choosing between the two values $m = 0$, 1 will typically suffice:

$$\hat{D}_m = \frac{\hat{C}_0 - \hat{C}_2 - \hat{v}_n}{\hat{C}_0 - \hat{C}_1 - \hat{v}_n} - \frac{B_{2m+2} - B_{2m+2}(2/n)}{B_{2m+2} - B_{2m+2}(1/n)}, \quad n \geq 4. \tag{1.30}$$

$$\text{For } m = 0, \frac{B_{2m+2}}{B_{2m+2} - B_{2m+2}(1/n)} = \frac{2(n-2)}{n-1}. \tag{1.31}$$

$$\text{For } m = 1, \frac{B_{2m+2} - B_{2m+2}(2/n)}{B_{2m+2} - B_{2m+2}(1/n)} = \frac{4(n-2)^2}{(n-1)^2}. \tag{1.32}$$

$$\hat{D}_0 = \frac{\hat{C}_0 - \hat{C}_2 - \hat{v}_n}{\hat{C}_0 - \hat{C}_1 - \hat{v}_n} - \frac{2(n-2)}{n-1}, \quad n \geq 4. \tag{1.33}$$

$$\hat{D}_1 = \frac{\hat{C}_0 - \hat{C}_2 - \hat{v}_n}{\hat{C}_0 - \hat{C}_1 - \hat{v}_n} - \frac{4(n-2)^2}{(n-1)^2}, \quad n \geq 4. \tag{1.34}$$

Input $m = 1$ and $m = 0$ into Equation 1.30 and if $|\hat{D}_0| \leq |\hat{D}_1|$, then $m = 0$ and otherwise $m = 1$. For $m = 0$, 1 use following Eq. (1.27)

$$\widehat{\text{var}_0}\left(\tilde{S}_n\right) = \max\left\{0, \frac{\pi T}{6(n-1)} \times \left(\hat{C}_0 - \hat{C}_1 - \hat{v}_n\right)\right\}, \quad n \geq 2,$$
$$\widehat{\text{var}_1}\left(\tilde{S}_n\right) = \max\left\{0, \frac{\pi T}{30(n-1)} \times \left(\hat{C}_0 - \hat{C}_1 - \hat{v}_n\right)\right\}, \quad n \geq 2. \tag{1.35}$$

We must compute $\hat{v}_n$:

$$\hat{v}_n = \sum_{i=1}^{n} \sigma_i^2. \tag{1.36}$$

After computating $\hat{v}_n$, we have to calculate σ_i^2 following Equation (1.37). σ_i^2 is the variance due to Cavalieri sampling in each orientation k:

$$\sigma_i^2 = \left(\frac{2}{\pi} \times \frac{a}{l}\right)^2 \times h^2 \times \left\{\alpha(q_i) \times \left[3\left(\hat{C}_{0i} - \hat{v}_{ni}\right) - 4\hat{C}_{1i} + 4\hat{C}_{2i}\right] + \hat{v}_{ni}\right\}, \quad n_i \geq 3,$$
$$\hat{C}_{ki} = \sum_{j=1}^{n_i-k} I_{ij} I_{i,j+2}, \quad k = 0, 1, \ldots, n_i - 1. \tag{1.37}$$

We assume that the measurement function has a smoothness constant $q_i \in [0,1]$ that

$$a(q) = \frac{\Gamma(2q+2)\zeta(2q+2)\cos(\tau q)}{2\tau^{2q+2}(1-2^{2q-1})}, \quad q \in [0,1]. \tag{1.7}$$

The gamma function (Γ) and the Reimann zeta function (ζ) are tabulated and available in most mathematical software packages. In particular, $\alpha(0) = 1/12$, $\alpha(1) = 1/240$, $\alpha(1/2) = \zeta(3)/(8\pi^2\log2)$.

To estimate $\alpha(q)$ we need the smoothness constant q, which in turn can be estimated from the data by Kiêu–Souchet's formula:

$$q = \max\left\{0, \frac{1}{2\log(2)} \cdot \log\left(\frac{3(\hat{C}_0 - \hat{v}_n) - 4\hat{C}_2 + \hat{C}_4}{3(\hat{C}_0 - \hat{v}_n) - 4\hat{C}_1 + \hat{C}_2}\right) - \frac{1}{2}\right\}, \quad n \geq 7 \tag{1.38}$$

Table 1.2 and Table 1.3 give us the results from the example data for CE.

After initial setup and preparation of the formula, the intersection counts and other data were entered for each scan, and the final data were obtained automatically using R program (Appendix B).

Table 1.2   Intersection counts for each section for brain surface area estimation (S1: first orientation; S2: second orientation, S3: third orientation; S4: fourth orientation)

Section number/ orientations	S1	S2	S3	S4
1	23	10	20	12
2	25	27	32	18
3	32	37	27	28
4	34	33	35	30
5	31	41	28	34
6	37	31	29	38
7	35	32	21	32
8	30	31	30	34
9	31	33	33	30
10	37	32	38	36
11	42	31	32	32
12	44	32	34	24
13	37	33	18	18
14	19	23	12	16
Total	457	426	389	382
$\hat{C}_0$	15,549	13,630	11,525	11,308
$\hat{C}_1$	14,819	12,976	10,856	10,916
$\hat{C}_2$	13,546	11,928	10,054	10,316
$\hat{C}_4$	10,748	9608	7873	8352
$\hat{q}$	0.38	0.303	0	0
$\widehat{\alpha(q)}$	0.03	0.037	0.08	0.08
$\widehat{\mathrm{var}_q(\tilde{S}_n)}$	191.96	167.36	159.04	136.47

Table 1.3   Intersection counts for each section for brain surface area estimation and function values

Orientation	Intersections	Function	f_i^2	$f_i f_{i+1}$	$f_i f_{i+2}$	$f_i f_{i+3}$
1	457	291.109	84,744.45	78,995.92	73,989.14	70,836.72
2	426	271.362	73,637.34	68,970.18	66,031.6	78,995.92
3	389	247.793	61,401.37	60,296.46	72,134.77	67,241.6
4	382	243.334	59,211.44	70,836.72	66,031.6	61,846.5
Total	1654	1,059.968	282,192.1	280,649.3	280,041.5	280,649.3
Cycloid length (cm)	0.637		**C0**	**C1**	**C2**	**C3**
A/L (cm)	1.00					
H (cm)	1					
Surface area CM^2	832.08					

Isotropic Cavalieri Design

According to Cruz-Orive et al. (2010), isotropic Cavalieri design has two stages:

(1)   Choose a sampling axis which isotropically orients with respect to the object.
(2)   Take Cavalieri sections through entire the object. The sections must be systematic and parallel a fixed distance thickness (T) apart with a random starting interval.

We rotated MR images at random on a horizontal plan, and then cut the series exhaustively with a Cavalieri stack of sections using ImageJ (Figure 1.5). The result is an isotropic Cavalieri stack of sections (Cruz-Orive et al., 2010).

All sections from one series were retained for the analyses, with $T = 1\,\text{cm}$ as the distance between midplane virtual slices. We used ImageJ software for surface area estimation with the following formula:

$$S = (4 / \pi) \times T \times (B_1 + B_2 + B_3 + \cdots + B_n). \tag{1.39}$$

Let B_i denote the boundary length ith planar sections:

$$S = (4 / \pi) \times 1 \times (20 + 42 + 49 + 62 + 69 + 98 + 129 + 112 + 32)$$
$$S = 915.92 \text{ cm}^3. \tag{1.40}$$

Sections Analyzed with Independent Grid Design

If the section parameters cannot be measured automatically using ImageJ, then a second-stage sampling design may be applied for the estimate, as described in the following according to Cruz-Orive et al. (2010).

A given planar test grid was superimposed isotropically and uniformly at random, and independently, on each of the n sections. For each brain, the grid was superimposed uniformly at random and independently on each section.

Figure 1.6 illustrates the independent grids design with $I_1 = 55$, $I_2 = 51$, $I_3 = 46$, . . . , $I_{10} = 90$. For either the independent or the registered grid designs, the unbiased estimator $\hat{S}$ in Equation 1.41 may be used with the two-stage unbiased estimator:

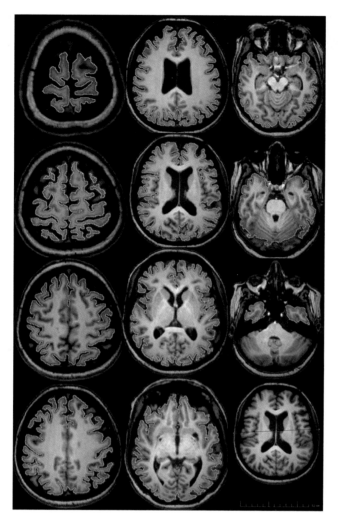

Figure 1.5   Isotropic Cavalieri sections.

$$S = T \times d \times (I_1 + I_2 + I_3 + \cdots + I_n) \tag{1.41}$$

$$S = 1 \times 1 \times (55 + 51 + 46 + 59 + 91 + 75 + 86 + 75 + 104 + 90)$$
$$S = 722 \text{ cm}^2. \tag{1.42}$$

A simple formula for variance of the surface area estimate was used according to Cruz-Orive et al. (2010):

$$Var_E(\tilde{V}) = \frac{\pi}{360} \times ST^4 + \frac{1}{4}\left(\frac{\zeta(3)}{2\pi^2} + \frac{1}{6}\right)STd^3$$
$$\text{var}(\tilde{V}) = 0.008727ST^4 + 0.056891STd^3. \tag{1.43}$$

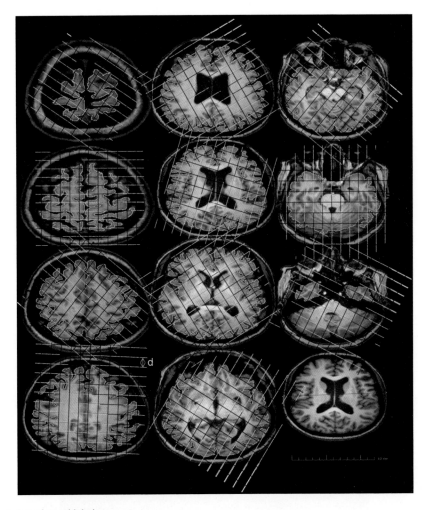

Figure 1.6   Independent grid design.

Surface Area Using the Invariator

The object of interest is a nonvoid, compact, and nonrandom subset Y of 3D Euclidean space with a piecewise smooth boundary ∂Y. The target parameters are the surface area $S(\partial Y)$ and the volume $V(Y)$ of Y. The classical construction of a motion invariant test line in 3D consists of choosing first a "pivotal" plane and then a motion invariant point z in this plane. Finally, a straight line normal to the pivotal plane through the point z is a motion invariant test line. The point z may be replaced with an IUR grid of points on the pivotal plane, as described by Cruz-Orive (2008). If a test line is drawn through each point of the grid and normal to the pivotal plane, the result is an IUR, the so-called unbounded "fakir probe" (Cruz-Orive, 1997; Cruz-Orive et al., 2010), a motion invariant test line in 3D. Using this construction to a uniform random grid of points in the pivotal plane, a "pivotal tessellation" is obtained (Cruz-Orive, 2009).

Figure 1.7a,b illustrates the unbiased estimation of the total surface area of the union of one section embedded in a ball with the invariator. In Figure 1.7a the equatorial pivotal section plane is isotropic around the ball center. The mentioned equatorial plane is shown in Figure 1.7a with

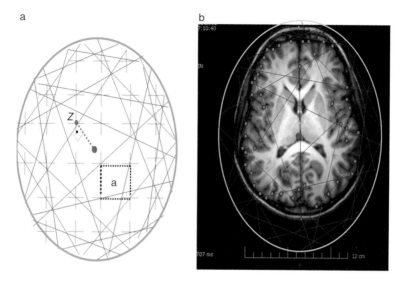

Figure 1.7   Invariator. (a) Construction of a *p*-line with respect to *O* through a uniform random point *z* in an isotropic equatorial section and randomly hitting point counting grid. (b) Invariator grid is superimposed for brain section.

a square grid of points superimposed on it. The grid has to be uniformly random, namely, the pivotal point must be uniformly random relative to a basic tile of the grid. Upon this grid, the corresponding invariator grid of test lines is constructed, and the raw data are then collected (Figure 1.7b). The estimators given by Equation (1.44) remain unbiased because the lines of the invariator grid are, in effect, motion invariant in 3D (Cruz-Orive et al., 2010).

$$S = 2 \times a \times I, \tag{1.44}$$

where *a* denotes the area of the fundamental tile of the grid (Figure 1.7b), and *I* is the (random) total number of intersections between the boundary ∂Y (Cruz-Orive et al., 2010).

The obvious advantage of this method is that the resulting probe may be applied on a pivotal section using a 2D device (Cruz-Orive et al., 2010).

We considered a new method to estimate surface area of variance according to Cruz-Orive et al. (2010). The mean for the object of var(*s/S*) can be estimated following the formula

$$mean\{\text{var}(s \: / \: S)\} = \text{var}(s) - \text{var}(\tilde{S}), \tag{1.45}$$

where var(*s*) is the observed sample variance among the r invariator estimators, whereas var($\tilde{S}$) refers to the observable sample variance (*S*) among the r accurate estimators (Cruz-Orive et al., 2010).

Volume and Surface Area Estimation Using Segmentation Method

The parameters of volume and surface area for cortical brain may be calculated using segmented images in combination with semiautomatic and automatic techniques such as the Fuzzy C-Means (FCM) algorithms. We used MATLAB software for segmenting MR images into parenchyma for brain volume and the surrounding line for the surface area of the cortex. After preprocessing (masking), the image matrix size was reduced, and segmentation was carried out using the FCM algorithm (Suckling et al., 1999; Mohamed et al., 2002; Tosun et al., 2004; Yu-Shen et al., 2010).

For calculation of total brain volume, the original brain image was converted to binary format. After defining a disc-shaped strell, morphological erode-and-dilate operations were performed and edge detection applied and collected with original brain image. The arithmetic process was done by filling in the area of brain as white such that only the brain region appears in the image. Finally, brain volume was obtained from the calculated area of each brain cross section.

Discussion

The Cavalieri principle has been frequently applied to the estimation of total intracranial volume, total brain volume, hippocampus, thalamus, and ventricles volume on MR images (Roberts et al., 2000; Keller et al., 2002, 2012; Ronan et al., 2006; Acer et al., 2007, 2008, 2011; Bas et al., 2009; Denby et al., 2009; Keller and Roberts, 2009). Many different methods exist for estimating brain volume using manual, semiautomated, and automated techniques. Manual approaches such as stereology are considered gold standard because it is assumed that human knowledge and perception is superior to computer algorithms that determine regional brain boundaries (Keller et al., 2012). However, manual segmentation is tedious, requires experiment and high attention to detail, and in many cases returns results with low interrater reliability.

As an alternative to manual approaches, automatic segmentation combined with the Cavalieri-point counting estimator has been widely applied to estimate volume of internal brain compartments, such as cerebellum, ventricle, and so on (Keller et al., 2002, 2012; Acer et al., 2007, 2008; Bas et al., 2009; Keller and Roberts, 2009). To assist in these procedures, various image analysis techniques have been developed in recent years to estimate the brain volume and surface area using automated and semiautomated segmentation algorithms, including freely available approaches for MR images (Fischl et al., 1999; Rajendra et al., 2009). Of these approaches, two popular fully automated segmentation and quantification software tools exist in the public domain. FreeSurfer performs subcortical and cortical segmentation and assigns a neuroanatomical label to each voxel based on probabilistic information automatically estimated from a large training set of expert measurements (Fischl et al., 2002). The second option, FSL/FIRST, performs subcortical segmentation using Bayesian shape and appearance models.

Fully automatic methods require minimal training and provide highly reproducible results for the same data. The disadvantage, however, is that fully automatic approaches do not allow for human intervention or manipulation, as well as place severe limits on choices available to users performing the segmentation. As a result of these limitations, semiautomatic methods have become the preferred approach for medical image segmentation (Keller and Roberts, 2009).

Semiautomatic segmentation can be divided into two major categories: region-based (region growing, region merging) and boundary-based techniques (Kevin et al., 2009). One example used the Cavalieri-point counting method of design-based stereology to estimate volume for a range of organs such as liver, prostate, and others (Sahin and Ergur, 2006; Acer et al., 2011). Stereology has been shown to be at least as precise as tracing and thresholding volumetry techniques and substantially more time efficient than other semiautomated techniques (Gundersen et al., 1981; Keller et al., 2012).

Quantification of brain MR image data using a semiautomated threshold has also been carried out using ImageJ, a public domain image processing and analysis package developed at the National Institutes of Health (NIH) software for scientific and medical usage. This software can be used to automatically measure areas of user-defined ROIs on MR sections according to the contrast and brightness of thresholded grayscale images. The segmented ROIs may be automatically exported to an Excel file with final volume calculated as the product of the area and the MRI slice thickness.

For isolated objects and individual particles embedded in a solid material, the invariator (Cruz-Orive, 2005) may be used to estimate surface area, membrane thickness, and volume, and eliminates the need for 3D scanning (Cruz-Orive, 2011). Although Cruz-Orive et al. (2010) demonstrated the invariator for small isolated or embedded objects such as estimation of the external surface and the volume of rat brains, there is no study for nonembedded objects.

In conclusion, we provide examples of point counting and vertical sectioning, isotropic Cavalieri, independent grid design, and invariator applications for the estimation of first-order parameter volume and surface area from MR images through human brains. Second, a new CE estimation procedure is given for brain surface using the vertical section design. These studies indicate that counting approximately 400–500 cycloid–brain surface intersections on 14 systematically sampled MR sections with 10-mm section thickness results in a reliable surface area estimate with a CE below 5%.

References

Acer, N., Sahin, B., Baş, O., Ertekin, T., Usanmaz, M. 2007. Comparison of three methods for the estimation of total intracranial volume: stereologic, planimetric, and anthropometric approaches. *Ann Plast Surg* **58** (1): 48–53.

Acer, N., Sahin, B., Usanmaz, M., Tatoğlu, H., Irmak, Z. 2008. Comparison of point counting and planimetry methods for the assessment of cerebellar volume in human using magnetic resonance imaging: a stereological study. *Surg Radiol Anat* **30** (4): 335–339.

Acer, N., Cankaya, M. N., Işçi, O., Baş, O., Camurdanoğlu, M., Turgut, M. 2010. Estimation of cerebral surface area using vertical sectioning and magnetic resonance imaging: a stereological study. *Brain Res* **1310**: 29–36.

Acer, N., Turgut, A., Özsunar, Y., Turgut, M. 2011. Quantification of volumetric changes of brain in neurodegenerative diseases using magnetic resonance imaging and stereology. In *Neurodegenerative Diseases—Processes Prevention, Protection and Monitoring*, edited by R. C. Chung Chang, pp. 1–26. Rijeka: InTech Open Access Publisher.

Allen, J. S., Damasio, H., Grabowski, T. J., Bruss, J., Zhang, W. 2003. Sexual dimorphism and asymmetries in the gray-white composition of the human cerebrum. *Neuroimage* **18** (4): 880–894.

Anbeek, P., Vincken, L., Floris, K., Koeman, G., Osch, A., Matthias, J. P., Grond, J. V. 2008. Probabilistic brain tissue segmentation in neonatal magnetic resonance imaging. *Pediatr Res* **63**: 158–163.

Baddeley, A. J., Gundersen, H. J. G., Cruz-Orive, L. M. 1986. Estimation of surface area from vertical sections. *J Microsc* **142** (3): 259–276.

Bas, O., Acer, N., Mas, N., Karabekir, H. S., Kusbeci, O. Y., Sahin, B. 2009. Stereological evaluation of the volume and volume fraction of intracranial structures in magnetic resonance images of patients with Alzheimer's disease. *Ann Anat* **191**: 186–195.

Cruz-Orive, L. M. 1997. Stereology of single objects. *J Microsc* **186**: 93–107.

Cruz-Orive, L. M. 2005. A new stereological principle for test lines in three-dimensional space. *J Microsc* **219**: 18–28.

Cruz-Orive, L. M. 2006. A general variance predictor for Cavalieri slices. *J Microsc* **222** (3): 158–165.

Cruz-Orive, L. M. 2008. Comparative precision of the pivotal estimators of particle size. *J Microsc* **27**: 17–22.

Cruz-Orive, L. M. 2009. The pivotal tessellation. *Image Anal Stereol* **28**: 101–105.

Cruz-Orive, L. M. 2011. Flowers and wedges for the stereology of particles. *J Microsc* **243** (1): 86–102.

Cruz-Orive, L. M., Gual-Arnau, X. 2002. Precision of circular systematic sampling. *J Microsc* **207**: 225–242.

Cruz-Orive, L. M., Ramos-Herrera, M. L., Artacho-Pérula, E. 2010. Stereology of isolated objects with the invariator. *J Microsc* **240** (2): 94–110.

Denby, C. E., Vann, S. D., Tsivilis, D., Aggleton, J. P., Montaldi, D., Roberts, N., Mayes, A. R. 2009. The frequency and extent of mammillary body atrophy associated with surgical removal of a colloid cyst. *AJNR Am J Neuroradiol* **30**: 736–743.

Ertekin, T., Acer, N., Turgut, A. T., Aycan, K., Ozçelik, O., Turgut, M. 2010. Comparison of three methods for the estimation of the pituitary gland volume using magnetic resonance imaging: a stereological study. *Pituitary* **14** (1): 31–38.

Evans, S. M., Janson, A. M., Nyengaard, J. 2004. Quantitative methods. In *Neuroscience: A Neuroanatomical Approach*, edited by S. M. Evans, A. M. Janson, and J. R. Nyengaard. Cary, NC: Oxford University Press.

Fischl, B., Sereno, M. I., Dale, A. M. 1999. Cortical surface-based analysis. II: Inflation, flattening, and a surface-based coordinate system. *Neuroimage* **9** (2): 195–207.

Fischl, B., Salat, D. H., Busa, E., Albert, M., Dieterich, M., Haselgrove, C., van der Kouwe, A., Killiany, R., Kennedy, D., Klaveness, S., Montillo, A., Makris, N., Rosen, B., Dale, A. M. 2002. Whole brain segmentation: automated labeling of neuroanatomical structures in the human brain. *Neuron* **33** (3): 341–355.

García-Fiñana, M. 2006. Confidence intervals in Cavalieri sampling. *J Microsc* **222** (3): 146–157.

García-Fiñana, M., Cruz-Orive, L. M., Mackay, C. E., Pakkenberg, B., Roberts, N. 2003. Comparison of MR imaging against physical sectioning to estimate the volume of human cerebral compartments. *Neuroimage* **18** (2): 505–516.

García-Fiñana, M., Keller, S. S., Roberts, N. 2009. Confidence intervals for the volume of brain structures in Cavalieri sampling with local errors. *J Neurosci Methods* **179** (1): 71–77.

Gokhale, A. M., Evans, R. A., Mackes, J. L., Mouton, P. R. 2004. Design-based estimation of surface area in thick tissue sections of arbitrary orientation using virtual cycloids. *J Microsc* **216**: 25–31.

Gual Arnau, X., Cruz-Orive, L. M. 1998. Variance prediction under systematic sampling with geometric probes. *Adv Appl Prob* **30**: 889–903.

Gundersen, H. J. G., Jensen, E. B. V. 1987. The efficiency of systematic sampling in stereology and its prediction. *J Microsc* **147** (3): 229–263.

Gundersen, H. J. G., Boysen, M., Reith, A. 1981. Comparison of semiautomatic digitizer-tablet and simple point counting performance in morphometry. *Virchows Arch B Cell Pathol Incl Mol Pathol* **37** (3): 317–325.

Gundersen, H. J. G., Jensen, E. B. V., Kieu, K., Nielsen, J. 1999. The efficiency of systematic sampling in stereology— reconsidered. *J Microsc* **193**: 199–211.

Gur, R. C., Gunning-Dixon, F., Bilker, W. B., Gur, R. E. 2002. Sex differences in temporo-limbic and frontal brain volumes of healthy adults. *Cereb Cortex* **12** (9): 998–1003.

Hall, P., Ziegel, J. 2011. Distribution estimators and confidence intervals for stereological volumes. *Biometrika* **98** (2): 417–431.

Henery, C. C., Mayhew, T. M. 1989. The cerebrum and cerebellum of the fixed human brain: efficient and unbiased estimates of volumes and cortical surface areas. *J Anat* **167**: 167–180.

Howard, C. V., Reed, M. G. 1998. *Unbiased Stereology*. Oxford: BIOS Scientific Publishers.

Howard, C. V., Reed, M. G. 2005. *Unbiased Stereology*, 2nd ed. Oxford: BIOS/Taylor & Francis.

Jovicich, J., Czanner, S., Han, X., Salat, D., van der Kouwe, A., Quinn, B., Pacheco, J., Albert, M., Killiany, R., Blacker, D., Maguire, P., Rosas, D., Makris, N., Gollub, R., Dale, A., Dickerson, B. C., Fischl, B. 2009. MRI-derived measurements of human subcortical, ventricular and intracranial brain volumes: reliability effects of scan sessions, acquisition sequences, data analyses, scanner upgrade, scanner vendors and field strengths. *Neuroimage* **46** (1): 177–192.

Keller, S. S., Roberts, N. 2009. Measurement of brain volume using MRI: software, techniques, choices and prerequisites. *J Anthropol Sci* **87**: 127–151.

Keller, S. S., Mackay, C. E., Barrick, T. R., Wieshmann, U. C., Howard, M. A., Roberts, N. 2002. Voxel-based morphometric comparison of hippocampal and extrahippocampal abnormalities in patients with left and right hippocampal atrophy. *Neuroimage* **16**: 23–31.

Keller, S. S., Gerdes, J. S., Mohammadi, S., Kellinghaus, C., Kugel, H., Deppe, K., Ringelstein, E. B., Evers, S., Schwindt, W., Deppe, M. 2012. Volume estimation of the thalamus using freesurfer and stereology: consistency between methods. *Neuroinformatics* **10** (4): 341–350.

Kevin, K., Qing, H., Ye, D. 2009. A fast, semi-automatic brain structure segmentation algorithm for magnetic resonance imaging. IEEE International Conference on Bioinformatics and Biomedicine, 297–302.

Kiêu, K. 1997. Three lectures on systematic geometric sampling. Memoirs 13/1997. Department of Theoretical Statistics: University of Aarush.

Knickmeyer, R. C., Gouttard, S., Kang, C., Evans, D., Wilber, K., Smith, J. K., Hame, R. M., Lin, W., Gerig, G., Gilmore, J. H. 2008. A structural MRI study of human brain development from birth to 2 years. *J Neurosci* **28** (47): 12176–12182.

Kubínová, L., Janácek, J. 2001. Confocal microscopy and stereology: estimating volume, number, surface area and length by virtual test probes applied to three-dimensional images. *Microsc Res Tech* **53**: 425–435.

Kubínová, L., Janácek, J., Albrechtová, J., Karen, P. 2005. Stereological and digital methods for estimating geometrical characteristics of biological structures using confocal microscopy. In *From Cells to Proteins: Imaging Nature across Dimensions*, edited by V. Evangelista, L. Barsanti, V. Passarelli, and P. Gualtieri, pp. 271–321. Dordrecht, The Netherlands: Springer.

Mayhew, T. M., Mwamengele, G. L., Dantzer, V. 1990. Comparative morphometry of the mammalian brain: estimates of cerebral volumes and cortical surface areas obtained from macroscopic slices. *J Anat* **172**: 191–200.

Mayhew, T. M., Mwamengele, G. L., Dantzer, V. 1996. Stereological and allometric studies on mammalian cerebral cortex with implications for medical brain imaging. *J Anat* **189**: 177–184.

Michel, R. P., Cruz-Orive, L. M. 1988. Application of the Cavalieri principle and vertical sections method to lung: estimation of volume and pleural surface area. *J Microsc* **150**: 117–136.

Mohamed, N. A., Sameh, M. Y., Nevin, M., Aly, A. F., Moriarty, T. 2002. A modified fuzzy c-means algorithm for bias field estimation and segmentation of MRI data. *IEEE Trans Med Imaging* **21** (3): 193–199.

Mouton, P. R. 2002. *Principles and Practices of Unbiased Stereology: An Introduction for Bioscientists*. Baltimore, MD: The Johns Hopkins University Press.

Mouton, P. R. 2011. *Unbiased Stereology: A Concise Guide*. Baltimore, MD: The Johns Hopkins University Press.

Nisari, M., Ertekin, T., Ozcelik, O., Çınar, S., Doğanay, S., Acer, N. 2012. Stereological evaluation of the volume and volume fraction of newborns' brain compartment and brain in magnetic resonance images. *Surg Radiol Anat* **April 18** (epub ahead of print).

Pache, J. C., Roberts, N., Vock, P., Zimmermanns, A., Cruz-Orive, L. M. 1993. Vertical LM sectioning and parallel CT scanning designs for stereology: application to human lung. *J Microsc* **170**: 9–24.

Rajendra, A. M., Petty, C. M., Xu, Y., Hayes, J. P., Wagner, H. R., Lewis, D. V., LaBar, K. S., Styner, M., McCarthy, G. 2009. A comparison of automated segmentation and manual tracing for quantifying hippocampal and amygdala volumes. *Neuroimage* **45** (3): 855–866.

Regeur, L., Pakkenberg, B. 1989. Optimizing sample design for volume measurement of components of human brain using a stereological method. *J Microsc* **155**: 113–121.

Roberts, N., Puddephat, M. J., McNulty, V. 2000. The benefit of stereology for quantitative radiology. *Br J Radiol* **73**: 679–697.

Ronan, L., Doherty, C. P., Delanty, N., Thornton, J., Fitzsimons, M. 2006. Quantitative MRI: a reliable protocol for measurement of cerebral gyrification using stereology. *Magn Reson Imaging* **24**: 265–272.

Sahin, B., Ergur, H. 2006. Assessment of the optimum section thickness for the estimation of liver volume using magnetic resonance images: a stereological gold standard study. *Eur J Radiol* **57** (1): 96–101.

Suckling, J., Sigmundsson, T., Greenwood, K., Bullmore, E. T. 1999. A modified fuzzy clustering algorithm for operator independent brain tissue classification of dual echo MR images. *Magn Reson Imaging* **17** (7): 1065–1076.

Tosun, D., Rettmann, M. E., Han, X., Tao, X., Xu, C., Resnick, S. M., Pham, D. L., Prince, J. L. 2004. Cortical surface segmentation and mapping. *Neuroimage* **23**: 108–118.

Weisenfeld, N., Warfield, S. K. 2009. Automatic segmentation of newborn brain MRI. *Neuroimage* **47** (2): 564–572.

Yu-Shen, L., Jing, Y., Hu, Z., Guo-Qin, Z., Jean-Claude, P. 2010. Surface area estimation of digitized 3D objects using quasi-Monte Carlo methods. *Pattern Recognit* **43** (11): 3900–3909.

Webliography

http://rsb.info.nih.gov/ij Image processing and analysis in Java
http://www.mccauslandcenter.sc.edu/mricro/mricro/index.html MRIcro for structural and functional analysis of MR images
http://www.liv.ac.uk/mariarc EasyMeasure for stereologic estimation of MR images

Appendix A: R Commands for Point Counting Method

```
library(VGAM)
est.ce<-function(sample,shapecoeff,N)  {
n<-length(sample)
cat('n',n,fill=T)
C0<-sum(sample*sample)
C=NULL
for(k in 1:(n-1))
C(k)=sum(sample(1:(n-k))*sample((k+1):n))
cat('C',c(C0,C),fill=T)
ss=sum(sample)
cat('sum of Pi',ss,fill=T)
Nugg<-0.0724*shapecoeff*sqrt(n*ss)
cat('vhat',Nugg,fill=T)
if(n<5)  {
ans=readline("Is it a regular object? Type y or n")
if(ans=="y")  q=1
if(ans=="y")  alphaq=1/240
if(ans=="n")  q=0
```

```
if(ans=="n")  alphaq=1/12
}
if(n>=5)  q=max(0,log((3*C0-4*C(2)+C(4))/(3*C0-4*C(1)+C(2))))/
(2*log(2))-0.5)
cat('q',q,fill=T)
if(n>=5)  alphaq=(gamma(2*q+2)*zeta(2*q+2)*cos(pi*q))/
(((2*pi)^(2*q+2))*(1-2^(2*q-1)))
cat('alphaq',alphaq,fill=T)
cev=alphaq*(3*C0-4*C(1)+C(2))/ss^2
sqrtcevp=sqrt(cev)*100
cat('sqrt of cev*100',sqrtcevp,fill=T)
cePC=Nugg/ss^2
sqrtcePCp=sqrt(cePC)*100
cat('sqrt of cePC*100',sqrtcePCp,fill=T)
ce=cev+cePC
sqrtcep=sqrt(ce)*100
cat('sqrt of ce*100',sqrtcep,fill=T)
Qhat=shapecoeff*ss*(d*SU/SL)^2
vQhat=alphaq*(3*C0-4*C(1)+C(2))*shapecoeff^2
lambda=function(rq,N){
if(rq==0)  sqrt(N)*5.49/sqrt(2)
else if(rq==0.1)  sqrt(N)*3.11/sqrt(2)
else if(rq==0.2)  sqrt(N)*3.05/sqrt(2)
else if(rq==0.3)  sqrt(N)*3.1/sqrt(2)
else if(rq==0.4)  sqrt(N)*3.14/sqrt(2)
else if(rq==0.5)  sqrt(N)*3.31/sqrt(2)
else if(rq==0.6)  sqrt(N)*3.4/sqrt(2)
else if(rq==0.7)  sqrt(N)*3.42/sqrt(2)
else if(rq==0.8)  sqrt(N)*3.38/sqrt(2)
else if(rq==0.9)  sqrt(N)*3.3/sqrt(2)
else  sqrt(N)*3.16/sqrt(2)
}
rq=round(q,1)
lambdaq=lambda(rq,N)
cat('lambdaq',lambdaq,fill=T)
citerm=shapecoeff*lambdaq*sqrt(alphaq*(3*C0-4*C(1)+C(2)))
lowerci=Qhat-citerm
upperci=Qhat+citerm
cat('Qhat',Qhat,fill=T)
cat('T',shapecoeff,fill=T)
cat('Var(Qhat)',vQhat,fill=T)
cat('CE(Qhat) %',(sqrt(vQhat)/Qhat)*100,fill=T)
cat('lower confidence limit',lowerci,fill=T)
cat('upper confidence limit',upperci,fill=T)
}
sample=c(26,66,98,132,156,163,158,150,115,85,22)
shapecoeff=1
d=1
SU=1
```

```
SL=1
est.ce(sample,shapecoeff,2)
```

Appendix B: R Commands for Vertical Section to Estimate Surface Area

```
require(VGAM)
est.ce<-function(sample,adivl,h) {
n<-nrow(sample)
I<-rowMeans(sample)*ncol(sample)
one <- rep(1, length(I))
sum.I <- t(one) %*% I
S=(2*h*adivl*sum.I)/n
g<-(2*adivl*h)/pi
f<-g*I
one2 <- rep(1, length(f))
sum.f <- t(one2) %*% f
C0<-sum(f*f)
C1<-f(1)*f(2)+f(2)*f(3)+f(3)*f(4)+f(4)*f(1)
C2<-f(1)*f(3)+f(2)*f(4)+f(3)*f(1)+f(4)*f(2)
C3<-f(1)*f(4)+f(2)*f(1)+f(3)*f(2)+f(4)*f(3)
xyzA<-sample(1,)
xyzB<-sample(2,)
xyzC<-sample(3,)
xyzD<-sample(4,)
sampleA<-xyzA(xyzA != 0)
sampleB<-xyzB(xyzB != 0)
sampleC<-xyzC(xyzC != 0)
sampleD<-xyzD(xyzD != 0)
cat('1.oryantasyon',fill=T)
nA<-length(sampleA)
cat('nA',nA,fill=T)
CA0<-sum(sampleA*sampleA)
CA=NULL
for(k in 1:(nA-1))
CA(k)=sum(sampleA(1:(nA-k))*sampleA((k+1):nA))
cat('CA',c(CA0,CA),fill=T)
if(nA<5) {
ans=readline("Is it a regular object? Type y or n")
if(ans=="y") qA=1
if(ans=="y") alphaqA=1/240
if(ans=="n") qA=0
if(ans=="n") alphaqA=1/12
}
if(nA>=5) qA=max(0,log((3*CA0-4*CA(2)+CA(4))/(3*CA0-
4*CA(1)+CA(2)))/(2*log(2))-0.5)
if(nA<7) qA=0
cat('qA',qA,fill=T)
```

```
if(nA>=5) alphaqA=(gamma(2*qA+2)*zeta(2*qA+2)*cos(pi*qA))/
(((2*pi)^(2*qA+2))*(1-2^(2*qA-1)))
cat('alphaq A',alphaqA,fill=T)
cat('. . . . . . . . . . . . . . .',fill=T)
cat('2.oryantasyon',fill=T)
nB<-length(sampleB)
cat('nB',nB,fill=T)
CB0<-sum(sampleB*sampleB)
CB=NULL
for(k in 1:(nB-1))
CB(k)=sum(sampleB(1:(nB-k))*sampleB((k+1):nB))
cat('CB',c(CB0,CB),fill=T)
if(nB<5) {
ans=readline("Is it a regular object? Type y or n")
if(ans=="y") qB=1
if(ans=="y") alphaqB=1/240
if(ans=="n") qB=0
if(ans=="n") alphaqB=1/12
}
if(nB>=5) qB=max(0,log((3*CB0-4*CB(2)+CB(4))/(3*CB0-
4*CB(1)+CB(2)))/(2*log(2))-0.5)
if(nB<7) qB=0
cat('qB',qB,fill=T)
if(nB>=5) alphaqB=(gamma(2*qB+2)*zeta(2*qB+2)*cos(pi*qB))/
(((2*pi)^(2*qB+2))*(1-2^(2*qB-1)))
cat('alphaq B',alphaqB,fill=T)
cat('. . . . . . . . . . . . . . .',fill=T)
cat('3.oryantasyon',fill=T)
nC<-length(sampleC)
cat('nC',nC,fill=T)
CC0<-sum(sampleC*sampleC)
CC=NULL
for(k in 1:(nC-1))
CC(k)=sum(sampleC(1:(nC-k))*sampleC((k+1):nC))
cat('CC',c(CC0,CC),fill=T)
if(nC<5) {
ans=readline("Is it a regular object? Type y or n")
if(ans=="y") qC=1
if(ans=="y") alphaqC=1/240
if(ans=="n") qC=0
if(ans=="n") alphaqC=1/12
}
if(nC>=5) qC=max(0,log((3*CC0-4*CC(2)+CC(4))/(3*CC0-
4*CC(1)+CC(2)))/(2*log(2))-0.5)
if(nC<7) qC=0
cat('qC',qC,fill=T)
if(nC>=5) alphaqC=(gamma(2*qC+2)*zeta(2*qC+2)*cos(pi*qC))/
(((2*pi)^(2*qC+2))*(1-2^(2*qC-1)))
cat('alphaq C',alphaqC,fill=T)
```

```
cat('. . . . . . . . . . . . . . . .',fill=T)
cat('4.oryantasyon',fill=T)
nD<-length(sampleD)
cat('nD',nD,fill=T)
CD0<-sum(sampleD*sampleD)
CD=NULL
for(k in 1:(nD-1))
CD(k)=sum(sampleD(1:(nD-k))*sampleD((k+1):nD))
cat('CD',c(CD0,CD),fill=T)
if(nD<5) {
ans=readline("Is it a regular object? Type y or n")
if(ans=="y") qD=1
if(ans=="y") alphaqD=1/240
if(ans=="n") qD=0
if(ans=="n") alphaqD=1/12
}
if(nD>=5) qD=max(0,log((3*CD0-4*CD(2)+CD(4))/(3*CD0-
4*CD(1)+CD(2)))/(2*log(2))-0.5)
if(nD<7) qD=0
cat('qD',qD,fill=T)
if(nD>=5) alphaqD=(gamma(2*qD+2)*zeta(2*qD+2)*cos(pi*qD))/
(((2*pi)^(2*qD+2))*(1-2^(2*qD-1)))
cat('alphaq D',alphaqD,fill=T)
T=pi/4
sigmaA=(((2/pi)*adivl)^2)*(h^2)*alphaqA*(3*(CA0-I(1))-
4*CA(1)+CA(2))+(((2/pi)*adivl)^2)*(h^2)*I(1)
sigmaB=(((2/pi)*adivl)^2)*(h^2)*alphaqB*(3*(CB0-I(2))-
4*CB(1)+CB(2))+(((2/pi)*adivl)^2)*(h^2)*I(2)
sigmaC=(((2/pi)*adivl)^2)*(h^2)*alphaqC*(3*(CC0-I(3))-
4*CC(1)+CC(2))+(((2/pi)*adivl)^2)*(h^2)*I(3)
sigmaD=(((2/pi)*adivl)^2)*(h^2)*alphaqD*(3*(CD0-I(4))-
4*CD(1)+CD(2))+(((2/pi)*adivl)^2)*(h^2)*I(4)
v=sigmaA+sigmaB+sigmaC+sigmaD
b2=1.3333
b4=1.7776
D0=((C0-C2-v)/(C0-C1-v))-b2
D1=((C0-C2-v)/(C0-C1-v))-b4
if(abs(D0)<=abs(D1))
varSn=(((8/9)*(pi^2)*(C0-C1-v))/64)+((T^2)*v)
if(abs(D0)>abs(D1))
varSn=(((128/135)*(pi^2)*(C0-C1-v))/1024)+((T^2)*v)
cat('Brain Surface Area >> . . . . . . . . . . . . . . . .')
cat('n',n)
cat('. . . . . . . . . . . . . . . .')
cat('S',S)
cat('. . . . . . . . . . . . . . . .')
cat('C',c(C0,C1,C2,C3))
cat('. . . . . . . . . . . . . . . .')
cat('varSn',varSn)
```

```
CESn=sqrt(varSn)/S
cat('. . . . . . . . . . . . . . .')
cat('CESn',CESn)
}
sample <-
matrix(c(23,10,20,12,25,27,32,18,32,37,27,28,24,33,35,
30,31,41,28,34,37,31,29,38,35,32,21,32,30,31,30,34,31,33,33,30,
37,32,38,36,42,31,32,32,44,32,34,24,37,33,18,18,19,23,12,16),
nrow = 4)
adivl=1
h=1
est.ce(sample,adivl,h)
```

2 Cell Proliferation in the Brains of Adult Rats Exposed to Traumatic Brain Injury

Sandra A. Acosta,[1] Naoki Tajiri,[1] Paula C. Bickford,[1,2] and Cesar V. Borlongan[1]

[1] Center of Excellence for Aging and Brain Repair, Department of Neurosurgery and Brain Repair, University of South Florida College of Medicine, Tampa, FL, USA
[2] James A. Haley Veterans Affairs Hospital, Tampa, FL, USA

Background

About 1.7 million people in the United States suffer from traumatic brain injury (TBI), with nearly 52,000 deaths per year accounting for roughly one-third of all injury-related deaths (Faul et al., 2010). The enormous cost of TBI-related expenses per year, estimated to be around 52 billion USD (Mammis et al., 2009; Glover et al., 2012), reflects the fact that disabilities in patients who survive head injuries often persist for decades following their injury (Liu, 2008). The severity of disabilities varies according to the seriousness of the injury, with the most common damage in loss of sensory-motor function, deficits in learning and memory, anxiety, and depression (Starkstein and Jorge, 2005; Yu et al., 2009). Notably, TBI appears to predispose long-term survivors to age-related neurodegenerative diseases such as Alzheimer's disease, Parkinson's disease, and posttraumatic dementia (Starkstein and Jorge, 2005; Goldman et al., 2006; Yu et al., 2009; Ho et al., 2012; Johnson et al., 2012; Mannix and Whalen, 2012).

Long-term neurological deficits from TBI include neuroinflammation that appears to intensify over time, leading to more severe secondary injuries (Faul et al., 2010; Potts et al., 2009; Wagner et al., 2007; Holschneider et al., 2011). At present, no well-characterized model exists for chronic TBI that includes brain atrophy involving proximal and distal subcortical regions vulnerable to injury (Dietrich et al., 1999; Rodriguez-Paez et al., 2005; Kelley et al., 2007; Onyszchuk et al., 2009; Shitaka et al., 2011). In this study, we used an *in vivo* model of chronic TBI to examine the neuroinflammatory responses in subcortical regions of gray matter (dorsal striatum, thalamus) and white matter (corpus callosum, hippocampal fimbria-fornix, and cerebral peduncle). Neuronal cell loss, cell proliferation, and neuronal differentiation in neurogenic niches were evaluated to assess progressive secondary injuries in these vital regenerative brain areas. Our overall findings support the concept that massive neuroinflammation following TBI leads to a second wave of cell death, creating a chronic TBI condition that impairs the proliferative capacity of cells and impedes neurogenesis.

Materials and Methods

Subjects

Male Sprague-Dawley rats were housed under normal conditions (20°C, 50% relative humidity, and a 12-hour light/dark cycle). Personnel blind to the treatment condition carried out these studies.

Surgical Procedures

The Institutional Animal Care and Use Committee (IACUC) at the University of South Florida (Tampa, FL) approved all experimental procedures in this study. Ten-week-old male rats ($n = 24$) were subjected to either TBI using a controlled cortical impactor (CCI) ($n = 12$) or sham control (no TBI) ($n = 12$) (Pittsburgh Precision Instruments, Inc., Pittsburgh, PA). In brief, rats were fixed in a stereotaxic frame (David Kopf Instruments, Tujunga, CA, USA) and administered deep anesthesia with 1–2% isoflurane maintained through a gas mask. The impactor rod was angled 15° degrees vertically to maintain a perpendicular position with reference to the tangential plane of the brain curvature at the impact surface. A linear variable displacement transducer (Macrosensors, Pennsauken, NJ) was connected to the impactor to ensure consistent velocity and duration. Using an electric drill, the skull was exposed by craniectomy to a depth of about 2.5-mm radius. Brains were impacted at the fronto-parietal cortex (coordinates −0.2 mm anterior, +0.2 mm lateral to the midline) with a velocity of 6.0 m/s. The impactor rod was located at a depth of 1.0 mm below the dura matter and maintained in place for 150 ms. Sham control injury surgery exposed rats to anesthesia followed by scalp incision, craniectomy, and suturing. All rats were closely monitored postoperatively with weight and health surveillance recording per IACUC guidelines. Rats were fed regular rodent diet (Harlan 2018, Harlan) during pre- and post-TBI and kept hydrated at all times with the analgesic ketoprofen administered after TBI surgery. An automated thermal blanket pad and a rectal thermometer supported body temperature within normal limits.

Hematoxylin and Eosin Analysis

Hematoxylin and eosin (H&E) staining was carried out to confirm the core impact injury of the TBI model. As reported in our earlier studies (Yu et al., 2009; Glover et al., 2012) and repeated in the present study, the primary damage produced by the CCI TBI model occurred in the fronto-parietal cortex. H&E staining revealed secondary cell loss in the hippocampus. Starting at coordinates AP-2.0 mm and ending at AP-3.8 mm from bregma, coronal brain sections (40 μm) covering the dorsal hippocampus were sampled. A series of six sections per rat was processed for staining. Using a low-power (20×) objective, neurons with nuclear and cytoplasmic staining were manually counted across the whole CA3 area, starting from the end of hilus to the beginning of curvature of the CA2 region in both the ipsilateral and contralateral side. Data are presented as mean values ±SEM, with statistical significance at $p < 0.05$.

Immunohistochemistry

Under deep anesthesia rats were sacrificed 8 weeks after TBI surgery and perfused through the ascending aorta with 200 mL of ice-cold phosphate buffer saline (PBS) followed by 200 mL of 4% paraformaldehyde (PFA) in PBS. Brains were removed and post-fixed in the same fixative for 24 hours followed by 30% sucrose in PBS for 1 week. Coronal sectioning by cryostat was carried out at a thickness of 40 μm with H&E staining on every sixth section through the dorsal hippo-campus. Staining for the cell cycle-regulating protein Ki67, DCX, and OX6 was done on every sixth section throughout the entire striatum and dorsal hippocampus. Sixteen free-floating coronal sections (40 μm) were incubated in 0.3% hydrogen peroxide (H_2O_2) solution followed by 1 hour of incubation in blocking solution (0.1 M PBS) supplemented with 3% normal goat serum and 0.2% Triton X-100). Sections were then incubated overnight with Ki67 (1:400 Nocastra), DCX (1:150 Santa Cruz), and OX6 (major histocompatibility complex or MHC class II; 1:750 BD) antibody markers in PBS supplemented with 3% normal goat serum and 0.1% Triton X-100. Sec-tions were washed and biotinylated secondary antibody (1:200; Vector Laboratories, Burlingame, CA) in PBS supplemented with 3% normal goat serum, and 0.1% Triton X-100 was applied for 1 hour. The sections were then incubated for 60 minutes in avidin–biotin substrate (ABC kit, Vector Laboratories, Burlingame, CA). Sections were incubated for 1 minute in 3,30-diaminobenzidine (DAB) solution (Vector Laboratories), mounted onto glass slides, dehydrated in ethanol and xylene, and cover-slipped using mounting medium.

Stereological Analysis

For all 24 rats, every sixth section through a distance of about 240 μm apart was sampled through stereotaxic coordinates AP-0.2 mm to AP-3.8 mm. Unbiased stereology was carried on sampled sections following immunostaining with OX6, Ki67, and DCX to visualize activated microglia, cell proliferation, and differentiation into immature neurons, respectively. A Nikon Eclipse 600 microscope integrated with computer-assisted stereology software. The estimated volume of OX6-positive cells was quantified in the cortex, striatum, thalamus, fornix, cerebral peduncle, and corpus callosum, while total numbers of cells immunopositive for Ki67 and DCX were estimated within the subgranular zone (SGZ) and the subventricular zone (SVZ) in both ipsilateral and contralateral hemispheres. Each counting frame (100×100 μm for OX6, Ki67, and DCX) was placed at an intersection of the lines forming a virtual grid (125×125 μm), which was randomly generated and placed by the software within the outlined structure. Sampling was optimized to count at least 300 cells per animal with coefficient of error (CE) of about 0.07.

Statistical Analysis

For data analyses, contralateral and ipsilateral corresponding brain areas were used as raw data providing two sets of data per treatment condition (TBI vs. sham control). One-way analysis of variance (ANOVA) was used for group comparisons, followed by subsequent pairwise compari-sons with Bonferonni correction for multiple comparisons. All data are represented as mean values with ±SEM. Statistical significance was set at $p < 0.05$ for all analyses.

Results

Preliminary analyses of the data with comparisons between sham control (ipsilateral) and sham control (contralateral) across all brain regions did not show significant differences. Afterward, data from both sides of the sham group were combined. Pairwise comparisons were carried out to evaluate the effects of chronic TBI on neuroinflammation in different regions of the brain, includ-ing cortex, striatum, thalamus, corpus callosum, cerebral peduncle, fornix, CA3 neuron loss, cell proliferation in SVZ and SGZ, as detailed later.

Upregulation of MHC II+-Activated Microglia Cells in Chronic TBI

To test the hypothesis that the chronic stage of TBI was accompanied by upregulation of activated microglia cells (MHC II+), gray and white matter areas were examined such as cortex, striatum, thalamus, olfactory bulb, dentate gyrus, corpus callosum, cerebral peduncle, and fornix (Figure 2.1 and Figure 2.2). Of note, the dentate gyrus and olfactory bulbs displayed no detectable

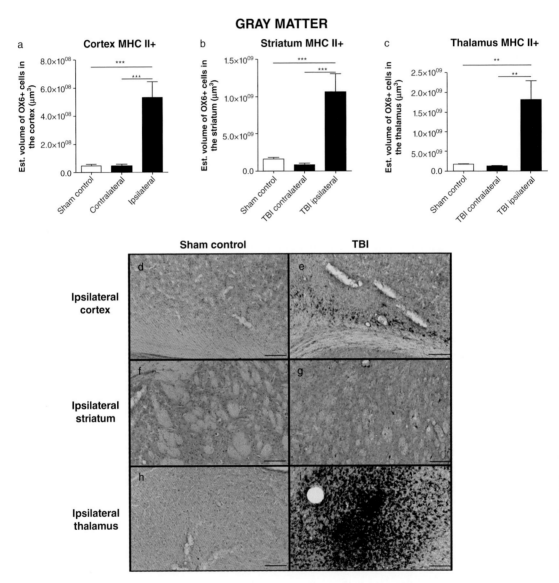

Figure 2.1 Upregulation of MHC II+ activated microglia cells in gray matter in chronic TBI. Results indicate that there is a clear exacerbation of activated microglia cells in ipsilateral side of subcortical gray matter regions in chronic TBI relative to contralateral side and sham control. After 8 weeks from initial TBI injury, asterisks denote significant upregulation on the volume of MHC II expressing cells in (a) cortex, (b) striatum, and (c) thalamus, while contralateral side presents an estimated volume of activated microglia cells similar to sham control animals. ANOVA revealed significant treatment effects as follows: cortex, $F_{2,45} = 18.49$, ***$p < 0.005$; striatum, $F_{2,45} = 15.71$, ***$p < 0.005$; and thalamus, $F_{2,45} = 12.23$, ***$p < 0.005$. Photomicrographs correspond to representative gray matter in coronal sections stained with OX6 (MHC II) from ipsilateral sham control and TBI rats, cortex (d and e), striatum (f and g), and thalamus (h and i). Scale bars for d, e, f, g, h, i = 1 μm.

OX6-immunoreactive cells. We calculated the volume of activated microglia cells (MHC II +) in the ipsilateral and contralateral areas using an anti-OX6 antibody. Chronic TBI produced a robust upregulation in the volume of MHC II-labeled activated microglia cells in gray matter areas ipsilateral to TBI, whereas the volume in the contralateral side was not significantly different to that in sham control (Figure 2.1a–c). There was a 12-, 7-, and a 10-fold increase in the volume of MHC Class II in cortex (Figure 2.1a,d,e), striatum (Figure 2.1b,f,g), and thalamus (Figure 2.1c,h,i), respectively: cortex, $F_{2,45} = 18.49$, $p < 0.005$; striatum, $F_{2,45} = 15.71$, $p < 0.005$; and thalamus, $F_{2,45} = 12.23$, $p < 0.005$. Similar analyses show that chronic TBI prompted an increase of activated MHC II-positive microglia cell volume in white matter areas ipsilateral and contralateral to TBI injury. Chronic TBI resulted in an upregulation of activated microglia cells in corpus callosum, cerebral peduncle, and fornix around the injury side (Figure 2.2a–c). There were no significant differences between ipsilateral and contralateral side of TBI animals, largely due to activation of microglia cells in corpus callosum in both hemispheres (p values > 0.05; Figure 2.2a). Additionally, significant increments in activated MHC II-positive microglia cells were detected in the ipsilateral cerebral peduncle (Figure 2.2a) and the ipsilateral hippocampal fornix (Figure 2.2c). ANOVA revealed significant treatment effects on MHC II-positive cells as follows: corpus callosum, $F_{2,45} = 5.656$, $p < 0.05$; cerebral peduncle, $F_{2,45} = 27.39$, $p < 0.0005$; fornix, $F_{2,45} = 5.541$, $p < 0.05$. A summary of all areas comparing sham control and chronic TBI is presented in Figure 2.2d. All data are represented as mean values ±SEM.

Chronic TBI Impairs Hippocampal Cell Survival and Proliferation

In order to test the hypothesis that neuronal cell loss and impaired cell proliferation accompanied long-term chronic TBI, the total number of surviving neurons in the hippocampal CA3 region and the estimated number of positive dividing cells within SVZ and SGZ were examined. We found that long-term chronic TBI significantly affected CA3 cell survival; $F_{2,9} = 10.78$, $p < 0.005$, characterized by decreased neurons in the CA3 area of the ipsilateral hippocampus relative to sham control; $p < 0.05$ (Figure 2.3a). There was no significant loss of neurons in the CA3 contralateral to chronic TBI animals compared to sham control ($p > 0.05$; Figure 2.3a). Additionally, cell proliferation was examined by quantifying the cell proliferation marker Ki67 (Figure 2.3). Chronic TBI significantly reduced cell proliferation in SVZ ($F_{2,45} = 10.45$, $p < 0.0005$) in both the ipsilateral and contralateral side compared with sham control (p's < 0.05; Figure 2.3b). Following this observation of chronic TBI-induced downregulation in the SVZ, we next inspected the cell proliferation in the SGZ, another neurogenic niche (Figure 2.3). Again, chronic TBI was found to disturb cell proliferation in the SGZ ($F_{2,45} = 3.755$, $p < 0.005$). Quantification of cell proliferation within the SGZ demonstrated that there was a significant decrease in cell proliferation only in the ipsilateral side of chronic TBI compared with sham control ($p < 0.05$). The contralateral SGZ did not show significant decrements in cell proliferation relative to sham control ($p > 0.05$). The dentate gyrus and olfactory bulb did not display overt cell loss.

Chronic TBI Does Not Affect Neuronal Differentiation in Neurogenic Niches

After showing chronic TBI-induced extensive downregulation of cell proliferation in the two main neurogenic niches (SVZ and SGZ), we examined neuronal differentiation. Although there appeared a general downregulation of DCX-positive cells, the fraction of new cells generated in the SVZ and SGZ initiating down the neuronal path seemed to be similar in the control compared to the TBI conditions (Figure 2.4a,b). Chronic TBI did not significantly impair cellular differentiation into neuronal lineage in the ipsilateral SVZ and SGZ when compared with the corresponding contralateral side or with sham control animals ($p > 0.05$).

WHITE MATTER

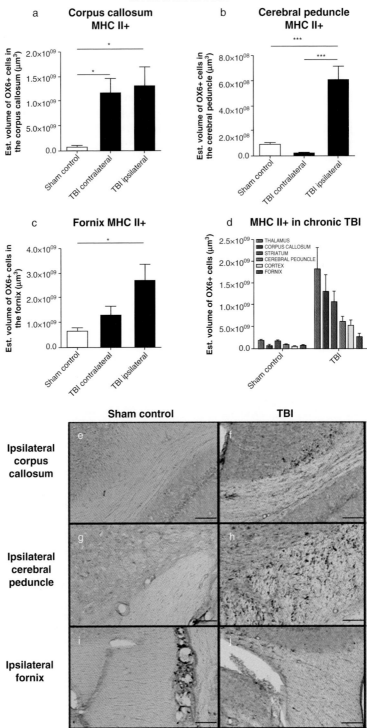

a **Corpus callosum MHC II+**

b **Cerebral peduncle MHC II+**

c **Fornix MHC II+**

d **MHC II+ in chronic TBI**

Sham control | TBI

Ipsilateral corpus callosum

Ipsilateral cerebral peduncle

Ipsilateral fornix

32

Figure 2.2   Upregulation of MHC II+-activated microglia cells in white matter in chronic TBI. Results indicate that there is an upregulation of activated microglia cells after 8 weeks post-TBI in proximal white matter areas. There is an upregulation of MHC II+ cells in the ipsilateral and contralateral side of corpus callosum relative to sham control (a). In contrast, upregulation of MHC II+-activated microglia cells in the cerebral peduncle (b) and fornix (c) is only present in the ipsilateral side as compared with the contralateral and sham control. There were no significant differences between contralateral side and sham control animals in panel b and panel c. ANOVA revealed significant treatment effects as follows: corpus callosum, $F_{2,45} = 5.656$, $*p < 0.05$; cerebral peduncle, $F_{2,45} = 27.39$, $***p < 0.0005$; and fornix, $F_{2,45} = 5.541$, $*p < 0.05$. Representative photomicrographs, ipsilateral corpus callosum, sham control panel e and TBI panel f, ipsilateral cerebral peduncle, sham control panel g and TBI panel h, and ipsilateral fornix, sham control panel i and TBI panel j. Scale bars for panels e–j = 1 μm. A summary of MHC II+ estimated volume is presented, capturing different subcortical regions, including those proximal and distal from TBI insult (panel d). Chronic TBI greatly upregulates the neuroinflammation in the thalamus expressing the highest upregulation of MHC II+-activated microglia cells, despite its distal subcortical location. Strong expression of MHC II+-activated microglia cells is also detected in the corpus callosum and striatum (panel d).

◀

Discussion

The present study demonstrated long-term neuroinflammation in the setting of chronic TBI, which was closely associated with neuronal cell loss and impaired cell proliferation in discrete brain structures adjacent to and even remote from the core-injured region. At 8 weeks post-TBI, directly TBI-impacted cortical site showed significant upregulation of activated microglia cells, as did proximal adjacent ipsilateral areas, as well as areas distal from the injury site. In parallel, a significant decrease of hippocampal neurons in the CA3 region ipsilateral to injury was detected relative to sham control. In the CA3 region, there was no cell loss in the contralateral side after chronic TBI. Examination of the neurogenic niches revealed significant declines in cell proliferation in both SVZ and SGZ ipsilateral to TBI. Of note, only the contralateral side of SVZ, but not the SGZ, seemed to be affected by chronic TBI, showing a 40% decrease in cell proliferation compared with sham control. The present location of chronic inflammation seems to correlate with the observed cell loss and impaired cell proliferation. The SVZ and the dorsal hippocampus are located proximal to the area of CCI in the cortex. In addition, the proximity of the fornix and corpus callosum and thalamus to the hippocampus might have affected the CA3 cell survival and SGZ cell proliferation due to the chronic activated microglia cells present in these regions.

Neurodegeneration after the initial TBI involves acute and chronic stages. Cell death during the acute, but not chronic, stages of TBI in the CCI model has been well characterized (Harting et al., 2008; Yu et al., 2009; Yang et al., 2010; Gao et al., 2011). Acute primary injury manifestations start to appear during the early stages of TBI, as evidenced by elevated intracerebral pressure, ruptured blood–brain barrier, brain edema, and reduced cerebral blood flow at the area of injury (Cernak, 2005; Cernak et al., 2005; Schmidt et al., 2005). In addition, a massive innate immune response at the molecular level appears within minutes to ease elimination of cellular debris (Harting et al., 2008). This wave of progressive injury contributes to long-term damage post-TBI in animals, as well as in patients even decades after the injury (Starkstein and Jorge, 2005; Goldman et al., 2006; Rogers and Read, 2007; Ho et al., 2012). Following acute head trauma, increased cell proliferation and neural differentiation were detected within the neurogenic niches (SVZ and SGZ), likely corresponding to an endogenous regenerative mechanism to provide neuroprotection at the site of injury (Parent, 2003; Richardson et al., 2007; Hayashi et al., 2009; Bye et al., 2010, 2011; Shojo et al., 2010; Glover et al., 2012). The recognition that the chronic stage of neuroinflammation alters endogenous reparative mechanism, that is, proliferative properties of neurogenic niches especially the SVZ (Pluchino et al., 2008), requires the development of new strategies to mobilize these proliferative cells to specific injured brain areas for regenerative purposes (Pluchino et al., 2008). Of note, only 10% of new cells in the SGZ survive for up to 4 weeks

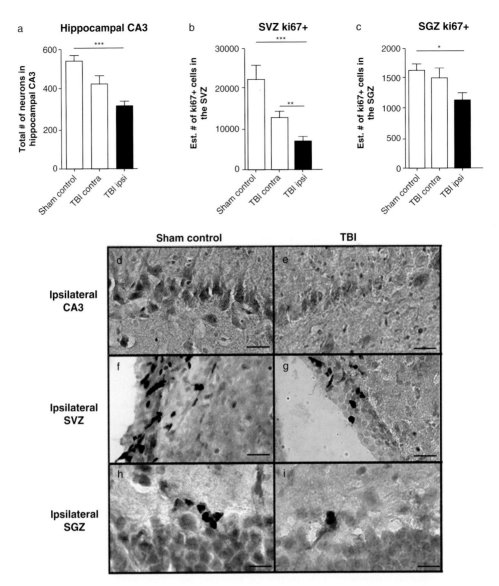

Figure 2.3 Hippocampal CA3 cell loss and downregulation of cell proliferation. H&E staining revealed a significant cell loss in the hippocampal CA3 region after chronic TBI (a). Ki67, a cell proliferation marker, revealed a significant chronic TBI-related decrease in the SVZ of cell proliferation only in the ipsilateral side relative to contralateral side and sham control animals (b). Contralateral measurements revealed that cell proliferation also decreases, but it does not show significant differences when compared with sham control animals (b). Also, Ki67 revealed a significant decrease in cell proliferation in the SGZ of the hippocampus in the ipsilateral side compared to sham control (c). In summary, ANOVA revealed significant treatment effects as follows: hippocampal CA3 neurons, $F_{2,9} = 10.78$, ***$p < 0.005$; SVZ, $F_{2,45} = 10.45$, ***$p < 0.005$; and SGZ, $F_{2,45} = 3.755$, ***$p < 0.005$. Representative photomicrographs from coronal sections ipsilateral CA3 region stained with hematoxylin/eosin in sham control and TBI rats (d and e). Ipsilateral SVZ from sham control and TBI rats (f and g) and ipsilateral SGZ from sham control and TBI rats (h and i) are shown. Scale bars for panels d–i = 50 μm.

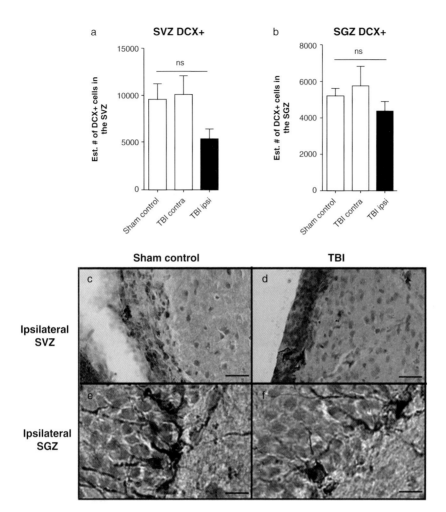

Figure 2.4   Neural differentiation is not affected by chronic TBI. DCX staining, a neural differentiation marker, revealed that there is no significant impairment in neural differentiation in either SVZ of the lateral ventricle (a) or the SGZ of the hippocampus relative to contralateral side and sham control animals (b). The "ns" denotes nonsignificant differences ($p > 0.05$). Representative coronal sections from ipsilateral SVZ stained with DCX in sham control and TBI rats (c and d) and SGZ from sham control and TBI rats (e and f) are shown. Scale bars for panels c–f = 50 μm.

postinjury in a close head injury mouse model of focal TBI, and 60% of new cells in the pericontusional cortex become astrocytes in response to brain injury (Bye et al., 2010, 2011). Additionally, a decreased survival of immature neurons can be seen as early as 7 days in a mouse model of moderate TBI. At 4 weeks post-TBI, both cell proliferation and neural differentiation greatly decrease relative to sham control mice (Rola et al., 2006). The observed preferential effect of TBI on cell proliferation, but not on neuronal differentiation, may be due to a fraction of new cells undergoing neurogenesis not affected by TBI, even though overall proliferation rates are substantially reduced. In particular, this fraction of new cells generated in the SVZ and SGZ committed toward the neuronal lineage remains active in both control and TBI conditions. The type of insult (TBI, radiation, neurotoxin) may affect the brain microenvironment with varying levels of signaling cues for cell proliferation and differentiation, in turn resulting in an imbalance of new dividing cells and cells differentiating to a neuronal phenotype. This hypothesis clearly warrants further investigations.

Progressive injury to hippocampal, cortical, and thalamic areas contributes to long-term cognitive damage post-TBI as noted in military men and in civilian patients even decades after the injury (Schmidt et al., 2005; Starkstein and Jorge, 2005; Goldman et al., 2006; Rogers and Read, 2007; Harting et al., 2008; Yu et al., 2009; Gao et al., 2011; Elder et al., 2012; Ho et al., 2012; Vasterling et al., 2012). It is well recognized that hippocampal cell loss is a consequence of TBI (Ariza et al., 2006). TBI patients have been shown to exhibit deficits in verbal declarative memory, which is modulated in part by the hippocampal formation and executive functioning (Mathias and Mansfield, 2005; Ge et al., 2009). Neuropsychological tests performed in U.S. Army soldiers after deployment revealed that TBI is closely associated with functional impairments, while TBI co-morbid with PTSD and depression presents with chronic long-lasting cognitive deficits (Vasterling et al., 2012). In addition, cognitive functions modulated by the thalamic-cortical areas of the brain are also affected by chronic TBI as revealed by high-resolution tensor magnetic resonance imaging (Little et al., 2010). Patients with a history of brain injury exhibit ventral thalamic atrophy, which correlates with impaired executive function, attention, and memory and learning deficits post-TBI (Little et al., 2010). Interestingly, cerebral blood flow to the thalamus is significantly reduced even by mild TBI and coincides with impairments in speech, learning, and memory (Ge et al., 2009). Taken together, impaired cognitive functions mediated by cortex, hippocampus, and thalamus may manifest in chronic TBI.

The present study suggests that chronic TBI causes cell proliferation through a cascade of events. Differences in these findings from previous studies (Parent, 2003; Rola et al., 2006; Bye et al., 2010, 2011) may relate to the timing of histological analyses (acute vs. chronic), varying models of TBI (mild vs. moderate), and choice of animal species (mice vs. rat). Despite the variability in experimental procedures and animal subjects, these studies, including our own, point to the susceptibility of newly formed cells within neurogenic niches, implicating the pivotal role for endogenous cells likely involved in the host reparative mechanism in response to TBI (Rola et al., 2006; Pluchino et al., 2008).

Similar comorbidity critical factors in the clinic, such as patient age, injury severity, and past medical history influence the outcomes of TBI; however, neuroinflammation as a key factor in cell death appears consistent following brain injury (Starkstein and Jorge, 2005; Goldman et al., 2006; Kelley et al., 2007; Laskowitz et al., 2010; Ramlackhansingh et al., 2011; Ho et al., 2012; Mannix and Whalen, 2012; Rovengno et al., 2012). Upregulation of neuroinflammation in the present study was depicted by exacerbation of activated microglia cells in gray matter structures, such as cortex, striatum, thalamus, and white matter, including corpus callosum, fornix, and cerebral peduncles. In the clinic, long-term microglia activation was visualized *in vivo* within the thalamus, putamen, occipital cortices, and white matter areas as the internal capsule, in patients exhibiting severe impairments in cognitive function up at least 11 months after moderate to severe TBI (Ramlackhansingh et al., 2011). Consequently, microglial cells pose as a candidate target for mitigating cell death in an effort to develop novel anti-inflammation-based therapeutic modalities in TBI (Starkstein and Jorge, 2005; Goldman et al., 2006; Liu, 2008; Ho et al., 2012; Johnson et al., 2012; Mannix and Whalen, 2012).

Our findings of white matter changes in chronic TBI agree with previous reports demonstrating the negative influences of activated microglial cells after TBI (Filley, 1998; Gunning-Dixon and Raz, 2000; Jia et al., 2012). White matter axonal injury is a very common feature in clinical setting after TBI, which accounts for impairments of cognitive function and may result in high mortality rate (Filley, 1998; Gunning-Dixon and Raz, 2000; Jia et al., 2012). Axonal degeneration, typical in white matter injury, interrupts the action potential throughout the cortex (Filley, 1998; Gunning-Dixon and Raz, 2000; Roher et al., 2002) and combined with overt activation of microglia cells in cortical and subcortical areas may lead to impaired cell survival and cell proliferation in both immediate and remote areas of the impacted brain region (Iijima et al., 1998; Grady et al., 2003;

Goldman et al., 2006; Yang et al., 2010; Ho et al., 2012). In the present study, there were 70% and 34% decrements in cell proliferation in the SVZ and SGZ, respectively, in comparison to sham control. These findings suggests that chronic neuroinflammation alters cell proliferation, but additional studies to elucidate this mechanism and its direct influence on impeding endogenous proliferation need to establish this point. Notwithstanding, these results advance the potential benefits of anti-inflammatory therapies during the chronic stage of TBI.

Taken together, these findings suggest that while TBI is generally considered an acute injury, the disease pathology over the long term includes both a chronic cell death perturbation (neuroinflammation) and a diminished endogenous repair mechanism (cell proliferation). The recognition of long-term pathological disturbances associated with chronic inflammation and neuropsychological diseases indicate vigilant follow-up monitoring of TBI patients is needed to better manage the disease progression. A multipronged treatment targeting inflammatory and cell proliferative pathways may diminish the chronic TBI pathological effects for afflicted patients.

Acknowledgments

C. V. B. is supported by the National Institutes of Health (1R01NS071956-01A1) and the James and Esther King Biomedical Research Program (1KG01-33966).

References

Ariza, M., Serra-Grabulosa, J. M., Junque, C., Ramirez, B., Mataro, M. et al. 2006. Hippocampal head atrophy after traumatic brain injury. *Neuropsychologia* **44**: 1956–1961.

Bye, N., Ng, S. Y., Morganti-Kossmann, M. C. 2010. Characterizing endogenous neurogenesis following experimental focal traumatic brain injury (TBI), and investigating the effect of treatment with minocycline. *Injury* **41** (Suppl 1): S42.

Bye, N., Carron, S., Han, X., Agyapomaa, D., Ng, S. Y. et al. 2011. Neurogenesis and glial proliferation are stimulated following diffuse traumatic brain injury in adult rats. *J Neurosci Res* **89**: 986–1000.

Cernak, I. 2005. Animal models of head trauma. *NeuroRx* **2**: 410–422.

Cernak, I., Stoica, B., Byrnes, K. R., Di Giovanni, S., Faden, A. I. 2005. Role of the cell cycle in the pathobiology of central nervous system trauma. *Cell Cycle* **4**: 1286–1293.

Dietrich, W. D., Truettner, J., Zhao, W., Alonso, O. F., Busto, R. et al. 1999. Sequential changes in glial fibrillary acidic protein and gene expression following parasagittal fluid-percussion brain injury in rats. *J Neurotrauma* **16**: 567–581.

Elder, G. A., Dorr, N. P., De Gasperi, R., Gama Sosa, M. A., Shaughness, M. C. et al. 2012. Blast exposure induces post-traumatic stress disorder-related traits in a rat model of mild traumatic brain injury. *J Neurotrauma* **29**: 2564–2575.

Faul, M., Xu, L., Wald, M. M., Coronado, V. G. 2010. *Traumatic Brain Injury in the United States: Emergency Department Visits, Hospitalizations and Deaths 2002–2006*. Atlanta, GA: Centers for Disease Control and Prevention, National Center for Injury Prevention and Control.

Filley, C. M. 1998. The behavioral neurology of cerebral white matter. *Neurology* **50**: 1535–1540.

Gao, X., Deng, P., Xu, Z. C., Chen, J. 2011. Moderate traumatic brain injury causes acute dendritic and synaptic degeneration in the hippocampal dentate gyrus. *PLoS ONE* **6**: e24566.

Ge, Y., Patel, M. B., Chen, Q., Grossman, E. J., Zhang, K. et al. 2009. Assessment of thalamic perfusion in patients with mild traumatic brain injury by true FISP arterial spin labelling MR imaging at 3T. *Brain Inj* **23**: 666–674.

Glover, L. E., Tajiri, N., Lau, T., Kaneko, Y., van Loveren, H. et al. 2012. Immediate, but not delayed, microsurgical skull reconstruction exacerbates brain damage in experimental traumatic brain injury model. *PLoS ONE* **7**: e33646.

Goldman, S. M., Tanner, C. M., Oakes, D., Bhudhikanok, G. S., Gupta, A. et al. 2006. Head injury and Parkinson's disease risk in twins. *Ann Neurol* **60**: 65–72.

Grady, M. S., Charleston, J. S., Maris, D., Witgen, B. M., Lifshitz, J. 2003. Neuronal and glial cell number in the hippocampus after experimental traumatic brain injury: analysis by stereological estimation. *J Neurotrauma* **20**: 929–941.

Gunning-Dixon, F. M., Raz, N. 2000. The cognitive correlates of white matter abnormalities in normal aging: a quantitative review. *Neuropsychology* **14**: 224–232.

Harting, M. T., Jimenez, F., Adams, S. D., Mercer, D. W., Cox, C. S., Jr. 2008. Acute, regional inflammatory response after traumatic brain injury: implications for cellular therapy. *Surgery* **144**: 803–813.

Hayashi, T., Kaneko, Y., Yu, S., Bae, E., Stahl, C. E. et al. 2009. Quantitative analyses of matrix metalloproteinase activity after traumatic brain injury in adult rats. *Brain Res* **1280**: 172–177.

Ho, L., Zhao, W., Dams-O'Connor, K., Tang, C. Y., Gordon, W. et al. 2012. Elevated plasma MCP-1 concentration following traumatic brain injury as a potential "predisposition" factor associated with an increased risk for subsequent development of Alzheimer's disease. *J Alzheimers Dis* **31**: 301–313.

Holschneider, D. P., Guo, Y., Roch, M., Norman, K. M., Scremin, O. U. 2011. Acetylcholinesterase inhibition and locomotor function after motor-sensory cortex impact injury. *J Neurotrauma* **28**: 1909–1919.

Iijima, T., Shimase, C., Sawa, H., Sankawa, H. 1998. Spreading depression induces depletion of MAP2 in area CA3 of the hippocampus in a rat unilateral carotid artery occlusion model. *J Neurotrauma* **15**: 277–284.

Jia, X., Cong, B., Wang, S., Dong, L., Ma, C. et al. 2012. Secondary damage caused by CD11b+ microglia following diffuse axonal injury in rats. *J Trauma Acute Care Surg* **73** (5): 1168–1174.

Johnson, V. E., Stewart, W., Smith, D. H. 2012. Widespread tau and amyloid-beta pathology many years after a single traumatic brain injury in humans. *Brain Pathol* **22**: 142–149.

Kelley, B. J., Lifshitz, J., Povlishock, J. T. 2007. Neuroinflammatory responses after experimental diffuse traumatic brain injury. *J Neuropathol Exp Neurol* **66**: 989–1001.

Laskowitz, D. T., Song, P., Wang, H., Mace, B., Sullivan, P. M. et al. 2010. Traumatic brain injury exacerbates neurodegenerative pathology: improvement with an apolipoprotein E-based therapeutic. *J Neurotrauma* **27**: 1983–1995.

Little, D. M., Kraus, M. F., Joseph, J., Geary, E. K., Susmaras, T. et al. 2010. Thalamic integrity underlies executive dysfunction in traumatic brain injury. *Neurology* **74**: 558–564.

Liu, C. Y. 2008. Combined therapies: national Institute of Neurological Disorders and Stroke funding opportunity in traumatic brain injury research. *Neurosurgery* **63**: N12.

Mammis, A., McIntosh, T. K., Maniker, A. H. 2009. Erythropoietin as a neuroprotective agent in traumatic brain injury review. *Surg Neurol* **71**: 527–531, discussion 531.

Mannix, R. C., Whalen, M. J. 2012. Traumatic brain injury, microglia, and beta amyloid. *Int J Alzheimers Dis* **2012**: 608732.

Mathias, J. L., Mansfield, K. M. 2005. Prospective and declarative memory problems following moderate and severe traumatic brain injury. *Brain Inj* **19**: 271–282.

Onyszchuk, G., LeVine, S. M., Brooks, W. M., Berman, N. E. 2009. Post-acute pathological changes in the thalamus and internal capsule in aged mice following controlled cortical impact injury: a magnetic resonance imaging, iron histochemical, and glial immunohistochemical study. *Neurosci Lett* **452**: 204–208.

Parent, J. M. 2003. Injury-induced neurogenesis in the adult mammalian brain. *Neuroscientist* **9**: 261–272.

Pluchino, S., Muzio, L., Imitola, J., Deleidi, M., Alfaro-Cervello, C. et al. 2008. Persistent inflammation alters the function of the endogenous brain stem cell compartment. *Brain* **131**: 2564–2578.

Potts, M. B., Adwanikar, H., Noble-Haeusslein, L. J. 2009. Models of traumatic cerebellar injury. *Cerebellum* **8**: 211–221.

Ramlackhansingh, A. F., Brooks, D. J., Greenwood, R. J., Bose, S. K., Turkheimer, F. E. et al. 2011. Inflammation after trauma: microglial activation and traumatic brain injury. *Ann Neurol* **70**: 374–383.

Richardson, R. M., Sun, D., Bullock, M. R. 2007. Neurogenesis after traumatic brain injury. *Neurosurg Clin N Am* **18**: 169–181, xi.

Rodriguez-Paez, A. C., Brunschwig, J. P., Bramlett, H. M. 2005. Light and electron microscopic assessment of progressive atrophy following moderate traumatic brain injury in the rat. *Acta Neuropathol* **109**: 603–616.

Rogers, J. M., Read, C. A. 2007. Psychiatric comorbidity following traumatic brain injury. *Brain Inj* **21**: 1321–1333.

Roher, A. E., Weiss, N., Kokjohn, T. A., Kuo, Y. M., Kalback, W. et al. 2002. Increased A beta peptides and reduced cholesterol and myelin proteins characterize white matter degeneration in Alzheimer's disease. *Biochemistry* **41**: 11080–11090.

Rola, R., Mizumatsu, S., Otsuka, S., Morhardt, D. R., Noble-Haeusslein, L. J. et al. 2006. Alterations in hippocampal neurogenesis following traumatic brain injury in mice. *Exp Neurol* **202**: 189–199.

Schmidt, O. I., Heyde, C. E., Ertel, W., Stahel, P. F. 2005. Closed head injury: an inflammatory disease? *Brain Res Brain Res Rev* **48**: 388–399.

Shitaka, Y., Tran, H. T., Bennett, R. E., Sanchez, L., Levy, M. A. et al. 2011. Repetitive closed-skull traumatic brain injury in mice causes persistent multifocal axonal injury and microglial reactivity. *J Neuropathol Exp Neurol* **70**: 551–567.

Shojo, H., Kaneko, Y., Mabuchi, T., Kibayashi, K., Adachi, N. et al. 2010. Genetic and histologic evidence implicates role of inflammation in traumatic brain injury-induced apoptosis in the rat cerebral cortex following moderate fluid percussion injury. *Neuroscience* **171**: 1273–1282.

Starkstein, S. E., Jorge, R. 2005. Dementia after traumatic brain injury. *Int Psychogeriatr* **17** (Suppl 1): S93–S107.

Vasterling, J. J., Brailey, K., Proctor, S. P., Kane, R., Heeren, T. et al. 2012. Neuropsychological outcomes of mild traumatic brain injury, post-traumatic stress disorder and depression in Iraq-deployed US Army soldiers. *Br J Psychiatry* **201**: 186–192.

Wagner, A. K., Kline, A. E., Ren, D., Willard, L. A., Wenger, M. K. et al. 2007. Gender associations with chronic methylphenidate treatment and behavioral performance following experimental traumatic brain injury. *Behav Brain Res* **181**: 200–209.

Yang, J., You, Z., Kim, H. H., Hwang, S. K., Khuman, J. et al. 2010. Genetic analysis of the role of tumor necrosis factor receptors in functional outcome after traumatic brain injury in mice. *J Neurotrauma* **27**: 1037–1046.

Yu, S., Kaneko, Y., Bae, E., Stahl, C. E., Wang, Y. et al. 2009. Severity of controlled cortical impact traumatic brain injury in rats and mice dictates degree of behavioral deficits. *Brain Res* **1287**: 157–163.

3   Age Effects in Substantia Nigra of Asian Indians

Phalguni Anand Alladi

Department of Neurophysiology, National Institute of Mental Health and Neurosciences, Bangalore, India

Background

Loss of melanized neurons of substantia nigra pars compacta (SNpc) is a prominent marker of neurodegeneration and is a consistent finding in Parkinson's disease (PD). A strong association between α-synuclein aggregation and Lewy body formation in the aging brain and PD points to the occurrence of endoplasmic reticular (ER) stress-mediated protein misfolding.

Independent epidemiological studies involving the different ethnic populations worldwide report higher prevalence of PD in Caucasians compared with the Asians and nonwhites of Africa (Muthane et al., 2001, 2007 for a review). Recent door-to-door studies conducted in India report relatively lower prevalence of PD in Asian Indians (Das et al., 2010). These findings may provide some evidence for ethnicity and cultural factors as important factors for the variable incidence of PD in different human populations.

The strong association between aging as a major risk factor for PD and the reduced numbers of melanized nigral neurons in PD has stimulated numerous studies to quantify age-related loss of nigral neurons. In studies of aging French and American subjects, there was a lack of age-related loss of nigral neurons seen in the British Caucasians. In the American subjects, numbers of melanized nigral neurons remained comparable during aging, though there was an exponential increase in α-synuclein expression and loss of colabeled tyrosine hydroxylase (TH), and Nurr1 immunoreactive neurons occurred from middle age and onward. Fearnley and Lees (1991) and Gibb and Lees (1991) reported that distinct mechanisms are responsible for SNpc neurodegeneration in aging and PD, negating the hypothesis that PD represents a condition of accelerated aging. A subsequent series of studies on primate and human brains equated aging with a pre-Parkinsonian state, with dopaminergic neuronal loss in the two conditions, albeit more severe in PD, as evidenced by the similarity of cellular mechanisms (Chu et al., 2002; Chu and Kordower, 2007; Collier et al., 2011).

Comparisons of nigral neuron loss in normal aging and PD is complicated by results from nonstereology and stereology approaches. Using a quantification method similar to that of Fearnley and Lees (1991), Muthane et al. (1998) reported on the absence of age-related loss of nigral neurons in Asian Indians, a population that is an ethnically distinct population from Caucasians. These studies on one 7-µm thick section counted profiles of melanized neurons at the emergence

Neurostereology: Unbiased Stereology of Neural Systems, First Edition. Edited by Peter R. Mouton.
© 2014 John Wiley & Sons, Inc. Published 2014 by John Wiley & Sons, Inc.

of the occulomotor nerve (cranial nerve III). Numerous subsequent studies have reported total numbers of neurons in aging brain using the principles of unbiased stereology on brains from different Caucasian populations. Except for a study from France (Kubis et al., 2000), which showed stability in number of dopaminergic SNpc neurons in normal adults between 44 and 100 years, three of these studies from Finland (Ma et al., 1999), Denmark (Cabello et al., 2002), and the United States (Chu et al., 2002) reported age-related degeneration in the number or dopaminergic phenotype of SNpc neurons. The study by Chu et al. (2002) analyzed differences in neurodegeneration patterns, with a stable number of melanized neurons during aging and a progressive decline in numbers of TH immunoreactivity after midlife. Hence, this study proposes age-related loss of the dopaminergic phenotype, that is, capacity to synthesize dopamine, but not neuron loss. A later study by the same group reported loss of dopaminergic phenotype after midlife accompanied by exponential increases in α-synuclein expression (Chu and Kordower, 2007).

To further explore the possibility of ethnic differences in the vulnerability of dopaminergic SNpc neurons, we revisited the Asian Indian population using stereology principles to assess the extent of melanization using cresyl violet stain and the qualitative expression of TH and nuclear-related receptor1 (Nurr1) on immunohistochemically stained cryosections. Qualitative examination revealed neuromelanin in the SNpc of fetal through 1 year of age and gradually increases to the adult levels. We found glial cell-derived neurotrophic growth factor (GDNF) receptors (GFRα1 and RET) expressed on the dopaminergic SNpc neurons through aging, suggesting GDNF responsiveness through life. There was stability in the total number of dopaminergic neurons, that is, the melanized and nonmelanized neurons, as well as the number of TH-Nurr1 colabeled neurons. Furthermore, none of the age groups, even the elderly, showed evidence of apoptosis (terminal deoxynucleotidyl transferase-mediated dUTP nick-end labeling [TUNEL] positivity) in dopaminergic SNpc neurons. The findings of relative stability in number and function of dopaminergic neurons may partly explain the lower prevalence of PD in the Asian Indian population compared with Caucasians.

Materials and Methods

We analyzed a total of 36 midbrain specimens from Asian Indians, including 35 (14 females, 21 males) from fatal traffic accidents and a single fetal midbrain obtained from medical termination of pregnancy at 28 weeks of gestation (28GW). This study had the approval of the institutional human ethics committee. The tissue pH increased with the duration of the postmortem interval; however, it did not affect the solubility of proteins, and no major abnormalities in tissue integrity were noted (Chandana et al., 2009). Exclusion criteria included large cerebral lacerations, cerebral edema, parenchymal hemorrhage, and tonsilar herniation. The ages ranged between 28 gestational weeks (28GW) to 80 years, and for the ease of analysis, the specimens were divided into groups by decades, for example, fetal, 1–9 years, 10–19 years, 20–29 years, and so on. As negative controls, we analyzed a few specimens ($n = 3$) archived in formalin of nonneurodegenerative diseases that do not affect the substantia nigra (SN) (metabolic encephalopathy, atherosclerotic cerebrovascular disease, and idiopathic meningeal thickening). These extra specimens were used only for quantification and morphometry of Nissl-stained tissue.

Processing of the Midbrain Tissue

We used chilled 4% paraformaldehyde as a fixative since the tissues were to be used for immunohistochemistry. Formalin (10%) was avoided as this may render proteins unavailable to antibody labeling in thicker sections. Each tissue specimen was fixed for at least 48 hours. Tissues were cryoprotected in sucrose gradients of 15% and 30%, serially cryosectioned at 40 μm, thawed on gelatin subbed slides, and cover-slipped for microscopic studies.

Reference Space

The tissue analyzed in this study included the caudal portion of the SNpc, including sections from the caudal level of the mammillary bodies to the rostral border of the corpus quadrigemini. The rostral-most portion of the SN was unavailable as it is generally detached from the brainstem block at the time of autopsy (Ma et al., 1999). The optic tract formed the rostral boundary, while the decussation of cerebellar peduncle formed the caudal limit of the SNpc. On the coronal plane, the oculomotor nerve emerged medial to the SNpc, with the substantia nigra pars reticulata located toward its ventral edge (Carpenter and Peter, 1972; Siddiqi et al., 1999; Siddiqi and Peters, 1999; Halliday et al., 2005). The anatomical extent of SNpc studied in our population was comparable to that studied in other populations (Ma et al., 1999; Kubis et al., 2000; Chu et al., 2002).

Nissl Stain

With cresyl violet histochemistry, the dark-colored neuromelanin pigment of the nigral neuron stains are distinct from the rich blue stain of the Nissl's granules (Figure 3.1a, arrows), while nonmelanized neurons lack the black pigment (Figure 3.1a, arrowheads). Sections were briefly dipped in chloroform followed by rehydration in descending series of alcohol (100%, 90%, 80%, 70% ethanol and double distilled water), stained in 1% buffered cresyl violet (0.1 M phosphate buffer) for 5 minutes at 55°C. Excess stain was differentiated by a brief dip in double distilled water followed by ascending grades of alcohol (70%, 80%, 90%, and 100%), cleared in xylene,

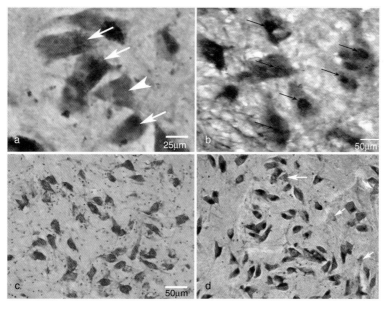

Figure 3.1 Photomicrographs of human substantia nigra pars compacta stained with Nissl's stain (a, c, and d) and colabeling of Nurr1 and TH (b). Note the granular staining of the neuromelanin in the majority of the cells (a, arrows). Some of the cells lack neuromelanin, which are termed as borderline/nonmelanized neurons (a, arrowhead). Compare panel c (nigra of a 1-year-old subject) with panel d (nigra of an 80-year-old subject). There are no obvious changes in the two other than the presence of melanin. Panel b shows the presence of Nurr1 (grayish black) in the nucleus of dopaminergic neurons (brown).

and mounted using distyrene plasticizer xylol (DPX). Total number of melanized and nonmelanized/borderline neurons were estimated using the optical disector method (Sterio, 1984).

Immunohistochemistry Protocols

Dopaminergic Neuronal Markers and GDNF Receptors

Antibodies to two markers were used to label and quantify dopaminergic neurons: TH, a cytoplasmic enzyme, and Nurr1, a nuclear transcriptional protein (Chu et al., 2002; Alladi et al., 2009). Neuromelanin was bleached using 0.6% potassium permanganate followed by 2% oxalic acid (Kastner et al., 1992) followed by endogenous peroxidase quenching in the presence of 70% methanol and 0.03% H_2O_2. The background staining was blocked with 3% skim milk protein solution for 4 hours, and then the sections were incubated in anti-Nurr1 antibody (1:1000, Santa Cruz Biotechnology Inc., USA) for 72 hours at 4°C. The initial 4 hours were at room temperature to facilitate the antigen–antibody binding reaction. The secondary antibody was biotinylated anti-rabbit IgG (4 hours) followed by application of avidin–biotin complex (1:200, Elite ABC kits; Vector Laboratories; USA). The reaction was visualized using 0.05% 3,3′-diaminobenzidine and 0.03% H_2O_2, with 3% Ni_2SO_4 as an enhancer. Using Ni_2SO_4, the reaction product appeared gray to black with Nurr1 localized to the nucleus (Figure 3.1b, black arrows). For TH immunostaining, the same sections were further blocked briefly and reincubated in second primary antibody (TH, 1:1000, Santa Cruz Biotechnology, Inc.) for 72 hours. After the application of biotinylated horse antimouse secondary antibody (1:200) and avidin–biotin complex (1:200, Vector Laboratories) for 4 hours each, the staining was detected using 3,3′-diaminobenzidine and 0.03% H_2O_2 as a chromogen, and the reaction product was brown and localized to the cytoplasm (Figure 3.1b). Labeling of GDNF receptors GFRα1 and RET was performed by single labeling method with appropriate primary and secondary antibodies and was detected using 3,3′-diaminobenzidine as a chromogen (Alladi et al., 2010a).

Immunofluorescence Labeling of α-Synuclein, GRP-78, Caspase 12, and Ubiquitin

From the series of adjacent midbrain sections, one series was used for colabeling with α-synuclein and caspase 12 and the second for GRP78 and TH. A third series of sections were stained for ubiquitin and TH. For each of the series, the nonspecific binding was blocked with 3% skimmed milk protein solution. The primary antibodies used in the study were procured from commercial vendors (α-synuclein and GRP78, Santa Cruz Biotechnology Inc, Santacruz, CA, USA; Caspase 12, Sigma-Aldrich USA; ubiquitin, Novacastra Laboratories ltd, Newcastle upon Tyne, UK) and were monospecific as confirmed on Western blots. The labeling was detected using appropriate fluorochromes tagged secondary antisera (Alladi et al., 2010b). Washing in between the steps was done using 0.01 M phosphate buffered saline containing Triton-X 100. Neuronal counts were done using a computerized stereology system with fluorescence microscopy equipped with a motorized stage for movement in the three directions (BX61, Olympus Microscopes, Japan). The immunofluorescence was also analyzed using laser confocal scanning microscope to ascertain the colabeling pattern, if any, and intensity measurements (Leica DMIRE-TCS, Germany). For this, the laser illumination was set at 488 nm for fluorescein isothiocyanate (FITC) and 514 nm for Cy3, respectively. The segregation of the bandwidths for FITC (490–550 nm) and Cy3 (560–640 nm) helped avoid nonspecific overlap of emission frequencies that would otherwise cause a false impression of colabeling (Alladi et al., 2010b).

Apoptosis Labeling

Age-related neuronal death in the SNpc was confirmed using the TUNEL method from commercially available kits (Chemicon International, Temecula, USA). Blocking with 3% BSA reduced

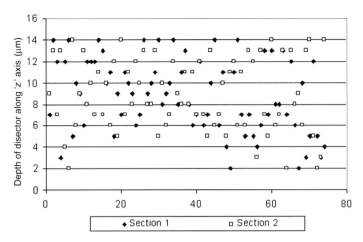

Figure 3.2 A plot from two representative sections shows the homogenous distribution of "profiles" along the *z*-axis, that is, the depth of the "disector," which suggests that the profiles were well stained throughout the depth of the section.

the nonspecific staining, then the sections were "equilibrated" and incubated with the TdT enzyme at 37°C for 4 hours. This was followed by incubation in FITC-conjugated digoxigenin for 2 hours, which was visualized by an excitation wavelength of 488 nm and an emission bandwidth of 495–540 nm using a Laser scanning confocal microscope (Leica-TCS-SL, Leica Microsystems, Germany). The TUNEL-stained sections were colabeled with TH to identify the dying dopaminergic neurons. TH (1:1000 dilution; Santa Cruz Biotechnology Inc, USA) labeling was detected using cyanine3 (CY3)-tagged antimouse secondary antibody (1:200 dilution; Sigma-Aldrich USA). Human rectal biopsy sections were used as positive controls.

Stereology Methods

The numbers of Nissl-stained (melanized, borderline/nonmelanized) and immunostained neurons (TH-Nurr1 colabeled, GRP-78, Caspase 12, α-synuclein, and ubiquitin immunoreactive) were estimated using the optical fractionator method. The stained sections were adjudged for the staining quality and the penetration of the primary antibody (Figure 3.2). Sections were cut at an instrument setting of 40 μm with the final processed thickness after all tissue processing in the range 24.6–25.4 μm.

Stereology was done on every tenth section of the coded specimens, with the SNpc outlined at low magnification (4×) and neuron counts under high-resolution oil immersion magnification (100× objective). The constants for the cell counting included disector height (14 μm) and guard zones (4 μm).

Stereological estimation of neurons with RET receptors, previously reported in primate and human substantia nigra (Walker et al., 1998; Dass et al., 2006), remained stable through aging (Figure 3.3a–d).

The expression of α-synuclein was localized to the cytoplasm and processes (Figure 3.4a,c; d,f). A few nigral neurons did not stain for α-synuclein (Figure 3.4a,c; d,f, white arrows).

Discussion

Aging, the single most important risk factor for PD, causes degeneration of dopaminergic neurons of the SNpc on a less severe scale than in PD (Hassler, 1939; Chu et al., 2002; Chu and Kordower,

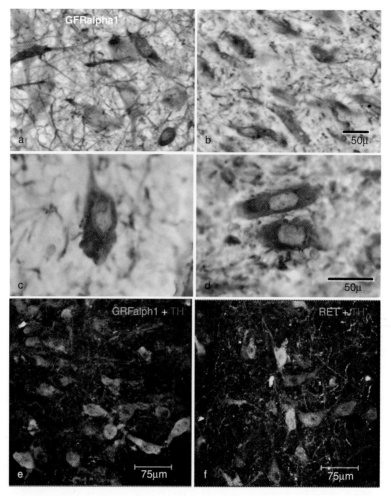

Figure 3.3 Representative photomicrographs of human substantia nigra pars compacta stained for GFRα1 (a, 4 years and b, 80 years) and RET (c, 4 years and d 80 years). Note the staining pattern is similar in the two age groups. Panel e shows a "merged image" of a section colabeled for GFRα1 (FITC, green) and TH (CY3, red). Panel f shows a "merged image" of a section colabeled for RET (FITC, green) and TH (CY3, red). Note the yellowish orange color is due to the mixing of green and red emissions by the fluorochromes, suggesting colocalization of the two proteins.

2007). The commonality of SNpc neuronal loss in aging and PD supports the hypothesis that PD may be a manifestation of accelerated aging. Epidemiological studies report a higher prevalence of PD in Caucasians (Schoenberg et al., 1988; Tanner and Goldman, 1994) than in Asian Indians (Razdan et al., 1994; Gourie-Devi et al., 1996; Das et al., 1998, 2010), with the exception of one ethnic group, that is, the Parsis (Bharucha et al., 1988). Nigral neurons in the middle and caudal nigra of Asian Indians were comparable to the Danish population and higher than the Finnish and American populations (Alladi et al., 2009). In line with the study from France, Asian Indians showed no evidence of age-related cell loss of dopaminergic neurons in PD (Kubis et al., 2000). The absolute numbers of melanized nigral neurons and their vulnerability in terms of cell loss differed in various populations (Table 3.1).

One factor governing the vulnerability of populations to develop PD could be the basal number of dopaminergic neurons, quantity of neuromelanin in these neurons, and the rate of age-related loss in SNpc. Since melanized neurons are selectively lost from the SN of primate models of PD

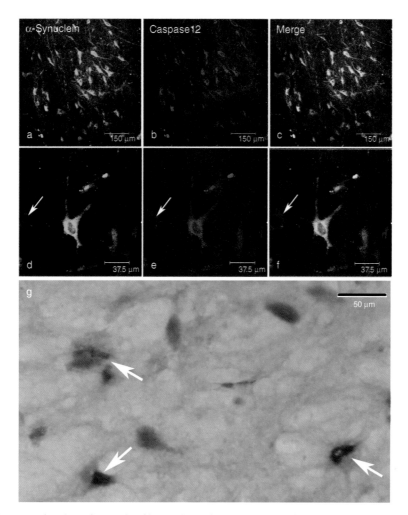

Figure 3.4 Representative photomicrographs of human (age = 4 years) substantia nigra pars compacta stained for α-synuclein (FITC, green) and caspase 12 (CY3, red). Note the staining in the processes and the neuropil. Panel c shows a "merged image" of panels a and b (yellowish green), suggesting colabeling of both proteins. Panels d–f show high magnification image showing clear nucleus. Note an unstained cell in the vicinity (arrow) which is probably a dopaminergic neuron not immunoreactive for these proteins. Note the aggregation of insoluble α-synuclein (arrows) in the nigral neurons of a 69-year-old subject.

(Herrero et al., 1993), similar to that in patients with PD (Fearnley and Lees, 1991), higher neuromelanin content could render the dopaminergic neurons more vulnerable to degeneration (Kastner et al., 1993).

A study in 1998 carried out on a single midbrain section from each brain reported the absence of age-related loss of nigral neurons in Asian Indians, with 40% fewer neurons than British Caucasians (Muthane et al., 1998). Although the results from a later study using a stereological approach differed from these findings with absolute counts higher in Asian Indians (Chu et al., 2002; Alladi et al., 2009), the lack of age-related loss of melanized neurons was consistent with the earlier findings (Figure 3.1, compare c and d). Thus, the lower prevalence of PD in Indians may be attributed to higher number of nigral neurons, supporting the hypothesis that populations with higher prevalence of PD may have fewer total numbers of nigral neurons (Fahn, 1989).

The question of why some dopaminergic neurons are nonmelanized in primates and humans remains unclear (Fedorow et al., 2005). Although nonmelanized neurons are involved in dopamine

Table 3.1 Comparison of neuronal numbers and the pattern of cell loss in different populations

Sl. no.	Country of study	Age range (years)	No. of melanized neurons	Age-related cell loss?	Other observations	Reference
1	Finland	70 ± 10	163,238 ± 42,372	Not documented	Cellular atrophy	Ma et al. (1996)
2	France	40–110	–	Dopaminergic neurons: no	No changes	Kubis et al. (2000)
3	Denmark	19–40	378,000	Yes	Cellular hypertrophy	Cabello et al. (2002)
		71–92	256,000			
4	USA	18–39	169,362 ± 4813	Melanized neurons: no;	Exponential increase in α-synuclein and insoluble α-synuclein, Marinesco bodies	Chu et al. (2002)
		44–68	180,778 ± 9488	Dopaminergic neurons: yes		
		76–102	164,304 ± 11,973			
5	India	28GW–80	262,732 ± 83,601	Melanized neurons: no; Dopaminergic neurons: no; Apoptosis: no	No changes in size, mild increase in α-synuclein; Increase in GRP78 and Marinesco bodies	Alladi et al. (2009, 2010b)

synthesis, they may be less vulnerable. Neuromelanin is a by-product of the oxidation of dopamine synthesized by borderline/nonmelanized nigral neurons (Kingsbury et al., 1999). The expression of TH mRNA is upregulated in nonmelanized neurons in idiopathic PD, whereas reduction in TH expression precedes the death of melanized neurons.

The higher number of nonmelanized neurons in Asian Indians may play a role in preserving nigral function. In our study, the number of borderline/nonmelanized neurons stabilized by midlife (approximately 10%) and remained constant through life, even in the elderly (Figure 3.1d, white arrowheads), and was relatively higher (5%) than that reported from the UK (Gibb, 1992). The number of Nurr1-TH colabeled neurons was stable through all the ages in Asian Indians, also supporting the preservation of dopaminergic phenotype. Expression of Nurr1, an essential transcription factor for dopaminergic phenotype expression (Zetterstrom et al., 1996, 1997), undergoes linear reduction in normal aging (Chu et al., 2002) and in PD (Chu and Kordower, 2007). In normal aging, the decline in Nurr1 expression begins earlier than the decline of TH immunoreactivity and precedes loss of dopaminergic function. In that study, the numbers of melanized neurons remained stable, while the number of Nurr1 and TH immunoreactive neurons declined gradually with age. This finding suggests that the neurons may not die but rather lose their capacity to synthesize dopamine, that is, lose their dopaminergic phenotype. These observations fit with the study of the French population (Kubis et al., 2000) and were further supported by Western blot studies showing no significant decline in these proteins with age. The marginal decrease in TH expression on Western blots could reflect a mild age-related decline in motor performance in older individuals (Chu et al., 2002; Alladi et al., 2009).

During normal aging, loss of neighboring cells occurs in approximately 2% of the melanized nigral neurons, along with other morphological and ultrastructural changes such as chromatin condensation and cell shrinkage associated with apoptosis (Anglade et al., 1997). Light and electron microscopic studies of nigral neurons in SN of normally aging American adults and PD patients also confirmed the occurrence of apoptosis (Tompkins and Hill, 1997; Tompkins et al., 1997). In the Asian Indian population, however, we found no evidence of nigral TUNEL positive dopaminergic neurons, similar to the findings in brains of Japanese adults (Mochizuki et al., 1997). In addition to the degeneration-induced loss, nigral neurons undergo morphological changes such as reduction in soma size in aging and PD (Ma et al., 1996; Itoh et al., 1997). In the Asian Indians, neuronal size did not show any changes, similar to that in the French population (Kubis et al., 2000). Another study observed that hypertrophy compensated for age-related loss of pigmented nigral neurons (Cabello et al., 2002). Neuronal size in the Indian and French brains may not have hypertrophied due to the absence of pronounced neurodegeneration or neuronal loss.

Use of GDNF, a potential neurotrophic factor for dopaminergic neurons, has been proposed for treatment of PD (Lin et al., 1993; Beck et al., 1995; Tomac et al., 1995; Gash et al., 1996; Lapchak, 1998; Kordower, 2003). Our study showed preserved expression of both GDNF receptors, that is, GFRα1 and RET, in human SNpc during aging. GFRα1 (Cik et al., 2000) and the signaling component RET tyrosine kinase (Trupp et al., 1996) are the components of multicomponent receptor complex through which GNDF confers neuroprotection to nigral neurons. The stable expression of cRet and GFRα1 may indicate compensatory changes in target-derived GDNF in response to extensive loss of dopaminergic neurons in the SNpc with concomitant loss of striatal dopamine (Bäckman et al., 2006). The GFRα1 protein is expressed in motor and nonmotor areas rostral to the midbrain (Serra et al., 2005), while RET mRNA expression is found exclusively in the motor areas. Our study provides evidence that GFRα1 and RET were colocalized on the nigral neurons and hence probably were part of the multireceptor complex (Alladi et al., 2010a, Figure 3.3e,f; NB: Cells show greenish orange color due to mixing of green [GFRalpha1/RET] and red [TH], suggesting colocalization), comparable to the findings in nonhuman primates (Dass et al., 2006). It has been documented that in the rodent habenula, spinal cord motor neurons and nigral neurons have the highest amounts of these receptors (Wang et al., 2008). Since the growth factor receptors are preserved, it may be possible to reverse the nigrostriatal dysfunction by GDNF or neurturin (Dass et al., 2006). In brain from humans with PD, Walker et al. (1998) demonstrated persistence of RET immunoreactivity in the nigra, suggesting that the GDNF administration could be a successful therapy for the surviving dopaminergic neurons.

Unbiased stereology allowed us to compare the number of neurons labeled with different proteins, which would have been impossible using qualitative analysis alone. For example, we observed that the total number of GFRα1 neurons was marginally higher than the RET immunoreactive neurons. It is highly likely that GFRα1 was also expressed on nondopaminergic neurons, for example, GABAergic interneurons (Sarabi et al., 2001), which can be further investigated in our samples.

Most studies agree with the notion that Lewy bodies present evidence of neurodegeneration. The major components of intraneuronal inclusions called Lewy bodies are lipids, neurofilaments, misfolded proteins, α-synuclein, synphilin-1, ubiquitin, and the ubiquitin-pathway-related enzymes (Irizarry et al., 1998; Spillantini et al., 1998; Gai et al., 2000; Gomez-Tortosa et al., 2000; Wakabayashi et al., 2000). Finding that the nucleolar volume in healthy cells and those without Lewy bodies were comparable, Gertz et al. (1994) reports that the presence of Lewy bodies does not affect neuronal metabolism adversely. Greffard et al. (2010) indicate that during the progression of PD, the number of neurons with Lewy bodies remains consistent. Thus, the presence of Lewy body may signal neuronal degeneration or death.

Among the misfolded and accumulated proteins of the Lewy bodies, α-synuclein appears to form a major component and may play a role in normal postnatal development (Jakowec et al., 2001; Chu and Kordower, 2007). A couple of studies have proposed mechanisms for the selective nigral neuronal loss in PD and their relationship to α-synuclein. One study proposed that accumulation of soluble α-synuclein protein complexes render endogenous dopamine toxic (Xu et al., 2002). Another study demonstrated that the accumulation of soluble α-synuclein was restricted to nigral and striatal, but not cerebellar mitochondria, of PD subjects (Devi et al., 2008). They also found a correlation between such accumulations with decreased complex I activity and enhanced reactive oxygen species generation. In the PD patients, the α-synuclein mRNA levels showed a fourfold increase (Chiba-Falek et al., 2006), whereas levels of two proteins, α-synuclein and parkin substrate SEPT4, show more than 10-fold upregulation (Shehadeh et al., 2009). It is therefore highly likely that a logarithmic increase could escalate the vulnerability of the neurons. There exists a robust correlation between age-related increase in α-synuclein protein and loss of α-synuclein positive dopaminergic neurons in humans and monkeys specifically in the SNpc but not in the ventral tegmental area (Chu and Kordower, 2007). The human population in this study was from the United States. Our finding that all nigral neurons did not stain for α-synuclein may account for the fewer number of α-synuclein positive neurons than TH-immunoreactive neurons. The increase in the number of α-synuclein expressing neurons with age in our Asian Indian cohort was statistically significant. But the increase in immunofluorescence intensity as a measure of protein expression in individual cells was approximately 19% over nine decades, with cytoplasmic aggregates of insoluble α-synuclein apparent after the sixth decade (Figure 3.4g, white arrows; Alladi et al., 2010b). Thus, the findings of soluble and insoluble α-synuclein, in some measure, differed in the two human studies. It may not be apposite to compare two studies directly, but since the methodology and software used were similar, it is possible that the differences in α-synuclein expression in these studies are due to ethnic differences between populations. The mild overexpression of α-synuclein seen in Asian Indian subjects may indicate subthreshold neurodegeneration, whereas a logarithmic increase may imply a more severe effect.

We found the caspase 12 expression was exclusively cytoplasmic (Figure 3.4b,c and e,f) and not nuclear in any of the age groups studied, suggesting the absence of ER stress-mediated cell death in these neurons (Alladi et al., 2010b). The absence of nuclear localization of caspase 12 in our samples correlates well with our earlier findings of lack of apoptosis in nigral dopaminergic neurons in our population (Alladi et al., 2009).

Our studies on Asian Indians, who have a lower prevalence of PD than several other populations, show preservation of dopaminergic neurons during aging. Second, the receptors of growth factor GDNF were also preserved. We also observed an increase in α-synuclein immunoreactivity, with absence of nuclear localization of caspase 12. Thus, neurodegeneration of dopaminergic neurons in SNpc may occur in a subthreshold manner, along with protective ER stress mechanisms and proteasomal function. Future studies may be worthwhile to investigate the role of calcium binding proteins, as well as effects on glia and synaptogenesis in this population. This neuroprotection during aging in the Asian Indians could be the result of genetic, environmental, dietary factors, or some combination of these. Among the dietary factors, the neuroprotective role of antioxidant curcumin has been reported in Alzheimer's disease (Lim et al., 2001) and PD. Curcumin is an active ingredient of turmeric, a traditional Indian food additive and herbal medicine. Curcumin and tetrahydrocurcumin reverse MPTP-induced depletion of dopamine and its metabolite DOPAC (Rajeswari and Sabesan, 2008). Chronic supplementation of turmeric protected against peroxynitrite-mediated inhibition of brain complex 1 via induction of the enzyme γ-glutamyl cysteine ligase and an increase in glutathione levels in MPTP-injected mice (Mythri et al., 2011). Thus, both curcumin and its metabolite may confer neuroprotection against MPTP-induced neurotoxicity. This and other dietary factors and lifestyle may protect the nigral neurons from age-related degeneration and may partly explain the lower prevalence of PD in Asian Indians.

Acknowledgments

The studies were funded by the Department of Science and Technology (SR/WOS-A/LS-268/2004), Government of India and Council for Scientific and Industrial Research (27(0226)/09-EMR-I) to

P.A.A. I am grateful to Prof. Shashi Wadhwa for introducing me to the wonderful world of Neuroscience and Stereology. I acknowledge the help of Prof. Gomathy Gopinath for the help on anatomy of substantia nigra. I am thankful to my mentors and collaborators, Dr. Uday Muthane, Dr. SK Shankar, Dr. TR Raju, and DR. BM Kutty.

References

Alladi, P. A., Mahadevan, A., Yasha, T. C., Raju, T. R., Shankar, S. K., Muthane, U. 2009. Absence of age-related changes in nigral dopaminergic neurons of Asian Indians: relevance to lower incidence of Parkinson's disease. *Neuroscience* **159**: 236–245.

Alladi, P. A., Mahadevan, A., Shankar, S. K., Raju, T. R., Muthane, U. 2010a. Expression of GDNF receptors GFRα1 and RET is preserved in substantia nigra pars compacta of aging Asian Indians. *J Chem Neuroanat* **40** (1): 43–52.

Alladi, P. A., Mahadevan, A., Vijayalakshmi, K., Muthane, U., Shankar, S. K., Raju, T. R. 2010b. Ageing enhances alpha-synuclein, ubiquitin and endoplasmic reticular stress protein expression in the nigral neurons of Asian Indians. *Neurochem Int* **57** (5): 530–539.

Anglade, P., Vyas, S., Javoy-Agid, F., Herrero, M. T., Michel, P. P., Marquez, J., Mouatt-Prigent, A., Ruberg, M., Hirsch, E. C., Agid, Y. 1997. Apoptosis and autophagy in nigral neurons of patients with Parkinson's disease. *Histol Histopathol* **12**: 25–31.

Bäckman, C. M., Shan, L., Zhang, Y. J., Hoffer, B. J., Leonard, S., Troncoso, J. C., Vonsatel, P., Tomac, A. C. 2006. Gene expression patterns for GDNF and its receptors in the human putamen affected by Parkinson's disease: a real-time PCR study. *Mol Cell Endocrinol* **252** (1–2): 160–166.

Beck, K. D., Valverde, J., Alexi, T., Poulsen, K., Moffat, B., Vandlen, R. A., Rosenthal, A., Hefti, F. 1995. Mesencephalic dopaminergic neurons protected by GDNF from axotomy-induced degeneration in the adult brain. *Nature* **373**: 339–341.

Bharucha, N. E., Bharucha, E. P., Bharucha, A. E., Bhise, A. V., Schoenberg, B. S. 1988. Prevalence of Parkinson's disease in the Parsi community of Bombay, India. *Arch Neurol* **45**: 1321–1323.

Cabello, C. R., Thune, J. J., Pakkenberg, H., Pakkenberg, B. 2002. Ageing of substantia nigra in humans: cell loss may be compensated by hypertrophy. *Neuropathol Appl Neurobiol* **28**: 283–291.

Carpenter, M. B., Peter, P. 1972. Nigrostriatal and nigrothalamic fibers in the rhesus monkey. *J Comp Neurol* **144**: 93–115.

Chandana, R., Mythri, R. B., Mahadevan, A., Shankar, S. K., Srinivas Bharath, M. M. 2009. Biochemical analysis of protein stability in human brain collected at different post-mortem intervals. *Indian J Med Res* **129** (2): 189–199.

Chiba-Falek, O., Lopez, G. J., Nussbaum, R. L. 2006. Levels of alpha-synuclein mRNA in sporadic Parkinson disease patients. *Mov Disord* **21**: 1703–1708.

Chu, Y., Kordower, J. H. 2007. Age-associated increases of alpha-synuclein in monkeys and humans are associated with nigrostriatal dopamine depletion: is this the target for Parkinson's disease? *Neurobiol Dis* **25**: 134–149.

Chu, Y., Kompoliti, K., Cochran, E. J., Mufson, E. J., Kordower, J. H. 2002. Age-related decreases in Nurr1 immunoreactivity in the human substantia nigra. *J Comp Neurol* **450**: 203–214.

Cik, M., Masure, S., Lesage, A. S., Van Der Linden, I., Van Gompel, P., Pangalos, M. N., Gordon, R. D., Leysen, J. E. 2000. Binding of GDNF and neurturin to human GDNF family receptor alpha 1 and 2. Influence of cRET and cooperative interactions. *J Biol Chem* **275**: 27505–27512.

Collier, T. J., Kanaan, N. M., Kordower, J. H. 2011. Ageing as a primary risk factor for Parkinson's disease: evidence from studies of non-human primates. *Nat Rev Neurosci* **126**: 359–366.

Das, S., Sanyal, K., Moitra, A. 1998. A pilot study on neuroepidemiology in urban Bengal. *Indian J Public Health* **42** (2): 34–36, 41.

Das, S. K., Misra, A. K., Ray, B. K., Hazra, A., Ghosal, M. K., Chaudhuri, A., Roy, T., Banerjee, T. K., Raut, D. K. 2010. Epidemiology of Parkinson's disease in the city of Kolkata, India: a community-based study. *Neurology* **75** (15): 1362–1369.

Dass, B., Kladis, T., Chu, Y., Kordower, J. H. 2006. RET expression does not change with age in the substantia nigra pars compacta of rhesus monkeys. *Neurobiol Aging* **27** (6): 857–861.

Devi, L., Raghavendran, V., Prabhu, B. M., Avadhani, N. G., Anandatheerthavarada, H. K. 2008. Mitochondrial import and accumulation of alpha-synuclein impair complex I in human dopaminergic neuronal cultures and Parkinson disease brain. *J Biol Chem* **283** (14): 9089–9100.

Fahn, S. 1989. The history of parkinsonism. *Mov Disord* **4** (Suppl 1): S2–S10.

Fearnley, J. M., Lees, A. J. 1991. Ageing and Parkinson's disease: substantia nigra regional selectivity. *Brain* **114** (Pt 5): 2283–2301.

Fedorow, H., Tribl, F., Halliday, G., Gerlach, M., Riederer, P., Double, K. L. 2005. Neuromelanin in human dopamine neurons: comparison with peripheral melanins and relevance to Parkinson's disease. *Prog Neurobiol* **75**: 109–124.

Gai, W. P., Yuan, H. X., Li, X. Q., Power, J. T., Blumbergs, P. C., Jensen, P. H. 2000. In situ and in vitro study of colocalization and segregation of alpha-synuclein, ubiquitin, and lipids in Lewy bodies. *Exp Neurol* **166**: 324–333.

Gash, D. M., Zhang, Z., Ovadia, A., Cass, W. A., Yi, A., Simmerman, L., Russell, D., Martin, D., Lapchak, P. A., Collins, F., Hoffer, B. J., Gerhardt, G. A. 1996. Functional recovery in parkinsonian monkeys treated with GDNF. *Nature* **380**: 252–255.

Gertz, H. J., Siegers, A., Kuchinke, J. 1994. Stability of cell size and nucleolar size in Lewy body containing neurons of substantia nigra in Parkinson's disease. *Brain Res* **637** (1–2): 339–341.

Gibb, W. R. 1992. Melanin, tyrosine hydroxylase, calbindin and substance P in the human midbrain and substantia nigra in relation to nigrostriatal projections and differential neuronal susceptibility in Parkinson's disease. *Brain Res* **581**: 283–291.

Gibb, W. R., Lees, A. J. 1991. Anatomy, pigmentation, ventral and dorsal subpopulations of the substantia nigra, and differential cell death in Parkinson's disease. *J Neurol Neurosurg Psychiatry* **54** (5): 388–396.

Gomez-Tortosa, E., Newell, K., Irizarry, M. C., Sanders, J. L., Hyman, B. T. 2000. alpha-Synuclein immunoreactivity in dementia with Lewy bodies: morphological staging and comparison with ubiquitin immunostaining. *Acta Neuropathol (Berl)* **99**: 352–357.

Gourie-Devi, M., Gururaj, G., Satishchandra, P., Subbakrishna, D. K. 1996. Neuro-epidemiological pilot survey of an urban population in a developing country: a study in Bangalore, south India. *Neuroepidemiology* **15** (207): 313–320, 1327–1337.

Greffard, S., Verny, M., Bonnet, A. M., Seilhean, D., Hauw, J. J., Duyckaerts, C. 2010. A stable proportion of Lewy body bearing neurons in the substantia nigra suggests a model in which the Lewy body causes neuronal death. *Neurobiol Aging* **31** (1): 99–103.

Halliday, G. M., Ophof, A., Broe, M., Jensen, P. H., Kettle, E., Fedorow, H., Cartwright, M. I., Griffiths, F. M., Shepherd, C. E., Doubl, K. L. 2005. Alpha-synuclein redistributes to neuromelanin lipid in the substantia nigra early in Parkinson's disease. *Brain* **128**: 2654–2664.

Hassler, R. 1939. Zur pathologischen anatomie des senilen und des parkinsonistichen tremor. *J Psychol Neurol* **49**: 13–55.

Herrero, M. T., Hirsch, E. C., Kastner, A., Ruberg, M., Luquin, M. R., Laguna, J., Javoy-Agid, F., Obeso, J. A., Agid, Y. 1993. Does neuromelanin contribute to the vulnerability of catecholaminergic neurons in monkeys intoxicated with MPTP? *Neuroscience* **56** (2): 499–511.

Irizarry, M. C., Growdon, W., Gomez-Isla, T., Newell, K., George, J. M., Clayton, D. F., Hyman, B. T. 1998. Nigral and cortical Lewy bodies and dystrophic nigral neurites in Parkinson's disease and cortical Lewy body disease contain alpha-synuclein immunoreactivity. *J Neuropathol Exp Neurol* **57**: 334–337.

Itoh, K., Weis, S., Mehraein, P., Muller-Hocker, J. 1997. Defects of cytochrome c oxidase in the substantia nigra of Parkinson's disease: and immunohistochemical and morphometric study. *Mov Disord* **12**: 9–16.

Jakowec, M. W., Donaldson, D. M., Barba, J., Petzinger, G. M. 2001. Postnatal expression of alpha-synuclein protein in the rodent substantia nigra and striatum. *Dev Neurosci* **23**: 91–99.

Kastner, A., Hirsch, E. C., Lejeune, O., Javoy-Agid, F., Rascol, O., Agid, Y. 1992. Is the vulnerability of neurons in the substantia nigra of patients with Parkinson's disease related to their neuromelanin content? *J Neurochem* **59**: 1080–1089.

Kastner, A., Hirsch, E. C., Herrero, M. T., Javoy-Agid, F., Agid, Y. 1993. Immunocytochemical quantification of tyrosine hydroxylase at a cellular level in the mesencephalon of control subjects and patients with Parkinson's and Alzheimer's disease. *J Neurochem* **61**: 1024–1034.

Kingsbury, A. E., Marsden, C. D., Foster, O. J. 1999. The vulnerability of nigral neurons to Parkinson's disease is unrelated to their intrinsic capacity for dopamine synthesis: an in situ hybridization study. *Mov Disord* **14**: 206–218.

Kordower, J. H. 2003. In vivo gene delivery of glial cell line-derived neurotrophic factor for Parkinson's disease. *Ann Neurol* **53** (Suppl 3): S120–S132.

Kubis, N., Faucheux, B. A., Ransmayr, G., Damier, P., Duyckaerts, C., Henin, D., Forette, B., Le Charpentier, Y., Hauw, J. J., Agid, Y., Hirsch, E. C. 2000. Preservation of midbrain catecholaminergic neurons in very old human subjects. *Brain* **123** (Pt 2): 366–373.

Lapchak, P. A. 1998. A preclinical development strategy designed to optimize the use of glial cell line-derived neurotrophic factor in the treatment of Parkinson's disease. *Mov Disord* **13** (Suppl 1): 49–54.

Lim, G. P., Chu, T., Yang, F., Beech, W., Frautschy, S. A., Cole, G. M. 2001. The curry spice curcumin reduces oxidative damage and amyloid pathology in an Alzheimer transgenic mouse. *J Neurosci* **21**: 8370–8377.

Lin, L. F., Doherty, D. H., Lile, J. D., Bektesh, S., Collins, F. 1993. GDNF: a glial cell line-derived neurotrophic factor for midbrain dopaminergic neurons. *Science* **260**: 1130–1132.

Ma, S. Y., Rinne, J. O., Collan, Y., Roytta, M., Rinne, U. K. 1996. A quantitative morphometrical study of neuron degeneration in the substantia nigra in Parkinson's disease. *J Neurol Sci* **140**: 40–45.

Ma, S. Y., Roytt, M., Collan, Y., Rinne, J. O. 1999. Unbiased morphometrical measurements show loss of pigmented nigral neurones with ageing. *Neuropathol Appl Neurobiol* **25**: 394–399.

Mochizuki, H., Mori, H., Mizuno, Y. 1997. Apoptosis in neurodegenerative disorders. *J Neural Transm Suppl* **50**: 125–140.

Muthane, U., Yasha, T. C., Shankar, S. K. 1998. Low numbers and no loss of melanized nigral neurons with increasing age in normal human brains from India. *Ann Neurol* **43**: 283–287.

Muthane, U., Jain, S., Gururaj, G. 2001. Hunting genes in Parkinson's disease from the roots. *Med Hypotheses* **57**: 51–55.

Muthane, U. B., Ragothaman, M., Gururaj, G. 2007. Epidemiology of Parkinson's disease and movement disorders in India: problems and possibilities. *J Assoc Physicians India* **55**: 719–724. Review.

Mythri, R. B., Veena, J., Harish, G., Shankaranarayana Rao, B. S., Srinivas Bharath, M. M. 2011. Chronic dietary supplementation with turmeric protects against 1-methyl-4-phenyl-1,2,3,6-tetrahydropyridine-mediated neurotoxicity in vivo: implications for Parkinson's disease. *Br J Nutr* **106** (1): 63–72.

Rajeswari, A., Sabesan, M. 2008. Inhibition of monoamine oxidase-B by the polyphenolic compound, curcumin and its metabolite tetrahydrocurcumin, in a model of Parkinson's disease induced by MPTP neurodegeneration in mice. *Inflammopharmacology* **16**: 96–99.

Razdan, S., Kaul, R. L., Motta, A., Kaul, S., Bhatt, R. K. 1994. Prevalence and pattern of major neurological disorders in rural Kashmir (India) in 1986. *Neuroepidemiology* **13**: 113–119.

Sarabi, A., Hoffer, B. J., Olson, L., Morales, M. 2001. GFRalpha-1 mRNA in dopaminergic and nondopaminergic neurons in the substantia nigra and ventral tegmental area. *J Comp Neurol* **441**: 106–117.

Schoenberg, B. S., Osuntokun, B. O., Adeuja, A. O., Bademosi, O., Nottidge, V., Anderson, D. W., Haerer, A. F. 1988. Comparison of the prevalence of Parkinson's disease in black populations in the rural United States and in rural Nigeria: door-to-door community studies. *Neurology* **38**: 645–646.

Serra, M. P., Quartu, M., Mascia, F., Manca, A., Boi, M., Pisu, M. G., Lai, M. L., Del Fiacco, M. 2005. Ret, GFRalpha-1, GFRalpha-2 and GFRalpha-3 receptors in the human hippocampus and fascia dentata. *Int J Dev Neurosci* **235**: 425–438.

Shehadeh, L., Mitsi, G., Adi, N., Bishopric, N., Papapetropoulos, S. 2009. Expression of Lewy body protein septin 4 in postmortem brain of Parkinson's disease and control subjects. *Mov Disord* **242**: 204–210.

Siddiqi, Z., Kemper, T. L., Killiany, R. 1999. Age-related neuronal loss from the substantia nigra-pars compacta and ventral tegmental area of the rhesus monkey. *J Neuropathol Exp Neurol* **58**: 959–971.

Siddiqi, Z. A., Peters, A. 1999. The effect of aging on pars compacta of the substantia nigra in rhesus monkey. *J Neuropathol Exp Neurol* **58**: 903–920.

Spillantini, M. G., Crowther, R. A., Jakes, R., Hasegawa, M., Goedert, M. 1998. alpha-Synuclein in filamentous inclusions of Lewy bodies from Parkinson's disease and dementia with Lewy bodies. *Proc Natl Acad Sci U S A* **95**: 6469–6473.

Sterio, D. C. 1984. The unbiased estimation of number and sizes of arbitrary particles using the disector. *J Microsc* **134** (Pt 2): 127–136.

Tanner, C. M., Goldman, S. M. 1994. Epidemiology of movement disorders. *Curr Opin Neurol* **7**: 340–345.

Tomac, A., Lindqvist, E., Lin, L. F., Ogren, S. O., Young, D., Hoffer, B. J., Olson, L. 1995. Protection and repair of the nigrostriatal dopaminergic system by GDNF in vivo. *Nature* **373**: 335–339.

Tompkins, M. M., Hill, W. D. 1997. Contribution of somal Lewy bodies to neuronal death. *Brain Res* **775**: 24–29.

Tompkins, M. M., Basgall, E. J., Zamrini, E., Hill, W. D. 1997. Apoptotic-like changes in Lewy-body-associated disorders and normal aging in substantia nigral neurons. *Am J Pathol* **150**: 119–131.

Trupp, M., Arenas, E., Fainzilber, M., Nilsson, A. S., Sieber, B. A., Grigoriou, M., Kilkenny, C., Salazar-Grueso, E., Pachnis, V., Arumae, U. 1996. Functional receptor for GDNF encoded by the c-ret proto-oncogene. *Nature* **381**: 785–789.

Wakabayashi, K., Engelender, S., Yoshimoto, M., Tsuji, S., Ross, C. A., Takahashi, H. 2000. Synphilin-1 is present in Lewy bodies in Parkinson's disease. *Ann Neurol* **47**: 521–523.

Walker, D. G., Beach, T. G., Xu, R., Lile, J., Beck, K. D., McGeer, E. G., McGeer, P. L. 1998. Expression of the proto-oncogene Ret, a component of the GDNF receptor complex, persists in human substantia nigra neurons in Parkinson's disease. *Brain Res* **792**: 207–217.

Wang, Y. Q., Bian, G. L., Wei, L. C., Cao, R., Peng, Y. F., Chen, L. W. 2008. Nigrostriatal neurons in rat express the glial cell line-derived neurotrophic factor receptor subunit c-RET. *Anat Rec (Hoboken)* **291**: 49–54.

Xu, J., Kao, S. Y., Lee, F. J., Song, W., Jin, L. W., Yankner, B. A. 2002. Dopamine-dependent neurotoxicity of alpha-synuclein: a mechanism for selective neurodegeneration in Parkinson disease. *Nat Med* **8** (6): 600–606.

Zetterstrom, R. H., Williams, R., Perlmann, T., Olson, L. 1996. Cellular expression of the immediate early transcription factors Nurr1 and NGFI-B suggests a gene regulatory role in several brain regions including the nigrostriatal dopamine system. *Brain Res Mol Brain Res* **41**: 111–120.

Zetterstrom, R. H., Solomin, L., Jansson, L., Hoffer, B. J., Olson, L., Perlmann, T. 1997. Dopamine neuron agenesis in Nurr1-deficient mice. *Science* **276**: 248–250.

4 Design-Based Stereology in the Brain Bank Setting

Mark W. Burke

Department of Physiology and Biophysics, College of Medicine, Howard University School of Medicine, Washington, DC, USA

Background

Design-based stereology refers to the use of standardized sampling schemes and unbiased geometric probes, without knowledge of particle size, shape, orientation, or distribution, to minimize or eliminate systematic errors in estimates of first- and second-order stereology parameters. The seminal 1984 paper by D. C. Sterio (1984) provides the foundation for design-based estimates of total numbers of arbitrary-shaped particles in biological tissue. This method replaced the simple determination of neuron densities based on profile counts on a few "representative" sections and the possibility of results that differ significantly from the true or expected total number of neurons, the so-called reference trap (Gundersen et al., 1988). Over the course of the past three decades, the optical disector technique has become the method of choice to quantify numbers of neurons in biological specimens (von Bartheld, 2002; West, 2002; Schmitz and Hof, 2005; Mouton, 2011), as applied pre- and postclinical changes in neurodegenerative and neurodevelopmental diseases (Pelvig et al., 2003; West et al., 2004; Joelving et al., 2006; Courchesne et al., 2011), age-related changes in neuronal populations (Pakkenberg et al., 2003; Stark et al., 2007; Jabes et al., 2011; Chareyron et al., 2012), assessing the effects of treatment versus control (Burke et al., 2009b; Mouton et al., 2009; Papia et al., 2010), and normal anatomy of specific brain areas (West and Gundersen, 1990; Mouton et al., 1997).

The objective of this chapter is to provide the reader with a practical guide for design of a stereology project that can be modified to address their specific hypothesis. Using the example of a monkey brain study from our brain bank tissue, this chapter takes into consideration specimen preparation, design of a stereology project, and presentation of results. This template is intended as a starting point for the reader to design their own pilot studies, an essential step for every project to maximize reliability and efficiency.

Specimen Preparation

A two-step design-based approach begins with statistical sampling with systematic collection of serial histological sections through the reference space (region of interest), followed by superimposing geometric probes to estimate the number or size of the particular cell population of interest.

Neurostereology: Unbiased Stereology of Neural Systems, First Edition. Edited by Peter R. Mouton.
© 2014 John Wiley & Sons, Inc. Published 2014 by John Wiley & Sons, Inc.

Systematic Sampling

Systematic random sampling (SRS) through an entire reference space is an essential starting point for statistically valid stereological estimates. To avoid sampling bias, the entire reference space must be available for sampling, a challenge for some studies of human brain tissue. In contrast, serial sectioning through the entire reference space is easily achieved for the typical study in experimental animals. In either case, prior to sectioning the brain, perfusion or immersion in paraformaldehyde, glutaraldehyde, or formalin minimizes autolytic degradation of tissue and preserves cellular morphology. A related requirement is that reference spaces must be anatomically well defined and delineated from adjacent structures. Specific brain areas may be subdivided according to cytoarchitecture characteristics defined in a specific plane of sectioning, for example, coronal.

SRS, an approach that ensures every structure an equal probability of being sampled, requires sectioning the entire reference space at regular fixed intervals, with the first cut random within the first interval.

Subsampling a total of about 8–12 sections from each reference space of interest produces a statistically valid sample through the region of interest (Gundersen et al., 1988; Mouton, 2011). The specific SRS design for each study depends on size of the brain area of interest. For example, a reference space about 6 mm (6000 μm) along a preferred sectioning axis, for example, coronal, sectioned at an instrument setting of 50 μm, produces a total of about 120 sections per brain.

For tissue sectioned by frozen microtomy, prior cryoprotection is required in graded phosphate buffered saline (PBS)-buffered sucrose solutions (10, 20, and 30%) at 4°C. Following overnight incubation in 10%, 1-cm blocks will typically sink in 2–3 days in 20% and additional 3–5 days in 30%. Complete sucrose infiltration is evident when the tissue blocks sink to the bottom of the container.

As tissue is sliced and processed for the desired stain or antibody, alternate sections may be systematically placed in antigen preserve (50% ethylene glycol, 1% polyvinyl pyrrolidone in PBS) at −20°C for future processing. For convenience, sections may be collected into 12- or 24-well plates or cups, with care taken to preserve their order (Figure 4.1). Sampling 1/12th of these sections yields 10 equidistant sections for analysis.

One of the series of sections on slides (series 1 in Figure 4.1) is used for cresyl violet staining with the remaining sections placed into standard 24-well plates containing antigen preserve. Once the block of tissue is serially sectioned and sections are placed into wells, the well is covered with the lid, labeled, wrapped with Parafilm, and placed in a −20°C freezer. The total number of sections taken for each series is logged, along with the section-sampling interval, and the number of series for each animal. This log is vital for tracking subsequent removal of sections from the brain bank for future studies. The benefits of a well-characterized brain bank include the possibility to collect data between funding decisions, ability for new students to rapidly collect data, and minimize the use and treatment of new animals. Our ongoing studies of development and aging in a nonhuman primate brain (*Chlorocebus sabeus*) involve sectioning each brain at 50 μm, generating over 1200 sections through a single hemisphere (Burke et al., 2009a; Zangenehpour et al., 2009). In any given year, our tissue bank sores over 60,000 SRS sections, with immunohistochemistry on sections stored in antigen preserve for up to 10 years (Figure 4.2).

Superimposing Geometric Probes

Optimal section thickness takes into account the first-order stereology parameter of interest (number, length, surface area, volume). The optical disector probe uses thin focal plane optical

Sampling Scheme

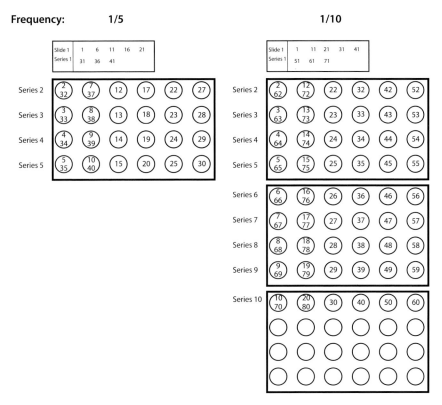

Figure 4.1   This systematic sampling scheme provides two section-sampling frequencies, 1/5 and 1/10 sections/series.

scanning through a known distance of a relatively thick section (Gundersen, 1986). The final section thickness after all tissue processing must be thick enough to allow for an adequate guard space to avoid the lost-cap error (Hedreen, 1998), yet thin enough to allow for the complete penetration of stains and antibodies. Typically, sections cut at an instrument setting of 40–50 μm produce a final, postprocessing tissue thickness in the range 17–24 μm, which allows for placement of a 10- to 12-μm high disector with penetration of antibodies by free-floating immunocytochemistry.

The total number of optical disectors analyzed depends on the *x-y* spacing across the reference area on each section. A pilot study will indicate the optimal spacing to obtain the goal of about 100–300 total intersections between the disector probe and cells of interest across all 8–12 sections through the reference space. Although the distribution of the cells of interest do not affect the accuracy of the stereological approach, a fewer number of disectors will provide an efficient estimate when the cells of interest have a relatively uniform distribution. Even for the most heterogeneous distribution of biological structures, however, increasing the number of disector–object intersections beyond 300 leads to poor efficiency due to negligible improvements in precision. Thus, the desired approach is "do more, less well," which means that light sampling with an unbiased estimator applied to a larger number of animals (subjects) is preferable to heavy sampling in a few animals.

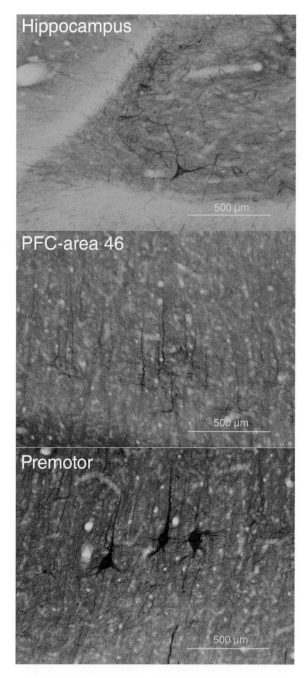

Figure 4.2 SMI-32 positive neurons in the hippocampus, prefrontal cortex, and premotor cortex. The tissues used for this immunohistochemistry stain were stored in antigen preserve for ~4 years after sectioning.

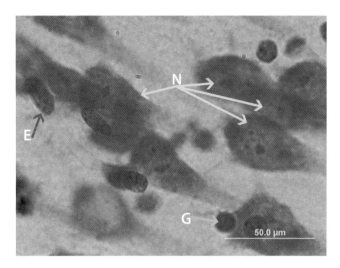

Figure 4.3 Microscopic image of the hippocampus stained with cresyl violet taken at 100× magnification. Neurons (N, yellow arrows) are defined as having visible centrally located nucleoli and clearly defined cytoplasm, whereas glial cells (G, green arrows), which are more heterogeneous than neurons, generally lacked visible nucleoli and cytoplasm. Endothelial cells (E, red arrow) appear rounded and slightly elongated when traversing the z-plane. At low magnifications (<60×), differentiating endothelia from glia cells become difficult, clearly identifying individual neurons in clusters is less accurate, and the measurement of tissue thickness is less accurate which may inadvertently skew the cell population estimate.

The optimal sampling size for an optical disector, where the disector volume is the product of area and height, allows for counting about 0 to 5 objects per disector. When focusing through the z-plane using a high-power objective, for example, 60–100× 1.4 N.A. oil objective, cells should be evident at every depth; if not, incomplete penetration of the stain or nonuniform dehydration of the tissue may be present. This precaution is especially important for immunostained tissue that requires penetration of antibodies through relatively thick tissue sections.

Avoiding error and uncertainty from recognition errors requires a standard definition for the particular biological object of interest (Figure 4.3). For example, neurons have a nuclear membrane, visible nucleolus, and clearly defined cytoplasm, whereas glial cells lack visible nucleoli and nuclear membrane, and have a small amount of cytoplasm (Joelving et al., 2006). The next section is a practical application of the design, implementation, and reporting of a design-based stereology project.

A Practical Application of Design-Based Stereology

The St. Kitts vervet (*Chlorocebus sabeus*) is an Old World primate with similar patterns and rates of cortical and subcortical brain development to that of humans. This species has been used to model human conditions such as anxiety (Palmour et al., 1997), hemispherectomy (Burke et al., 2012), Parkinson's disease (Elsworth et al., 1990), Alzhemier's disease (Lemere et al., 2004), and alcohol abuse (Juarez et al., 1993). This study describes a recent series of experiments to study the neuroanatomical effects of naturalistic fetal alcohol exposure (FAE) on the neuronal population of the cortex. Pregnant vervets were given access to a maximum of 3 gm ethanol/kg body weight (or an isocaloric sucrose control mixture) four times per week during the third trimester (Burke et al., 2009c; Papia et al., 2010). All subjects were housed in enriched environments in the laboratories of Behavioral Sciences Foundation, St Kitts, under protocols approved by the local Animal Care and Use Committee.

At about 2 years of age, that is, approximately equivalent to 8 years for a human being, four juvenile alcohol-exposed (three males, one female) and three juvenile sucrose-control (two males, one female) animals were sacrificed for neuroanatomical evaluation. After euthanasia and thoracotomy, each animal was perfused transcardially with PBS followed by 4% paraformaldehyde in phosphate buffer, pH 7.4.

Brains were extracted, blocked into 1-cm slabs in the coronal plane, cryoprotected in 30% buffered sucrose and frozen at −80°C until further processing. Ten parallel series of coronal sections (50 μm) were obtained for each animal. One series was Nissl stained with cresyl violet for volumetric quantification and qualitative microscopic examination, with each cresyl violet-stained section dehydrated in graded alcohols and cleared with xylenes. The other series were placed in antigen preserve (50% ethylene glycol, phosphate buffer solution, and 1% polyvinyl pyrrolidone) and stored at −20°C for future studies in our vervet brain bank (Burke et al., 2009d).

The Optical Fractionator

Total neuron numbers were estimated using the optical fractionator method (Gundersen, 1986). In this study the cortex was defined as the isocortex (frontal, parietal, temporal, and occipital lobes) and mesocortex (cingulate gyrus and the insula; see Figure 4.4) and excluded the allocortex (hippocampal formation) and subcallosal areas. Images of the reference space at low power (2.5×) with disectors superimposed at 100× were generated using a software program (see Figure 4.4, for example).

Table 4.1 gives the stereological parameters used in this study. Every 100th section was selected with a random starting section within 5 mm of the frontal pole to yield a systematic uniform sample

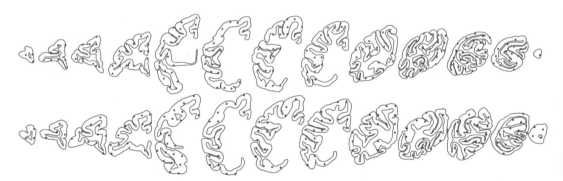

Figure 4.4 Schematic drawing of an FAE (top panel) and control (bottom panel) subject showing systematic uniform-random sampling as well as representative disector placement on the cut surface (+). For each subject, sampling randomly started within 5 mm of the frontal pole (left side of the panel) and spanned the entire cortex. Adapted from Burke et al. (2009a).

Table 4.1 Stereology parameters

	Sampling fraction	Number of sections	Disector volume μm³	Fraction sampled	CE ΣQ-	CE (ΣQ-)	ΣF	CE (ΣF-)	V (cm³)	N (in millions)	CE (N)
Control	1/100	12.7	25,000	1/355,482	315	0.024	162	0.024	16.2 ± 3.3	414 ± 36	0.042
FASD	1/100	12.3	25,000	1/579,244	228	0.052	198	0.024	11.5 ± 1.4	260 ± 20	0.067

of 12–13 sections per brain. An average of 180 optical disectors distributed over ~12 sections according to a systematic random sampling scheme was sampled. The frame area of each disector was $2500\,\mu m^2$ with a disector height of $10\,\mu m$. After tissue processing, the average measured thickness was $17.31\,\mu m$, and thus the upper and lower guard for each disector was set at an average of $3.65\,\mu m$. The volume of the disector was chosen to allow counting an average of 0 to 5 neurons per counting frame in the FAE subjects.

The total cell numbers (Ncell) were calculated by the optical fractionator equation (Gundersen, 1986):

$$\mathrm{Ncell} = \mathrm{ssf}^{-1} \times \mathrm{asf}^{-1} \times \mathrm{tsf}^{-1} \times SQ^{-}, \tag{4.1}$$

where ssf is the section sampling fraction, asf is the sampling fraction, tsf is the thickness-sampling fraction (where the measured thickness of the tissue is divided by the disector height), and ΣQ^{-} is the total number of cells counted within the disector. Coefficients of error (CE) were calculated for mean number of neurons (Nneu, total number of disectors [Ndis], and total number of cells [Ncells]) to assess the reliability of measurements (Gundersen and Jensen, 1987; West and Gundersen, 1990). The average CE for the number of disectors, neurons, and sections was well below 0.10, indicating an acceptable variation for this sampling scheme (Table 4.1). Since the CE represents intrinsic methodological error due to sampling (error variance), its contribution to observed variation (CV) should be less than its contribution to biological variation (BCV). The ratio BCV^2/CV^2, where $BCV^2 = CV^2 - \text{mean } CE^2$ and $CV^2 = BCV^2 + CE^2$, was used to determine the precision of the estimates. A ratio BCV^2/CV^2 of more than 0.5 indicates acceptable stereological precision (Joelving et al., 2006).

Results

The mean number of cortical neurons was 2.60×10^8 (CV = 0.31) in FAE subjects and 4.14×10^8 (CV = 0.19) in the control group (Figure 4.5). The estimation of neurons produced a ratio BCV^2/CV^2 of 0.91 for both groups, indicating a low error variance for these estimates of cells in vervet monkey neocortex.

To determine if neuronal reduction was uniform across the entire cortex or isolated to a specific region, the density of neurons was determined by taking the average number of neurons

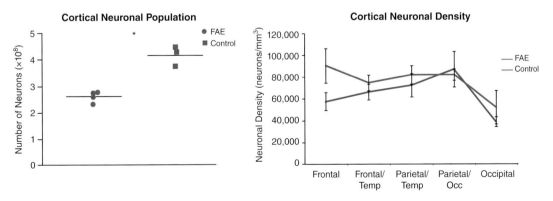

Figure 4.5   FAE subjects display a 37% reduction in cortical neuronal population. $*p < 0.05$ FAE versus control. The density of neurons suggested that the frontal cortex had a disproportionate reduction in neurons.

counted/mm^2 (i.e., mean cells per disector). The results suggested that neuronal density in the frontal cortex is particularly affected, which led us to a stereological investigation to test the effects of FAE on neuronal population in this region.

For stereology data, the reference volume and superimposed counting frames (disectors) were generated using an integrated hardware software system under 2.5× (topography) and 100× oil immersion (counting) objectives. In this study, the frontal lobe was defined as the region from the tip of the frontal pole (anterior) to the central sulcus (posterior) and the lateral sulcus (ventral), excluding the insula (Figure 4.4). Every 60th section was selected with a random starting point within 3 mm of the frontal pole that yielded an SRS set sample of 11–12 sections.

A standard grid size of 2500 μm^2 was generated through the computerized stereology system to yield an average of 179 and 186 disectors for the FAE and control group, respectively. An average of 398 neurons in the control group and 270 neurons in the FAE group were counted across the disectors. After tissue processing, the mean tissue thickness was about 19.1 μm with a guard distance of 4.5 μm with an average tsf of 0.518 for control subjects and 0.549 for FAE subjects. The average asf and ssf for each group was 0.0002 and 0.0168, respectively. The total number of neurons in the FAE group was determined to be 1.52×10^8 (CV = 0.16) and 2.34×10^8 (CV = 0.18) for the control subjects. The average CE for the number of neurons was 0.052 for control group and 0.062 for the FAE group, indicating an acceptable variation for this sampling scheme. The estimation of neurons produced a ratio BCV^2/CV^2 of 0.92 for the control group and 0.85 for the FAE group, indicating low error variance and a precise estimate of neuron number in the frontal lobe.

This study using natural ethanol consumption pattern (Ervin et al., 1990) of the vervet monkey indicates that prenatal ethanol exposure resulted in a 37% reduction in the total number of neurons in the frontal lobe ($p = 0.004$). These findings indicate that relatively moderate and naturalistic alcohol consumption during the third trimester results in an overall loss of cortical neurons. Regional variations of neuronal density suggest that the frontal cortex might account for much of the neuronal loss. Prior to sectioning of these brains, it was determined that the smallest potential region of interest would require a section sampling fraction of 1/10. As a result, the number of sections available for cortical analysis was over 100, and for the frontal lobe there were ~60 sections available. This sampling scheme offered the flexibility to investigate the effects of FAE on hippocampal neuronal populations (Burke et al., 2011), neuronal size and population of lateral geniculate nucleus, and glial population of the lateral geniculate nucleus (Papia et al., 2010) in cresyl violet-stained sections. The cataloged brain bank for this project now exceeds 45,000 serial sections, offering further flexibility to investigate the mechanisms of FAE-induced neuron loss, as well as its effects on neurogenesis and development via immunohistochemistry and design-based stereology.

Conclusion

Among the advantages of design-based stereological approaches over previous methods is the avoidance of all known sources of systematic (nonrandom) error arising from faulty assumptions and nonverifiable models (Gundersen et al., 1988; Mouton, 2011). Similar to most techniques in science, the validity of reported stereological data rests with the investigator. Common errors may arise from improperly calibrated imaging systems, the use of inappropriate objectives (e.g., using low instead of high-resolution objectives to count cells), recognition errors, for example, mistaking an endothelial cell as a glia cell), improper or ill-defined reference spaces, and other design-related issues. When sufficient care is taken to avoid these sources of bias, design-based stereology provides the most reliable and accepted method available for assessing number, size, and distributions of cells in biological specimens.

References

Burke, M., Zangenehpour, S. et al. 2009a. Knowing what counts: unbiased stereology in the non-human primate brain. *J Vis Exp* **27**. doi: 10.3791/1262.

Burke, M., Palmour, R. M. et al. 2011. Dose-related reduction in neuronal and doublecortin positive cell number in the hippocampus following prenatal ethanol exposure in the vervet monkey. *National Hispanic Science Network*. Miami, Fl. 11.

Burke, M. W., Palour, R. M. et al. 2009b. Neuronal reduction in frontal cortex of primates after prenatal alcohol exposure. *Neuroreport* **20** (1): 13–17.

Burke, M. W., Zangenehpour, S. et al. 2009c. Dissecting the non-human primate brain in stereotaxic space. *J Vis Exp* **29**: 1–5.

Burke, M. W., Zangenehpour, S. et al. 2009d. Brain banking: making the most of your research specimens. *J Vis Exp* **29**. doi: 10.3791/1260.

Burke, M. W., Kupers, R. et al. 2012. Adaptive neuroplastic responses in early and late hemispherectomized monkeys. *Neural Plast* **2012**: 852423.

Chareyron, L. J., Lavenex, P. B. et al. 2012. Postnatal development of the amygdala: a stereological study in macaque monkeys. *J Comp Neurol* **520** (9): 1965–1984.

Courchesne, E., Mouton, P. R. et al. 2011. Neuron number and size in prefrontal cortex of children with autism. *JAMA* **306** (18): 2001–2010.

Elsworth, J. D., Deutch, A. Y. et al. 1990. MPTP-induced parkinsonism: relative changes in dopamine concentration in subregions of substantia nigra, ventral tegmental area and retrorubral field of symptomatic and asymptomatic vervet monkeys. *Brain Res* **513** (2): 320–324.

Ervin, F. R., Palmour, R. M. et al. 1990. Voluntary consumption of beverage alcohol by vervet monkeys: population screening, descriptive behavior and biochemical measures. *Pharmacol Biochem Behav* **36** (2): 367–373.

Gundersen, H. J. 1986. Stereology of arbitrary particles: a review of unbiased number and size estimators and the presentation of some new ones, in memory of William R. Thompson. *J Microsc* **143** (Pt 1): 3–45.

Gundersen, H. J., Bendtsen, T. F. et al. 1988. Some new, simple and efficient stereological methods and their use in pathological research and diagnosis. *APMIS* **96** (5): 379–394.

Gundersen, H. J. G., Jensen, E. B. 1987. The efficiency of systematic sampling in stereology and its prediction. *J Microsc* **147**: 229–263.

Hedreen, J. C. 1998. Lost caps in histological counting methods. *Anat Rec* **250** (3): 366–372.

Jabes, A., Lavenex, P. B. et al. 2011. Postnatal development of the hippocampal formation: a stereological study in macaque monkeys. *J Comp Neurol* **519** (6): 1051–1070.

Joelving, F. C., Billeskov, R. et al. 2006. Hippocampal neuron and glial cell numbers in Parkinson's disease—a stereological study. *Hippocampus* **16** (10): 826–833.

Juarez, J., Guzman-Flores, C. et al. 1993. Voluntary alcohol consumption in vervet monkeys: individual, sex, and age differences. *Pharmacol Biochem Behav* **46** (4): 985–988.

Lemere, C. A., Beierschmitt, A. et al. 2004. Alzheimer's disease abeta vaccine reduces central nervous system abeta levels in a non-human primate, the Caribbean vervet. *Am J Pathol* **165** (1): 283–297.

Mouton, P. R. 2011. *Unbiased Stereology: A Concise Guide*. Baltimore, MD: The Johns Hopkins University Press.

Mouton, P. R., Price, D. L., Walker, L. C. 1997. Empirical assessment of synapse numbers in primate neocortex. *J Neurosci Methods* **75** (2): 119–126.

Mouton, P. R., Chachich, M. E., Quigley, C., Spangler, E., Ingram, D. K. 2009. Caloric restriction attenuates amyloid deposition in middle-aged dtg APP/PS1 mice. *Neurosci Lett* **464** (3): 184–187.

Pakkenberg, B., Pelvis, D. et al. 2003. Aging and the human neocortex. *Exp Gerontol* **38** (1–2): 95–99.

Palmour, R. M., Mulligan, J. et al. 1997. Of monkeys and men: vervets and the genetics of human-like behaviors. *Am J Hum Genet* **61** (3): 481–488.

Papia, M. F., Burke, M. W. et al. 2010. Reduced soma size of the M-neurons in the lateral geniculate nucleus following foetal alcohol exposure in non-human primates. *Exp Brain Res* **205** (2): 263–271.

Pelvig, D. P., Pakkenberg, H. et al. 2003. Neocortical glial cell numbers in Alzheimer's disease. A stereological study. *Dement Geriatr Cogn Disord* **16** (4): 212–219.

Schmitz, C., Hof, P. R. 2005. Design-based stereology in neuroscience. *Neuroscience* **130** (4): 813–831.

Stark, A. K., Toft, M. H. et al. 2007. The effect of age and gender on the volume and size distribution of neocortical neurons. *Neuroscience* **150** (1): 121–130.

Sterio, D. 1984. The unbiased estimation of number and sizes of arbitrary particles using the disector. *J Microsc* **134** (Pt 2): 9.

von Bartheld, C. 2002. Counting particles in tissue sections: choices of methods and importance of calibration to minimize biases. *Histol Histopathol* **17** (2): 639–648.

West, M. J. 2002. Design-based stereological methods for counting neurons. *Prog Brain Res* **135**: 43–51.

West, M. J., Gundersen, H. J. 1990. Unbiased stereological estimation of the number of neurons in the human hippocampus. *J Comp Neurol* **296** (1): 1–22.

West, M. J., Kawas, C. H. et al. 2004. Hippocampal neurons in pre-clinical Alzheimer's disease. *Neurobiol Aging* **25** (9): 1205–1212.

Zangenehpour, S., Burke, M. W. et al. 2009. Batch immunostaining for large-scale protein detection in the whole monkey brain. *J Vis Exp* **29**: 1–5.

5 Practical Stereology for Preclinical Neurotoxicology

Mark T. Butt

Tox Path Specialists, LLC, Frederick, MD, USA

The nervous system offers numerous opportunities for the accurate detection of morphologic disturbances. While organs such as the liver, kidney, and skin are relatively homogeneous in structure, the brain presents the extreme level of heterogeneity and complexity. Each nuclear group in the brain and spinal cord, as well as ganglia outside the CNS, may respond in a unique manner when exposed to a drug, lesion, or chemical toxin.

Microscopic examination of cellular morphology in the brain and spinal cord provides a specific window into damage at a set point in time, perhaps when prior morphologic changes are no longer detectable. Preclinical toxicology studies are typically carried out according to established regulatory guidelines (FDA Redbook, 2000) that involve the microscopic examination of tissues, including the brain and spinal cord, from animals exposed to various drugs/chemicals and sacrificed after single or multiple dosing regimens, typically 2 weeks, 4 weeks, 13 weeks, 26 weeks, 52 weeks, or 104 weeks. However, when exposed to a neurotoxic chemical, many neurons show a peak time of death in approximately 24–72 hours (Switzer, 2001). Within 7 days, the evidence of neuronal necrosis is largely cleared via phagocytic activity of resident macrophages (microglial cells). Administration of certain N-methyl-D-aspartate (NMDA) antagonists to rats produces a characteristic vacuolation of neurons visible 6–24 hours following chemical exposure, followed by occasional neuronal necrosis in a very specific area of the brain (Fix et al., 2004). Unless the brain is examined in the proper time frame, neuron loss from transient necrosis may be undetected and the tissue erroneously assessed as normal.

The toxicology literature is filled with morphological analyses of the so-called representative section, a single section sampled from a specific tissue or region of interest (such as a liver, or kidney, or dorsal root ganglion [DRG]) presumed to exemplify the full heterogeneity of the tissue. Various objects may be counted or measured, including cells, mitotic figures, nuclei, or nucleoli. The representative section offers several nonscientific advantages: convenience, low costs, and speed. Emerging consensus, however, calls for more thorough investigation of drug safety, including quantitative assays to reliably detect changes in number and/or size of various brain cells (neurons, glia), as well as other neural structures (nerve fibers, synapses, blood vessels, etc.). Quantitation is not always needed to determine the significance of a particular morphologic

Neurostereology: Unbiased Stereology of Neural Systems, First Edition. Edited by Peter R. Mouton.
© 2014 John Wiley & Sons, Inc. Published 2014 by John Wiley & Sons, Inc.

finding. For example, neuronal necrosis in the Purkinje cell layer of the cerebellum is a frequent target of morphologic evaluation. Such changes could be quantified if a percentage loss is important, but usually the presence of necrosis and an estimate of the severity of that necrosis (typically in the form of a severity grade of minimal, mild, moderate, or severe) will suffice. In contrast, a loss of neurons in a large brain region or DRG, or a change in the average neuronal size or the average nucleolar size, may require more than qualitative morphologic examination.

This chapter reports on the perspective from our extensive use of design-based stereology to investigate quantitative changes in the nervous system as applied to drug safety studies. The experience described here does not include the theoretical background or full range of design-based approaches available for toxicology studies. For discussion of stereological approaches applied to neurotoxicology, see reviews by Mouton and Gordon (2010) and Mouton (2011a,b).

Specimen Quality

A major part of the effort of a stereology investigation typically goes into the production of quality specimens. Quality specimens increase the probability of generating reliable results that address the hypothesis of the study. A pilot study completed prior to the start of data collection helps to optimize tissue preparation with particular attention to clear visualization of biological objects of interest in the reference space (region of interest). The following section outlines some of the critical factors that contribute to producing tissue slides of sufficient high quality for stereology.

Necropsy/Tissue Harvest

For design-based stereology, the reference space must be available in its entirety for sampling. Structures such as DRG, the trigeminal ganglia, and sympathetic ganglia require greater expertise to harvest than well-defined brain regions. The superior cervical ganglia are often destroyed if the head is removed; therefore, the head should stay attached if the reference space includes this tissue. Other sympathetic ganglia are easily damaged at necropsy or missed entirely. The DRG are distributed along the spinal column and are relatively easy to locate; however, removing the same DRG from each subject for comparisons between groups and animals may be difficult. A mid-thoracic DRG from one animal and the C7 or L6 ganglion in another could yield vastly different neuron numbers because some ganglia are associated with the limbs and others are not.

Fixation

Many tissues are fixed by immersion in 10% neutral buffered formalin, which may not provide satisfactory preservation of tissue structure for quantitative studies. To reduce autolysis and improve antigen preservation in experimental studies, particularly rats and mice, animals should be deeply anesthetized and perfused *in situ* with intracardial injection of saline followed by fixation with 4% paraformaldehyde. While fixation via perfusion improves overall tissue preservation, it may be incompatible with some neurochemical analyses, for example, protein levels by enzyme linked immunosorbent assay (ELISA) or levels of specific neurotransmitters. To save resources, one common practice involves splitting the brain into hemispheres at necropsy: one side (right or left) used for diagnostic and morphologic pathology or neurochemical studies, and the other side for stereology. Splitting brains into hemispheres requires special attention if the reference space lies on the medial/ventral aspects of the brain to avoid unequal sampling of midline structures, for example, medial septal nucleus.

Storage and Shipping

Shipping tissues on ice may freeze portions of tissue that are in too close apposition to the ice. Freezing artifacts in tissues renders them useless for stereology.

Sectioning

Many histology technicians are adept at preparing specimens suitable for diagnostic evaluation, though this expertise may not extend to stereologic investigations. In the majority of diagnostic settings, small parts of a ganglion, nerve, or the brain may be excluded without causing a major problem. For stereology studies, however, a critically important prerequisite is to make all parts of the reference volume available for sampling. When stereology is carried out on frozen sections, the freezing procedure must be done with care and attention to several factors. For example, cryoprotection of tissues during frozen sectioning is essential.

Staining

Traditional stains such as hematoxylin and eosin (H&E) stain sections from the brain and spinal cord into a somewhat monotonous sea of pink fiber pathways, with numerous islands of blue cellular nuclei. Since differentiation of individual cell populations of neurons, glia, and other brain structure is not always possible with these stains, the addition of special stains greatly assist with the morphologic evaluation of the nervous system. Examples of such stains are listed in Table 5.1.

Specific staining protocols help to identify the particular cells and subpopulations and other neural structure. General histochemical stains, such as Nissl and H&E, require only general attention to fixation and other tissue processing steps, while immunohistochemistry for specific structures or amino-cupric-silver procedure for necrotic neurons require greater attention to fixation. In order to preserve myelin sheaths, nerve sections may be postfixed in osmium. Because osmium penetrates poorly into tissue, tissue blocks for staining are typically limited to 1 mm in depth from the middle to the edge of the specimen. For nerve fibers, the ideal sectioning scheme allows for visualization of the entire nerve cross section through transverse sections.

Embedding

Stereology may be done on sections obtained from paraffin, plastic/resin, and frozen blocks. For cell counting studies, the primary goal is to produce specimens of sufficient thickness to allow for a true three-dimensional (3D) evaluation, that is, examination of multiple optical planes in the z-axis, while allowing for complete staining of the biological objects of interest. Frozen sections

---

Table 5.1   List of common special stains used for the morphologic evaluation of the nervous system

- Silver stains: stains neurofilamentous processes
- Cresyl violet and other Nissl stains: stain the rough endoplasmic reticulum (Nissl substance) common to some neuronal types
- Immunohistochemical stains: for specific cell types and neuronal populations
- Fluoro-Jade B: for the detection of necrotic neurons
- Selective (neurodisintegration) silver stains: extremely sensitive detection of disintegrating (necrotic) neuron cell bodies and appendages (axons, dendrites, synaptic terminals)

can be cut either from tissue embedded in gelatin or from frozen tissue without embedding. In either case, the sections must be either snap-frozen or cryoprotected prior to freezing to avoid freezing artifacts such as lysis of cell membranes.

Some studies may be optimal for the physical disector (Sterio, 1984) applied to thin sections, usually 10 μm or less, typically cut from paraffin or plastic sections. For the optical disector method, the sections must be sufficiently thick to allow for examination of multiple optical planes in the z-axis (Mouton, 2011a,b). Most paraffin sections are limited to about 50 μm in thickness by rotary microtomy while frozen sections allow for cutting sections up to 80 μm. Note that for routine neurostereology studies, section thickness is reported after all tissue processing is complete, that is, the final or postprocessing section thickness, rather than as the instrument setting when cutting sections from a paraffin or frozen block (also known as the "block advance").

Microtomy

Although a reasonable section quality is acceptable for diagnostic/morphologic evaluation, stereology requires sections of uniformly high quality, especially the avoidance of artifacts in the reference space. Folds and tears may render sections unsuitable for stereology, which in turn complicates the calculation of sampling fractions. For the stereologic calculations, it is important to track sections produced through a given reference space. Frozen sections placed into wells for later staining/mounting may be useful to maintain the section order.

Staining

Paraffin and cryostat sections are typically mounted to slides prior to staining, which may limit stain penetration to a single surface of the tissue sections, while thick frozen sections are stained free-floating, allowing for penetration of staining from both upper and lower section surfaces.

Complete penetration usually occurs without difficulty with histocytochemical protocols that use water-soluble reagents such as cresyl violet or H&E. Immunohistochemical stains provide a powerful tool for identifying subpopulations of neurons that express specific proteins. However, many antibody-based immunohistochemical stains are associated with limited penetration into tissue sections depending on the physical size of the antibodies and concentration of antigen within the objects of interest. If the stain penetrates, say, 8 μm through from each surface of free-floating sections cut at an instrument setting of 20 μm, then the inner four microns of the section will not stain. Penetration of thick sections may be improved by the use of detergents, for example, Triton X. Use of a pilot study together with a stereology program that records the depth in the section where each object is counted allows the user to confirm whether the stain penetrates the full thickness of the section.

Drying

Shrinkage of tissue sections is difficult to control when preparing specimens for stereologic investigation. Paraffin sections, which are typically limited to about 40- to 50-μm cut thickness, tend to shrink less than frozen sections. Thicker cut frozen sections tend to undergo greater tissue shrinkage, usually up to 50% or more. For example, frozen sections stained with a histochemical or immunohistochemical method typically shrink from a cut thickness of 50 μm to a final, postprocessing thickness of 15–20 μm. One way to minimize shrinkage is to use aqueous mounts and aqueous mounting media, such as Apathy's media (Bonthius et al., 2004) or Fluoro-Gel with TRIS buffer (Catalog number 17985-10, Electron Microscopy Sciences, Hatfield, PA).

Aqueous mounts maintain tissue hydration and prevent much of the shrinkage caused by dehydration, improving the overall 3D quality of the section, allowing for the delineation of multiple optical planes, and increasing the assessment of section thickness. However, aqueous mounts present a problem for histocytochemical stains, including Nissl stains, which tend to "bleed" out of the section over time. After the first 24 hours, the staining begins to fade out of the section, which is a substantial problem in preclinical safety studies where peer review of slides is often required. In this case, specimens used to produce the data must be archived for 5 or more years. Though tissue in nonaqueous mounts shrink more than in aqueous mounts, they may be coverslipped for a permanent mount with no loss of stain and preserved for decades without degradation. Because of tight antibody–antigen binding, immunohistochemical stains tend not to fade substantially even with aqueous mounting media (although this may vary).

Reference Space (Region of Interest)

Stereology studies typically include a detailed description of the anatomical boundaries of the reference space. It is essential to predefine the limits of the reference space, which is best determined during a pilot study prior to the definitive investigation. Structures such as the substantia nigra pars compacta, although easily identified by immunohistochemical stains for dopaminergic neurons, may be difficult to define at its rostral and caudal limits. Another example of irregular borders of a reference space is the cholinergic neurons in the nucleus basalis of Meynert of the basal forebrain (Figure 5.1).

Regarding the definition of the reference space for any particular study, consistency is more important than accuracy. Lack of consistency in the definition of reference spaces contributes to the difficulty in making comparisons of stereology data between different laboratories, as well as different studies from the same laboratory.

Total Myelinated Nerve Fibers

One valuable use of computerized stereology is the investigation of myelinated fibers in a single nerve cross section (Larsen, 1998; Perry et al., 2004; Urso-Baiarda and Grobbelaar, 2006). Nerves

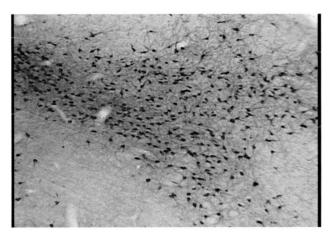

Figure 5.1   Low magnification image of nucleus Basalis of Meynert stained with antibodies to choline acetyltransferase (ChAT). Green line delineates the reference space (region of interest) for counting ChAT-pos neurons in this section.

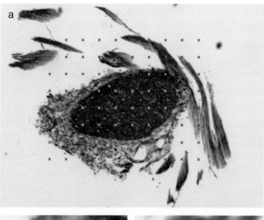

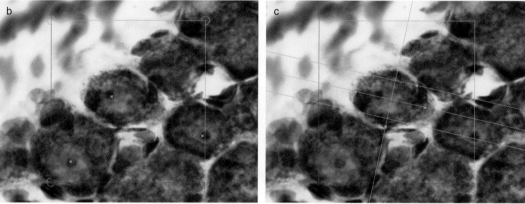

Figure 5.2 (a) Low magnification image of Nissl-stained DRG neurons. The well-defined reference space is easily outlined using the software. Points (+) indicate the location of disector frames to be analyzed. (b) High magnification image of DRG Nissl-stained neurons. Three marked nucleoli (=three neurons) within a single disector frame would be counted. (c) High magnification image of Nissl-stained neurons in dorsal root ganglion. The rotator method estimates the mean neuron volume based on the random orientation of lines across cells.

are collections of elongated structures (nerve fibers) consisting of myelinated axons and unmyelinated axons, as well as connective tissue and blood vessels. Some nerve fibers extend from the brain/spinal cord to the tissue/organ being innervated. For example, the sural nerve has long been used in human medicine as a site for biopsy because it is relatively accessible from the skin on the lateral aspect of the distal hindlimb. For diagnostic purposes, the sural nerve provides an excellent source for examination of sensory nerve fibers from which distal sensory neuropathies arise. Nerve cross sections are the exception to the philosophy that a single representative section may give misleading results for quantifying structures in a 3D structure. See Figure 5.2

A common preparation of nerve sections for optimal light microscopic evaluation, and the approach used in the author's laboratory for stereology studies of nerve fibers, involve nerve sections postfixed in osmium, embedded in resin, sectioned at approximately 1 μm, and stained with toluidine blue. Similar investigations are possible on paraffin embedded sections using stains specific to identify axons, typically silver or neurofilament stains combined with a myelin stain such as Luxol fast blue (Perry et al., 2004).

Neuron Counts in Ganglia

Compared with brain tissue, greater attention and expertise is required to produce quality tissue sections from ganglia, an aggregation of neurons outside the CNS (Avendaño and Lagares, 1996; Schiønning and Larsen, 1997; Williams et al., 2003; Ribeiro et al., 2004; Noorafshan et al., 2005). In particular, small ganglia from rodents are difficult to work with at every step of specimen preparation. Most necropsy technicians accomplished in the extraction of brain and spinal cord samples often require additional practice and training to harvest DRG, the trigeminal ganglion, and various sympathetic ganglia. Compared with large brain regions, small ganglia may be easily embedded and sectioned in a manner that allows for the proper production of isotropic uniform random sections required for some parameters, such as mean cell volume using the nucleator or rotator methods.

For frozen sections, embedding the ganglia in gelatin improves visualization during microtomy if using a sliding microtome. A deceptively complex structure, ganglia are quite cellular with classical neurons that show a clear and distinct nucleolus, and satellite cells surrounding the neurons. Resolving neurons, glia, satellite cells, Schwann cells, and endothelial cells require high magnification objectives with the ability to resolve stacks of optical planes in 3D. While neurons in the brain, spinal cord, and ganglia vary greatly in size, the size of nucleoli varies less. For this reason, nucleoli work well as the counting item for neurons in DRG and other reference spaces of the brain and spinal cord where each neuron contains a single nucleolus. Figure 5.2 shows an example of nucleoli as the counting object for estimating the total number of neurons in DRG.

If nucleoli cannot be identified in a reliable manner, the next best option is the nucleus, which stains well using Nissl stains.

Neuron Counts in the Brain

Neurons in the brain are organized into nuclei and layered cortices, for example, the cerebral cortex and cerebellar cortex. Most investigations use coronal sections, though sagittal sections provide a broad view of a wide range of brain structure, which may be useful for qualitative visualization of many nuclei on the same sections. The substantia nigra, subthalamus, and basal ganglia are examples of nuclei often analyzed by stereology studies (Ookschot, 1996; Scott et al., 2007). Many users find that easy access to a detailed atlas for the desired orientation helps them stay within the desired reference space during stereology studies.

Accurate estimation of total neuron number requires a reproducible and unambiguous definition of the volume of tissue sampled, that is, reference space, as well as the specific criteria for inclusion and exclusion of the neural objects of interest. For example, the substantia nigra is clearly located in the ventral midbrain, bilateral and dorsal to the crus cerebri (ventral portions of the cerebral peduncles), with dopaminergic neurons of the pars compacta region of the substantia nigra that stain for tyrosine hydroxylase (TH). However, some investigators include non-TH positive neurons (Baquet et al., 2009), and there is often variation in the precise definition of the medial boundaries, inclusion of the ventral tegmental area, and so on. The responsibility falls on each laboratory to establish the reference space boundaries and counting rules, remain consistent to these criteria, and then convey this information to readers in reports and publications.

Study Design

The goal for a well-optimized stereology study (e.g., total number of neurons) is 1 hour per reference space for a single brain or spinal cord, including technician time plus input from the principal investigator. Time to analyze multiple parameters (e.g., the ganglion volume, total neuron count, and average neuron size) for a single reference space will take more time, typically about 3–4 hours. The study design may also include provisions for making the stereology technician unaware (blinded) to the treatment status, as well as defining the boundaries of the reference space. As for many aspects of a well-designed stereology study, estimating time for completion is best assessed by a pilot study prior to the start of actual data collection.

Practical Stereology

Stereologic investigations may be carried out using manual or computer-assisted approaches. Computerized systems typically combine a digital/video imaging system with a software program that drives a motorized state mounted on a quality microscope with a range of low- and high-resolution lenses. Techniques for sampling tissue sections in an unbiased and systematic manner without using a motorized stage have been reported (Kaplan et al., 2005; Melvin et al., 2007).

Software Validation/Verification

Validation of personnel training and verification of a computerized stereology system, including hardware, software, data collection procedures, etc., ensures that the performance meets or exceeds the study's expectations for accuracy, precision, and reporting of results. The Food and Drug Administration (FDA) provides General Principles of Software Validation (www.fda.gov/medical devices/deviceregulationandguidance/guidancedocuments/vcm08528/.htm) to ensure the output (typically data/results) is consistent with the input. Software validation is "confirmation by examination and provision of objective evidence that software specifications conform to user needs and intended used, and that the particular requirements implemented through software can be consistently fulfilled." Validation of an integrated hardware–software system includes the following:

- Defined user requirements including the information to be collected and analyzed.
- Is the design consistent with the user's needs?
- Does the installation conform to user needs?
- Does the performance of the system conform to user needs?
- Implementation of standard operating procedures stating how the system will be used, how personnel will be trained, and the various forms/data outputs that will be used to collect and/or report/analyze data.
- How will issues/deficits/errors be documented, recorded, and corrected?
- How will software changes be made, and how will software versions be documented and tested?

Full validation of a computerized stereology system may not always be possible in academic settings with limited resources. However, the following steps are within the ability and resources of most investigating laboratories to ensure continued accurate data collection using a computerized stereology system.

z-Axis Movement

This can be done by physically measuring the thickness of a known standard (such as a high-quality coverslip) or preferably by measuring stage movement in the z-axis and comparing the result to the result recorded by the stereology program. Such verification may be conducted with high precision, accurate calipers (preferably calipers that have also been verified for accuracy).

Lens Tracking

Usually, a stereologic investigation requires the use of a low power objective (2× to 6×) to define a reference space such as a ganglion, nerve, or nuclear area in the brain, and then a higher power objective (40× to 100×) to count and/or measure objects of interest. Most microscopes have objectives placed into a revolving turret. The exact center of these lenses varies by a factor known as offset, which arises from imprecise alignment of the light path. Software systems contain routines that allow users to compensate for offset.

Linear and Area Measurements

Line-based measurements such as the nucleator and rotator can be verified using a set of circles and/or lines on a reference slide that includes a micrometer and/or other inserts that have been verified against a standard certified by the National Institutes of Standards and Technology (NIST). Such devices are available from a variety of vendors. Basically, the known reference lines or shapes are measured with the program, and the result is recorded by the software verified against the actual value. This technique can be used to verify disector size, region point counting area measurements (Cavalieri method), nucleator and rotator radius measurements, and distance between disectors.

Calculations

Not all stereology programs carry out calculations; for those that do, these calculations should be checked for accuracy along with secondary programs (e.g., Microsoft® Excel) for subsequent data processing.

Coefficient of Error (CE)

The CE is the difference between the stereology estimate and the expected (true) value, that is, the amount of error arising from all sources of sampling. The primary use of the CE is to determine the level of sampling required to achieve a reproducible result. Computerized stereology software programs either report the CE as part of the results, provide the user with the raw data to calculate this value, or give a range of CE values for users to select. An acceptable CE value is typically obtained with 100 to 300 probes spaced in a systematic-random manner across 8–12 sections through the entire reference space.

In conclusion, stereologic investigations may produce accurate and consistent results if care is taken to avoid all known sources of systematic error (bias), beginning with a protocol designed by a principal investigator with a thorough understanding of the nuances of stereology theory and the specific anatomical reference space of interest. While results generated by one laboratory for a given study may be accurate and informative, the wide range of differences for preparation of specimens, reference space definitions, and data collection methods make comparison of results between different laboratories neither possible nor constructive.

References

Avendaño, C., Lagares, A. 1996. A stereological analysis of the numerical distribution of neurons in dorsal root ganglia C_4-T_2, in adult macaque monkeys. *Somatosens Mot Res* **13**: 59–66.

Baquet, Z. C., Williams, D., Brody, J., Smeyne, R. J. 2009. A comparison of model-based (2D) and design-based (3D) stereological methods for estimating cell number in the substantia nigra pars compacta (SNpc) of the C57BL/6J mouse. *Neuroscience* **2161**: 1082–1090.

Bonthius, D. J., McKim, R., Koele, L., Harb, H., Karacay, B., Mahoney, J. et al. 2004. Use of frozen sections to determine neuronal number in the murine hippocampus and neocortex using the optical disector and optical fractionator. *Brain Res Protoc* **14**: 45–57. Center for Biologics Evaluation and Research. Available at http://www.fda.gov/downloads/RegulatoryInformation/Guidances/ucm126955.pdf

FDA Redbook. 2000. *Toxicological Principles for the Safety Assessment of Food Ingredients*. Silver Spring, MD: Neurotoxicity Studies. Available at http://www.fda.gov/Food/GuidanceComplianceRegulatoryInformation/GuidanceDocuments/FoodIngredientsandPackaging/Redbook/ucm078323.htm

Fix, A., Long, G., Wozniak, D., Olney, J. 2004. Pathomorphologic effects of N-methyl-D-aspartate antagonists in the rat posterior cingulate/retrosplenial cerebral cortex: a review. *Drug Dev Res* **32**: 147–152.

Kaplan, S., Gökyar, A., Ünal, B., Tunç, A. T., Bahadır, A., Aslan, H. 2005. A simple technique for localizing consecutive fields for disector pairs in light microscopy: application to neuron counting in rabbit spinal cord following spinal cord injury. *J Neurosci Methods* **145**: 277–284.

Larsen, J. O. 1998. Stereology of nerve cross sections. *J Neurosci Methods* **85**: 107–118.

Melvin, N. R., Poda, D., Sutherland, R. J. 2007. A simple and efficient alternative to implementing systematic random sampling in stereological designs without a motorized microscope stage. *J Microsc* **228**: 103–106.

Mouton, P. R. 2011a. *Unbiased Stereology: A Concise Guide*. Baltimore, MD: Johns Hopkins Press.

Mouton, P. R. 2011b. Applications of unbiased stereology to neurodevelopmental toxicology . In *Developmental Neurotoxicology Research*, Principles, Models, Techniques, Strategies and Mechanisms, edited by C. Wang and W. Slikke, pp. 53–77. Hoboken, NJ: John Wiley & Sons.

Mouton, P. R., Gordon, M. 2010. Stereological and image analysis techniques for quantitative assessment of neurotoxicology. In *Neurotoxicology*, 3rd ed, Target Organ Toxicology Series, edited by G. Jean Harry and H. A. Tilson, pp. 243–267. London and New York: Taylor & Francis.

Noorafshan, A., Azizi, M., Aliabadi, E., Karbalay-Doust, S. 2005. Stereological study on the neurons of superior cervical sympathetic ganglion in diabetic rats. *Iran J Med Sci* **30**: 24–27.

Ookschot, D. E. 1996. Total number of neurons in the neostriatal, pallidal, subthalamic, and substantia nigral nuclei of the rat basal ganglia: a stereological study using the cavalieri and optical disector methods. *J Comp Neurol* **366**: 580–599.

Perry, T. A., Weerasuriya, A., Mouton, P. R., Holloway, H. W., Greig, N. H. 2004. Pyridoxine-induced toxicity in rats: a stereological quantification of the sensory neuropathy. *Exp Neurol* **190**: 133–144.

Ribeiro, A. A., Davis, C., Gabella, G. 2004. Estimate of size and total number of neurons in superior cervical ganglion of rat, capybara and horse. *Anat Embryol* **208**: 367–380.

Schiønning, J. D., Larsen, J. O. 1997. A stereological study of dorsal root ganglion cells and nerve root fibers from rats treated with inorganic mercury. *Acta Neuropathol* **94**: 280–286.

Scott, S. A., Diaz, N. M., Ahmad, S. O. 2007. Stereologic analysis of cell number and size during postnatal development in the rat substantia nigra. *Neurosci Lett* **419**: 34–37.

Sterio, D. C. 1984. The unbiased estimation of number and sizes of arbitrary particles using the disector. *J Microsc* **134** (Pt 2): 127–136.

Switzer, R. C. 2001. Fundamentals of Neurotoxicity Detection. In *Fundamental Neuropathology for Pathologists and Toxicologists: Principles and Techniques*, edited by B. Bolon and M. T. Butt, pp. 139–156. Hoboken, NJ: John Wiley & Sons, Inc.

Urso-Baiarda, F., Grobbelaar, A. O. 2006. Practical nerve morphometry. *J Neurosci Methods* **156**: 333–341.

Williams, R. W., von Bartheld, C. S., Rosen, G. D. 2003. Counting cells in sectioned material: a suite of techniques, tools, and tips. *Curr Protoc Neurosci* **24**: 1.11.1–1.11.29.

6   An Overabundance of Prefrontal Cortex Neurons Underlies Early Brain Overgrowth in Autism

Eric Courchesne,[1] Peter R. Mouton,[2] Michael E. Calhoun,[1]
Clelia Ahrens-Barbeau,[1] Melodie J. Hallet,[1] Cynthia Carter Barnes,[1]
Karen Pierce,[1] and Katarina Semendeferi[3]

[1] *Department of Neuroscience, NIH-UCSD Autism Center of Excellence, University of California San Diego, La Jolla, CA, USA*
[2] *Department of Pathology and Cell Biology, Byrd Alzheimer's Disease Institute, University of South Florida, Tampa, FL, USA*
[3] *Department of Anthropology, University of California San Diego, San Diego, CA, USA*

Background

Autism is a developmental disorder involving early brain overgrowth (Courchesne et al., 2001, 2003, 2007; Sparks et al., 2002; Redcay and Courchesne, 2005; Dawson et al., 2007; Amaral et al., 2008). Overgrowth and dysfunction are strongly evident at young ages in prefrontal and temporal cortices (Carper et al., 2002; Carper and Courchesne, 2005; Webb et al., 2006; Courchesne et al., 2007; Amaral et al., 2008; Redcay and Courchesne, 2008; Schumann et al., 2010; Hazlett et al., 2011), two brain areas that regulate higher-order social, emotional, communication, and cognitive development. However, the average age of postmortem cases analyzed in more than fifty studies of the autistic brain is 22 years (Courchesne et al., 2007; Amaral et al., 2008). No single postmortem study of the young autistic brain has provided quantitative evidence to support or refute any current hypotheses. The results from postmortem studies of the older autistic brain show decreases in neuron numbers in cortex, amygdale, and cerebellum; proapoptotic and neuro-imflammatory molecular signals; and reduction in cortical minicolumn size, while MRI studies of the older autistic brain often report cortical thinning, reduction in the corpus callosum, reduced FA values in white matter fiber tracts, and either reduced brain size or absence of difference in size compared to normal (Courchesne et al., 2007, 2011a,b; Amaral et al., 2008). Such findings in the adult autistic brain do not explain why the infant and toddler with autism display early overgrowth.

The first speculation about the neural basis of early brain overgrowth proposed that dysregulation of cell proliferation and/or apoptosis might be the culprit (Courchesne et al., 2001, 2003; Courchesne and Pierce, 2005). This proposal, like all others since, has not been quantitatively tested. Neuropathological impressions of individual cases have described instances of heterotopias, focal laminar disorganization (Bailey et al., 1998; Hutsler et al., 2007), and subependymal dysplasia in older autistic brains, but lack quantitative information on the young autistic brain. A recent analysis of copy number variation in the DNA of living autistic patients raises the possibility of cell proliferation abnormality (Gohlke et al., 2007), but again direct evidence from the brain is lacking.

A proper number of neurons is fundamental to subsequent normal brain development and function. Following neural tube formation, the next major step in brain formation is the genesis of neurons. The rate of proliferation of neurons is exponential between human fetal weeks 10 and 20, leading to a net overabundance of neurons. This excess is normally pared away via prenatal apoptosis (Rabinowicz et al., 1996; Samuelsen et al., 2003; Bhardwaj et al., 2006) and near-adult numbers of cortical neurons around the time of birth (Rabinowicz et al., 1996; Samuelsen et al., 2003; Bhardwaj et al., 2006). A disruption in these processes could cause too many or too few neurons at birth, and abnormal connectivity and behavioral dysfunction during life.

We used computerized stereology to examine the neural basis of early brain overgrowth in autism. Our findings indicate that autism does involve a substantial overabundance of prefrontal neurons, and the greater the excess, the greater the overall deviant brain size (Courchesne et al., 2011c).

Methods

Autistic and Control Cases

Brains were obtained from the National Institute of Child Health and Human Development (NICHD) University of Maryland Brain and Tissue Bank or the Autism Tissue Program (ATP). Brains were from $n = 9$ autistic and $n = 7$ control males (for details, see Courchesne et al., 2011c) aged 2 to 16 years, which represents all young control male cases available at the time of the study and nearly all known young autism cases sectioned through the entire PFC. The extreme scarcity of young control and autistic postmortem cases is widely recognized. This paucity is even more pronounced with regard to tissue suitable for modern stereological study of the entirety of DL-PFC and M-PFC. The use of tissue sectioned as required for modern unbiased cell counting procedures ensures valid counts of total neuron number in PFC that cannot be obtained from estimates of neuron density from small blocks of cortical tissue (Braendgaard and Gundersen, 1986; Mouton, 2011).

All autism diagnostic classifications were based on either the results of postmortem ADI-R, the standard method for autism postmortem research; ADOS administered prior to death; or supporting clinical information available on the ATP Portal. For control cases, little information was available from brain and tissue bank records or the ATP Portal.

Anatomical Delineations of DL-PFC and M-PFC for Stereology Analyses

We analyzed two major prefrontal divisions: dorsolateral (DL-PFC) and mesial (M-PFC) prefrontal cortex (Figure 6.1). Landmarking was carried out blind to diagnostic membership, age of case, and the purpose, literature, and theories behind this study to ensure completely unbiased anatomic decisions. Anatomical delineation of the medial and dorsolateral PFC regions throughout their rostrocaudal extent was based on previous definitions (Semendeferi et al., 1997; Carper and Courchesne, 2005). Reliable anatomical boundaries were based on overall gross anatomy including tracking of sulci, and reliable boundaries were further refined/verified based on cytoarchitectonic criteria, including layer IV granularity, and, for instance, the presence of Betz cells indicating where precentral cortex should be differentiated from DL-PFC. Because these criteria were not

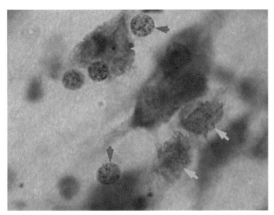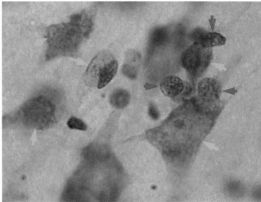

Figure 6.1 Morphological differences between neurons and microglia. Differences in neuron and microglia morphology are visible in 3D microscopic examination and are evident even in 2D images such as the ones shown here that were deliberately chosen to illustrate the most challenging cases with small neurons and/or large microglia. Neurons, some of which are as small as the biggest microglia, are labeled in green and microglia in red.

always present/sufficient (note the inclusion of young cases), the overall cortical width, layer VI/white-matter transition, and density/clarity of cortical columns were also used. These definitions were aided by the publications referenced above and by prior descriptions of cytoarchitectonic differentiation (Bucy, 1949; Rajkowska and Goldman-Rakic, 1995). Previous definitions (Semendeferi et al., 1997; Carper and Courchesne, 2005) were used for anatomical delineation of the M-PFC and DL-PFC regions throughout their rostrocaudal extent.

In brief, medial PFC included the entire medial surface of one hemisphere starting at the most rostral section and extending caudally until the paracentral lobule (PCL) had replaced PFC dorsally, the cingulate (CG) at mid dorsoventral levels, and the subcallosal area most ventrally. The medial PFC thus included the medial portion of the superior frontal and gyrus rectus, and the inferior and superior rostral gyrus. The most rostral sections also included medial portions of the frontopolar gyri.

For lateral PFC, the regions included were the lateral portion of the superior frontal gyrus, the middle frontal gyrus, the inferior frontal gyrus, and the frontal operculum. The most rostral sections also included lateral portions of the frontopolar gyri. The dorsolateral surface was thus included starting rostrally and extending to a ventral termination at orbital PFC regions followed caudally by the insula/insular gyrus, and, within this gross definition, precentral and postcentral gyri were excluded. To simplify border delineation at each transition, a straight line was drawn normal to the curvature of the cortical surface.

As these cases varied in intrinsic cytoarchitectonics (as would be expected given the range of ages and the potential for diagnosis-related differences), it was not possible to apply a single criterion across all cases. Generally speaking, without full reconstruction, the unambiguous identification of individual sulci is not feasible on histological sections, and cortical regions often transcend these boundaries; thus, the inclusion of cytoarchitectonic criteria is both necessary and useful. In some cases, however, particularly when many rostrocaudal levels were available and other criteria were only suggestive, sulci were followed over multiple levels and used for definition. The following lists the various transitions/borders and the most prominent features typically used to differentiate:

- In the case of the lateral-orbital frontal cortex transition at rostral levels, because the transition is from two similar frontal cortex regions, the most reliable criteria are gross anatomical features, and included the fronto-marginal, lateral-orbital, and lateral sulci.
- In the case of medial cortex-cingulate transitions, the gross anatomy (shape of CG gyrus, presence of deep CG sulci) provided the initial primary criteria, followed by granularity of layer IV, the clarity of the IV/V transition, and the density of layer II. In some cases, the cytoarchitectonics indicated cingulate extending slightly beyond or not quite reaching the bottom of the CG sulcus, but in the vast majority of cases, these criteria were in sync. The SCA ventrally had both clear cytoarchitectonic differences from the gyrus rectus, and differences in shape/curvature, and the first sulcus below the genu of the corpus callosum generally corresponded to the end of the cingulate.
- The frontal operculum always started medially at the insula border with the most medial-dorsal inflection of the circular insular sulcus, and continued laterally to the precentral gyrus transition, which was marked by clear cytoarchitectonic features.
- The border of frontal regions with the precentral gyrus was the most complex/variable. Identifying the border typically involved identifying a set of criteria specialized for each case that included identifying the cytoarchitectonics in the order below for regions that were clearly still frontal and comparing that to regions that were clearly not (e.g., more caudal parts of the precentral gyrus). The criteria were then mapped across sections and around the cortical layers until all criteria indicated the border location. The criteria were generally used in the following order:
  - granularity of layer IV
  - packing density of cortical columns
  - cortical thickness
  - white-matter/layer VI transition
  - layer IV/V transition
  - layer II thickness.

The presence of Betz cells was the only unambiguous in a minority of cases, but when present would be among the primary criteria.

Stereology Procedures

To avoid all known sources of bias, stereological analyses of neuron number and mean cell volume (MCV) within the DL-PFC and M-PFC were also carried out with assistance from a computerized stereology system (*Stereologer*, Stereology Resource Center, Tampa, FL) by a trained technician blind to diagnostic membership, age of case, as well as the purpose, literature, and theories behind this study.

Total Cell Number

Unbiased stereological methods independent of volumetric tissue shrinkage were used to quantify the total number of neurons in the entire DL-PFC and M-PFC volumes, according to methods detailed elsewhere (for more details, see Mouton, 2011). In this study the optical disector method was combined with the fractionator sampling method, the so-called optical fractionator design (West et al., 1991). The optical disector method involves the application of the unbiased disector principle (Sterio, 1984) to thin focal-plane z-axis scanning through a thick tissue section at 40×–100× oil immersion magnification (Braendgaard and Gundersen, 1986; Gundersen, 1986). On each Nissl-stained section, neurons were counted when the topmost nucleolus first came into focus within the 3D disector probe. Neurons were distinguished from glia on the basis of size and morphological features such as a prominent nucleolus, clear nuclear membrane, and high ratio of cytoplasm-to-nucleus. Neurons with nucleoli touching the exclusion planes of the disector frame or in first focus within the guard zones were not counted. The guard zone was $>8\,\mu m$ at the top and bottom of the section and the optical disector height was $10\,\mu m$. Sampling was carried out at a minimum of 100 locations in the x–y axes across 8–12 sections per region. The spacing between disectors was between 2.3 and 5 mm, depending on region size (typically 5 mm for lateral and 3.2 mm for mesial, with a smaller distance used for some of the smaller brains to ensure sufficient sampling). The total neuron number was estimated using the product of the total number of neurons counted within all disectors and the reciprocals of the area sampling fraction, the thickness sampling fraction, and the section sampling fraction. Sampling of tissue was continued to a coefficient of error of less than 10% (CE < 0.10). The neuronal density (Nv) for each reference space was calculated as the total number of neurons counted (ΣQ-) divided by the product of total number of disectors (N) and the volume of one disector (V_{dis}).

Volume Measurement

After sampling and counting neurons using the optical fractionator method, the MCV of neurons was estimated using the rotator method (Jensen and Gundersen, 1993). The data collector clicked at the boundary between the cell membrane and six lines generated at random across each sampled neuron. Due to the random placement these line lengths, their average length was directly proportional to the MCV for each neuron. Since MCV estimates were by necessity carried out on tissue sectioned in a single (coronal) plane, that is, rather than planes selected at random across all possible orientations, a small orientation bias could be present in the MCV estimates though this bias is negligible with respect to the findings in this study.

Distinguishing Neurons from Microglia

Distinguishing neurons and microglia on Nissl-stained sections requires detailed morphological examination and characterization in 3D. Cell size alone is not a suitable criterion for distinguishing neurons from microglia. Neurons were distinguished from glia on the basis of size and morphological features such as a prominent nucleolus, clear nuclear membrane, and high ratio of cytoplasm-to-nucleus. In this study about 1:250 randomly sampled cells were difficult to categorize, which would contribute to a rather insignificant percentage of about <0.4% of cells counted. To illustrate this point here, we searched for a set of small neurons or large microglia (i.e., targeted sampling rather than random) and had considerable difficulty finding truly ambiguous examples. Figure 6.1 demonstrates that morphological differences are seen even in these 2D images deliberately chosen to illustrate the most challenging cases. The ability to distinguish neuron vs. glial cell morphology is clearer in 3D, as used throughout this study.

Statistical Analyses

Analyses used SPSS software (SPSS Inc., Chicago IL) to assess within-case, between-case, and main and interaction effects of region (DL-PFC, M-PFC) and diagnosis (autism, control). A multivariate analysis of covariance (MANCOVA) was carried out using diagnosis as the independent variable, age as a covariate, and brain data (i.e., deviation of brain weight from age norms, neuron counts, microglia counts, neuron volume) as the dependent variables. A full model with age, diagnosis, and their interaction was initially evaluated. Diagnosis remained in the model as a significant factor; age and the interaction term were not significant. Pearson correlations were used to examine the relationship between neuron counts for the two regions, brain weight deviance, and age.

Results

Prefrontal Neuron Counts

As shown in Figure 6.2, there were 65% more neurons in DL-PFC in the autistic cases compared to the age- and gender-matched control group [1.45 ± 0.280 billion vs. 0.88 ± 0.143 billion; $F(1, 14) = 10.5$, $p = 0.006$] and 29% more neurons in M-PFC [0.356 ± 0.025 billion vs. 0.284 ± 0.035 billion; $F(1, 14) = 11.2$, $p = 0.005$]. Significant group differences remained after controlling for PMI. There was a strong and significant correlation between the number of DL-PFC neurons and

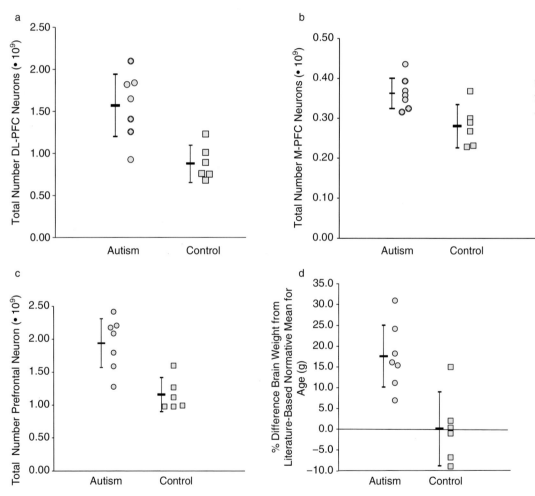

Figure 6.2 Results for autism ($n = 7$, male) and age-matched controls ($n = 6$, male) showing (a) 79% more DL-PFC neurons in autism cases ($p < 0.006$); (b) 29% more total number of M-PFC neurons in autism cases ($p < 0.005$); (c) 65% more PFC neurons in autism cases ($p < 0.002$); and 18% greater mean brain weight ($p < 0.01$) in autism cases compared to literature-based mean for age. There was a significant correlation (results not shown) between total number of PFC neurons and magnitude of deviation from normal brain weight for age ($r = 0.53$, $p < 0.035$). For further details, see Courchesne et al. (2011c).

the number of M-PFC neurons across autistic and control cases (r = 0.59, p = 0.016) (Figure 6.2c). This global neuron excess suggests that molecular mechanisms that ordinarily regulate neuron numbers are globally abnormal in prefrontal regions in autism. Finally, as hypothesized, there was a significant age-related decline in total number of DL-PFC neuron numbers in the autistic cases (r = −0.63, p = 0.033, 1-tailed) as predicted, but not in controls (r = −0.07, ns) (Figure 6.2a). Neuron counts in DL-PFC among the youngest autistic cases was nearly twice control levels (Figure 6.2a). M-PFC displayed a nonsignificant decline in the autistic group (r = −0.19, ns).

Postmortem Brain Weight

Figure 6.2d shows that brain weight strongly increased with age in controls (r = 0.85, p = 0.008, 1-tailed) but did not change in autistic cases (r = 0.4, ns), as predicted by previous literature (Redcay and Courchesne, 2005). Thus, at young but not older ages the autistic brain was substantially heavier than controls. The seven young 2- to 16-year-old autism cases exceeded normal age means by 212 grams, while the two adult autism cases had brain weights slightly less than (−51 grams or −3%) normal mean for age. These autism and control brain weights are therefore reasonably representative of the larger population of autistic and control cases reported in the literature (Redcay and Courchesne, 2005). Importantly, our cases were not selected on the basis of autopsy brain weight, but rather on the basis of being the only young male cases with whole frontal cortex sections available from the Autism Tissue Program, the Autism Brain Atlas set, and the UCSD ACE Center suitable for stereological measurements at the time of this study.

Prefrontal Neuron Counts and Brain Weight

There was a significant correlation between total number of prefrontal neurons and magnitude of deviation from normal mean brain weight for age (r = 0.53, p = 0.035) (Figure 6.2d) driven primarily by DL-PFC (r = 0.69, p = 0.003) and, to a lesser degree, M-PFC effects (r = 0.48, p = 0.057). The higher total number of prefrontal cortex neurons vis-à-vis the larger postmortem brain weights further validates the blinded stereological analyses reported here for autism cases and controls.

Neuron Volume and Microglia Counts

In order to consider the question of the impact of neuron size on interpretations of brain tissue in autism an ANCOVA was performed using age as a covariate. Although neuron volume was reduced slightly in autistic cases in both reference volumes, these differences from normal were not statistically significant [DL-PFC, $F(1, 12) = 0.34$. p = 0.572; M-PFC, $F(1, 12) = 0.18$, p = 0.6772].

Examining the groups as a whole, there was no significant correlation between mean neuron volume vs. difference from age matched average brain weight (DL-PFC, r = −0.092; M-PFC, r = −0.127, p > 0.05). There was also no significant correlation if the autism and control groups were considered as separate groups (all p values > 0.05). Likewise, there were no significant correlations between neuron volumes in either region of interest and neuron counts.

Microglia counts in DL-PFC [$F(1, 15) = 1.751$, ns] and M-PFC ($F(1, 15) = 0.202$, ns] did not differ between groups and were not correlated with neuron counts. Further analyses revealed that null effects of microglia counts remained after controlling for PMI, autopsy brain weight, neuron numbers and neuron size (all p values > 0.05).

Discussion

Normal brain growth and functional development in humans depend on a variety of foundational properties one of which is establishing a near-adult number of healthy neurons around the time of birth (Gohlke et al., 2007). Our results support the view that near-adult numbers of prefrontal neurons are indeed established during early development in humans. In our 2- and 3-year-old control cases, we found a near-adult number of prefrontal neurons; thus from age 2 through young adulthood, neuron numbers were unchanged in controls. From this base of neurons, elaboration of connectivity through axon growth, synaptogenesis occurs in a gradual manner from the first postnatal years when frontal circuits are sparse through eight years of age when connectivity is highly established (Conel, 1939–1967; Huttenlocher, 2002). During this age interval, experience and learning play a critical role in guiding axon growth and synapse selection (Quartz and Sejnowski, 1997).

Here we provide the first quantitative evidence that autism deviates sharply from this normal pattern in two major ways. By age 2–4 years in autism, there is nearly twice the normal number of PFC neurons. This overabundance indicates autism arises from defects in prenatal mechanisms that govern the number of neurons generated in the second trimester and/or removed later by prenatal or perinatal apoptosis. Figure 6.3 schematically depicts this theory. An overabundance of PFC neurons will produce more, not fewer, connections (axons, dendrites, and synapses) during early development. By one calculation (Ringo, 1991) the near doubling of neuron numbers could produce as many as four times the normal number of axons in the very young autistic brain. Autism, we argue, begins as a disorder of both excess neuron numbers and aberrant overabundant connectivity, not disconnectivity. It is important for future studies to assay neuron numbers in other cortical regions in autism using similarly rigorous stereological methods.

Our findings point to a second critical neuropathological phenomenon in autism: excess neuron numbers in the brains of young males with autism appear to be removed across decades, unlike the normal brain in which naturally occurring apoptosis removes excess rapidly across just a few months of prenatal and perinatal life. The child with autism therefore faces years of neuronal

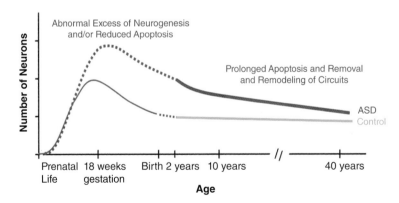

Figure 6.3   Schematic shows abnormal overabundance of prefrontal neuron numbers in autism found in the present study (red solid line) must have occurred in prenatal life (red dotted line). This is because (a) data and modeling (blue thin line) of normal prenatal development indicate that the dual counterbalancing processes of excess neurogenesis and corrective apoptosis play out in the second and third trimesters and establish a near-adult number of neurons by around the time of birth, and (b) our evidence (blue thick line) shows no changes in prefrontal neuron numbers in controls from toddler to adolescent and adult ages. We conclude that autism must be due to defects in developmental mechanisms that regulate this balance: that is, defects in regulation of neuron proliferation, apoptosis or both. The present evidence additionally indicates removal of abnormal excess and therefore circuit remodeling in autism may take years or decades. Blue dotted line is age range where there is an absence of quantitative evidence on neuron numbers in humans (Figure by Eric Courchesne and Kathleen Campbell).

apoptosis and substantial connectivity disassembly and, in the best of circumstances, a prolonged period of remodeling in an attempt to achieve improved circuit functioning. This abnormally slow age-related decline in PFC neuron number in autism must necessarily be accompanied by substantial removal and remodeling of axonal connections and synapses. Postmortem studies of older children, adolescents, and adults with autism commonly point to degenerative and remodeling processes including microglia activation, age-related increases in haphazard neuron-to-neuron spatial organization, neuron loss, reduced minicolumn size, molecular and gene expression signals of proapoptosis, reduced long- but increased short-distance axons, synaptic remodeling, and neuroinflammation (Araghi-Niknam and Fatemi, 2003; Vargas et al., 2005; Buxhoeveden et al., 2006; Schumann and Amaral, 2006; Garbett et al., 2008; van Kooten et al., 2008; Morgan et al., 2010, 2012; Zikopoulos and Barbas, 2010). These findings, we suggest, reflect not the origins of autism but rather the response to the original neurodevelopmental defects consequent to pathologically overabundant neurons, axons and synapses. Thus, it may be interesting to ask whether defects in synapse-relevant genes, several of which are risk-factors for autism, would place an autistic child at a much greater disadvantage during circuit remodeling. For this reason, further research is needed to understand the genetics of recovery from autism, as well as possible genetic mutations that may cause autism in the first place.

These findings may also give insight into why early intervention is essential and beneficial: Removal and remodeling earlier in life when connectivity is still limited and malleable could preemptively reduce the number of abnormal connections and guide more functional connectivity among the excess neurons (Dawson et al., 2010). Conversely, interventions begun later would entail the much more for difficult task of undoing and remodeling of far more extensive networks of embedded dysfunctional connectivity. Given the reduced neuroplasticity in older children and adults compared to early development, later interventions could lead to less than optimal clinical outcomes.

Autism, therefore, must be seen, studied and treated from a lifespan perspective. However, to our knowledge there is but a single paper that specifically addresses lifespan changes in the neurobiology of autism, and it provides new evidence as well as literature support for viewing autism as a multistage disorder: prenatal dysregulation of establishing the normal number of healthy neurons and cortical organization, early brain overgrowth, arrest of growth, and finally, removal and remodeling of aberrant cortical connectivity and excess neurons (Courchesne et al., 2011a). Animal and stem cell models of the neurobiology of autism should also be considered from the same vantage point. For such models to be successful, however, the genetic or nongenetic causes of neuronal overabundance need to be tracked down.

In conclusion, early brain overgrowth in autism (Courchesne et al., 2001, 2003) has at its roots a pathological overabundance of cortical neurons, and this pathology very possibly stands at the root cause of autism. This discovery opens new avenues for research into prenatal genetic and nongenetic causes of excess proliferation, the bases of abnormal connectivity, the reasons for neuroinflammation, proapoptosis, and synaptic remodeling across the life span, recovery genetics, and how early identification and intervention may improve clinical outcome for affected babies and toddlers. In short, identification of the prenatal causes of pathological excess of neurons in autism and the neurobiological sequelae hold promise for discovery of treatments that may lead to early recovery and an optimal clinical outcome for each baby with autism.

Acknowledgments

The authors of this chapter wish to acknowledge the contributions to the original work published in the November 9, 2011 issue of the *Journal of the American Medical Association*, including

Michael E. Calhoun (Sinq Systems, Columbia, MD), Katerina Semendeferi (Department of Anthropology at the University of California San Diego, La Jolla, CA), and Clelia Ahrens-Barbeau, Cynthia Carter Barnes, and Karen Pierce (Department of Neuroscience, NIH-UCSD Autism Center of Excellence, School of Medicine, University of California San Diego, La Jolla, CA). We would also like to thank Drs. Chet Sherwood and Muhammad Spocter (George Washington University) for their insight and review of PFC cytoarchitectonic features and regional borders. The research for this chapter was supported by funds from Autism Speaks, Cure Autism Now, The Peter Emch Family Foundation, The Thursday Club Juniors and the Rady Children's Hospital of San Diego and the UCSD-NIH Autism Center of Excellence (P50-MH081755) awarded to Eric Courchesne. We send our appreciation to all parents who made the difficult choice to support brain research through the donation of brain tissue from their loved ones. Tissue was provided by the National Institute of Child Health and Development (NICHD) Brain and Tissue Bank for Developmental Disorders (Baltimore, MD) under contracts N01-HD-4-3368 and N01-HD-4-3383, the Brain and Tissue Bank for Developmental Disorders (Miami, FL), Autism Tissue Program (Princeton, NJ), and direct donations to the Courchesne laboratory. We thank Dr. Ronald Zielke at the NICHD Brain and Tissue Bank for Developmental Disorders, Dr. Jane Pickett and Dr. Daniel Lightfoot at the Autism Tissue Program, Dr. Patrick Hof at Mt. Sinai SOM, and Dr. Jerzy Wegiel at IBR for facilitation of case acquisition. We also thank Melodie Hallett for statistical advice.

References

Amaral, D., Schumann, C. M., Nordahl, C. W. 2008. Neuroanatomy of autism. *Trends Neurosci* **31**: 137–145.

Araghi-Niknam, M., Fatemi, S. H. 2003. Levels of Bcl-2 and P53 are altered in superior frontal and cerebellar cortices of autistic subjects. *Cell Mol Neurobiol* **23**: 945–952.

Bailey, A., Luthert, P., Dean, A. et al. 1998. A clinicopathological study of autism. *Brain Res* **121**: 889–905.

Bhardwaj, R. D., Curtis, M. A., Spalding, K. L. et al. 2006. Neocortical neurogenesis in humans is restricted to development. *Proc Natl Acad Sci U S A* **103** (33): 12564–12568.

Braendgaard, H., Gundersen, H. J. G. 1986. The impact of recent stereological advances on quantitative studies of the nervous system. *J Neurosci Methods* **18**: 39–78.

Bucy, P. C. 1949. *The Precentral Motor Cortex*. Champaign, IL: The University of Illinois Press.

Buxhoeveden, D. P., Semendeferi, K., Buckwalter, J. et al. 2006. Reduced minicolumns in the frontal cortex of patients with autism. *Neuropathol Appl Neurobiol* **32** (5): 483–489.

Carper, R. A., Courchesne, E. 2005. Localized enlargement of the frontal cortex in early autism. *Biol Psychiatry* **57**: 126–133.

Carper, R. A., Moses, P., Tigue, Z. D. et al. 2002. Cerebral lobes in autism: early hyperplasia and abnormal age effects. *Neuroimage* **16**: 1038–1051.

Conel, J. L. 1939–1967. *The Postnatal Development of the Human Cerebral Cortex*, Vols. 1–8. Boston: Harvard University Press.

Courchesne, E., Pierce, K. 2005. Brain overgrowth in autism during a critical time in development: implications for frontal pyramidal neuron and interneuron development and connectivity. *Int J Dev Neurosci* **23**: 153–170.

Courchesne, E., Karns, C., Davis, H. R. 2001. Unusual brain growth patterns in early life in patients with autistic disorder: an MRI study. *Neurology* **57**: 245–254.

Courchesne, E., Carper, R., Akshoomoff, N. 2003. Evidence of brain overgrowth in the first year of life in autism. *JAMA* **290** (3): 337–344.

Courchesne, E., Pierce, K., Schumann, C. M. et al. 2007. Mapping early brain development in autism. *Neuron* **56**: 399–413.

Courchesne, E., Webb, S. J., Schumann, C. M. 2011a. From toddlers to adults: the changing landscape of the brain in autism. In *Autism Spectrum Disorders*, edited by D. G. Amaral, G. Dawson, and D. H. Geschwind. Oxford, UK: Oxford University Press.

Courchesne, E., Campbell, K., Solso, S. 2011b. Brain growth across the life span in autism: age-specific changes in anatomical pathology. *Brain Res* **1380**: 138–145.

Courchesne, E., Mouton, P. R., Calhoun, M. E., Semendeferi, K., Ahrens-Barbeau, C., Carter, C., Pierce, K. 2011c. Neuron number and size in prefrontal cortex of children with autism. *JAMA* November 9.

Dawson, G., Munson, J., Webb, S. J. et al. 2007. Rate of head growth decelerates and symptoms worsen in the second year of life in autism. *Biol Psychiatry* **61**: 458–464.

Dawson, G., Rogers, S., Munson, J. et al. 2010. Randomized, controlled trial of an intervention for toddlers with autism: the Early Start Denver Model. *Pediatrics* **125** (1): 17–23.

Garbett, K., Ebert, P. J., Mitchell, A. et al. 2008. Immune transcriptome alterations in the temporal cortex of subjects with autism. *Neurobiol Dis* **30**: 303–311.

Gohlke, J. M., Griffith, W. C., Faustman, E. M. 2007. Computational models of neocortical neuronogenesis and programmed cell death in the developing mouse, monkey, and human. *Cereb Cortex* **17**: 2433–2442.

Gundersen, H. J. G. 1986. Stereology of arbitrary particles: a review of unbiased number and size estimators and the presentation of some new ones, in memory of William R. Thompson. *J Microsc* **143** (Pt 1): 3–45.

Hazlett, H. C., Poe, M. D., Gerig, G. et al. 2011. Early brain overgrowth in autism associated with an increase in cortical surface area before age 2 years. *Arch Gen Psychiatry* **68** (5): 467–476.

Hutsler, J. J., Love, T., Zhang, H. 2007. Histological and magnetic resonance imaging assessment of cortical layering and thickness in autism spectrum disorders. *Biol Psychiatry* **61**: 449–457.

Huttenlocher, P. 2002. *Neural Plasticity: The Effects of Environment on the Development of Cerebral Cortex.* Boston: Harvard University Press.

Jensen, V. E. B., Gundersen, H. J. G. 1993. The rotator. *J Microsc* **170**: 35–44.

Morgan, J., Chana, G. et al. 2010. Microglial activation and increased microglial density observed in the dorsolateral prefrontal cortex in autism. *Biol Psychiatry* **68**: 368–376.

Morgan, J. T., Chana, G., Abramson, I. et al. 2012. Abnormalities in microglial and neuronal spatial organization in the dorsolateral prefrontal cortex in autism. *Brain Res* **1456**: 72–81.

Mouton, P. R. 2011. *Unbiased Stereology: A Concise Guide*, pp. 20–21. Baltimore, MD: The Johns Hopkins University Press.

Quartz, S. R., Sejnowski, T. J. 1997. The neural basis of cognitive development: a constructivist manifesto. *Behav Brain Sci* **20** (4): 537–556.

Rabinowicz, T., de Courten-Myers, G. M., Petetot, J. M. et al. 1996. Human cortex development: estimates of neuronal numbers indicate major loss late during gestation. *J Neuropathol Exp Neurol* **55** (3): 320–328.

Rajkowska, G., Goldman-Rakic, P. S. 1995. Cytoarchitectonic definition of prefrontal areas in the normal human cortex: I. Remapping of areas 9 and 46 using quantitative criteria. *Cereb Cortex* **5** (4): 307–322.

Redcay, E., Courchesne, E. 2005. When is the brain enlarged in autism? A meta-analysis of all brain size reports. *Biol Psychiatry* **58**: 1–9.

Redcay, E., Courchesne, E. 2008. Deviant functional magnetic resonance imaging patterns of brain activity to speech in 2–3-year-old children with autism spectrum disorder. *Biol Psychiatry* **64** (7): 589–598.

Ringo, J. L. 1991. Neuronal interconnections as a function of brain size. *Brain Behav Evol* **38**: 1–6.

Samuelsen, G. B., Larsen, K. B., Bogdanovic, N. et al. 2003. The changing number of cells in the human fetal forebrain and its subdivisions: a stereological analysis. *Cereb Cortex* **13** (2): 115–122.

Schumann, C. M., Amaral, D. G. F. 2006. Stereological analysis of amygdala neuron number in autism. *J Neurosci* **26** (29): 7674–7679.

Schumann, C. M., Bloss, C. S., Barnes, C. C. et al. 2010. Longitudinal magnetic resonance image study of cortical development through early childhood in autism. *J Neurosci* **30**: 4419–4427.

Semendeferi, K., Damasio, H., Frank, R., Van Hoesen, G. W. 1997. The evolution of the frontal lobes: a volumetric analysis based on three-dimensional reconstructions of magnetic resonance scans of human and ape brains. *J Hum Evol* **32** (4): 375–388.

Sparks, B. F., Friedman, S. D., Shaw, D. W. et al. 2002. Brain structural abnormalities in young children with autism spectrum disorder. *Neurology* **59**: 184–192.

Sterio, D. C. 1984. The unbiased estimation of number and sizes of arbitrary particles using the dissector. *J Microsc* **134**: 127–136.

van Kooten, I. A., Palmen, S. J., von Cappeln, P. et al. 2008. Neurons in the fusiform gyrus are fewer and smaller in autism. *Brain* **131**: 987–999.

Vargas, D. L., Nascimbene, C. et al. 2005. Neuroglial activation and neuroinflammation in the brain of patients with autism. *Ann Neurol* **57** (1): 67–81.

Webb, S. J., Dawson, G., Bernier, R., Panagiotides, H. 2006. ERP Evidence of atypical face processing in young children with autism. *J Autism Dev Disord* **36** (7): 881–890.

West, M. J., Slomianka, L., Gundersen, H. J. 1991. Unbiased stereological estimation of the total number of neurons in the subdivisions of the rat hippocampus using the optical fractionator. *Anat Rec* **231** (4): 482–497.

Zikopoulos, B., Barbas, H. 2010. Changes in prefrontal axons may disrupt the network in autism. *J Neurosci* **30** (44): 14595–14609.

7   Order in Chaos: Stereological Studies of Nervous Tissue

Peter Dockery

Anatomy School of Medicine, National University of Ireland, Galway, Ireland

Background

Our understanding of the functional anatomy of the nervous system has been transformed by advances in new technologies in imaging and microscopy. Medical imaging technologies such as magnetic resonance imaging (MRI), positron emission tomography (PET), ultrasonography, and optical imaging generate noninvasive, functionally relevant images that allow insight into structure–function relations in the living nervous system.

A good example of these advances is the development of diffusion tensor magnetic resonance imaging (DT-MRI, Beaulieu, 2010), an approach that provides *in vivo* visualization of certain aspects of white matter tracts. Like all methods, these imaging techniques have resolution limits and do not yet provide adequate access to the fine microanatomical organization of nervous tissue. With remarkably higher spatial and temporal resolution, novel developments in microscopy have improved our understanding of the cellular and molecular milieu of the nervous system. Areas of great potential include the continued development of super-resolution fluorescence microscopy (Hell, 2007; Testa et al., 2012) and developments in various label-free approaches (Witte et al., 2011).

Modern stereological methods represent an important breakthrough for the quantitative description of both the macro- and microanatomy of the CNS (for reviews, see Mayhew, 1991; Howard and Reed, 2005; Schmitz and Hof, 2005; Nyengaard and Gundersen, 2006; Mouton and Gordon, 2010; Mouton, 2011a,b). With a strong scientific hypothesis in mind, the power of these new stereology approaches leads to a key question—what to measure out of the apparently chaotic mass of anatomical structure of the nervous system, including the neurons, axons, dendrites, attending glia, vasculature, and extracellular elements. Of course, good data depend on good images, which is another topic outside the scope of this text. However, once the investigator is able to unambiguously visualize his/her structure of interest, the next step toward quantification leads directly to design-based (unbiased) stereology.

The Stereological Approach

Through systematic-random sampling, the stereological approach gathers detailed quantitative information on structural parameters of neural tissue, including volume (3D), surface area (2D), length (1D), and number (0D), without assumptions about the geometrical properties of the

---

Neurostereology: Unbiased Stereology of Neural Systems, First Edition. Edited by Peter R. Mouton.
© 2014 John Wiley & Sons, Inc. Published 2014 by John Wiley & Sons, Inc.

structures (Gundersen et al., 1988; Howard and Reed, 2005; Schmitz and Hof, 2005; Avendano, 2006; Mouton, 2011b; Kristiansen and Nyengaard, 2012). Unbiased sampling of the tissue ensures all parts of the tissue have an equal chance of being selected. This requirement is central for the quality, accuracy, and reliability of all unbiased estimators (Mouton, 2011b; Howard and Reed, 2005). Once unbiased sampling of tissue is ensured, the next step involves the systematic-random positioning of unbiased probes (estimators) such as points (0D), lines (1D), surfaces (2D), and disectors (3D). Because three equals the number of dimensions in the tissue, when the sum of dimensions in the parameter of interest and the probe equals at least 3D, the stereology design is considered theoretically unbiased.

The accuracy and precision of parameter estimates depends on two factors, bias and error, respectively. Common causes of sampling bias include failure to identify structures of interest (recognition bias), failure to sample in an unbiased manner (sampling bias), and faulty instrument calibration. There should also be an awareness of different forms of tissue deformation such as shrinkage and swelling since these can influence the accuracy of stereological estimates. Many sources of bias, the systematic difference between the parameter estimate and the true value, are not detectable from observations, cannot be removed or minimized, and do not diminish with further sampling. When all known sources of methodological bias are avoided or minimized to a negligible level, stereology provides theoretically unbiased (accurate) estimates of both relative ratios, such as volume density (Vv), surface density (Sv), length density (Lv), and number density (Nv), and absolute estimates of total volume (V), total surface (S), total length (L), and total number (N).

In contrast to bias (nonrandom error), random error in parameter estimates arises from two sources: biological variability (between-subject variation) from the real differences between subjects and method error (within-subject variation) from random fluctuation in expected estimates for repeated sampling within a given subject. Increased sampling can reduce these sources of random error, though the amount of sampling required in most cases is small relative to previous approaches using so-called "biased" stereology (Mouton, 2002, 2011a,b; Schmitz and Hof, 2005; Mouton and Gordon, 2010). According to the adage, "do more, less well," a high degree of variability with a low bias is preferable to a low degree of variability with a high bias (Mouton, 2002, 2011a,b; Baddeley and Vedel Jensen, 2004; Howard and Reed, 2005).

Reference Volume Estimation

Reference volume for an entire organ or subregion may be found using weight/density via water displacement (Archimedes principle). For material that may be cut into either physical or virtual sections, the stereology approach known as the Cavalieri method (Gundersen and Jensen, 1987) may be applied. This approach is highly efficient and has been shown to correlate with results from the water displacement method (Subbiah et al., 1996; Howard and Reed, 1998).

The Cavalieri principle provides a simple, efficient, and unbiased method to estimate the volume of an arbitrarily shaped object from the sum of the areas on systematic-random parallel sections through the object. In combination with point counting to estimate areas on cut surfaces, the Cavalieri method is often used for efficient estimation of total brain volume and various regions/nuclei of interest (Mayhew, 1992; Mouton et al., 1998; Fraher et al., 2007). The following example illustrates the Cavalieri-point counting method applied to estimation of human brain volumes from MRI images and physical sections (some material presented previously by Tuohy et al., 2004).

Brain volumes were estimated from T2-weighted images collected from normal subjects ($n = 5$ female, $n = 5$ male) using a 1.5 Tesla Seimens Magnetron Impact MRI scanner at the Cork Regional Hospital in Cork, Ireland. This study was carried out with full approval of the ethics committee at the Cork Regional Hospital. A series of 5-mm thick coronal slices were sampled

Table 7.1   Human brain dimensions from MRI images using the Cavalieri method and point counting[a-c]

Parameter	Male	Female
Total brain cm^3	1111 (5%)	1047 (6%)
Vv (%) Cerebellum	10 (6%)	11 (9%)
Vv (%) Thalamus	0.5 (11%)	0.5 (36%)
Vv (%) Caudate	0.3 (23%)	0.3 (15%)
Vv (%) Putamen	0.4 (35%)	0.4 (34%)

[a]Estimates of human brain volumes and volume fractions obtained for MRI.
[b]Values represent mean and interindividual coefficient of variation expressed as a percentage for five subjects in each group.
[c]Some of these data were presented by Tuohy et al. (2004).

Table 7.2   Brain dimensions obtained using the Cavalieri method

Species	Brain volume cm^3
Sheep	48
Manatee	165
Chimpanzee	205
Human	825

through the entire brain with a random start point for each series. Simple point counting was used to estimate sectional areas, and the sums of these areas were multiplied by 5 mm, the interslice distance.

The results showed a mean brain volume of 1048 ± 65 for female and 1111 ± 49 cm^3 (Table 7.1), findings which closely agree with a previous study by Mayhew and Olsen 1991.

The coefficient of error (CE) for the Cavalieri method (male CE = 2.45%, female CE = 2.49%) was calculated using a predictive formula, the quadratic approximation (Gundersen and Jensen, 1987) that takes into account the systematic nature of the sampling. The volume fraction and subsequent volumes of subregions were estimated (Table 7.1) for the cerebral hemispheres, cerebellum, putamen, caudate, thalamus, and the ventricles.

As shown in Table 7.2, we also applied the Cavalieri-point counting method to estimate volume mammalian brains from physical slices for the following species: sheep (*Ovis aries*), manatee (*Trichechus manatus latirostris*), chimpanzee (*Pan troglodytes*), and human (*Homo sapiens*). The material for this study was obtained from the University of Wisconsin and Michigan State Comparative Brain Collection (http://www.brainmuseum.org). Note that shrinkage due to tissue processing was not taken into account, which explains the about 25% lower estimate for total brain volume in the physical sections from human brain as compared to the same parameter estimated from *in vivo* imaging (Table 7.1).

Cell Volume Estimation

There are many situations where estimation of total volume of an entire organ or compartment is not feasible. A number of estimators have been developed to provide numerical adjectives that describe total volume of "particles," which in a biological context may be applied to cells or nuclei (Mayhew, 1992). Indirect methods of estimating mean particle volume involve either dividing total particle volume (V) by total number (N) or dividing volume density (Vv) by numerical density (Nv). More efficient alternatives use a so-called local size estimator, which involves direct estimation of mean particle volume using the disector or fractionator methods to estimate total N, followed by the application of isotropic test lines to estimate the number-weighted mean particle volume using the nucleator (Gundersen, 1986), rotator (Jensen and Gundersen, 1993), or optical rotator (Tandrup et al., 1997) approaches. Another local size estimator, the point sampled intercept (PSI method), uses a point-grid to preferentially sample larger particles, followed by calculation of volume-weighted mean particle volume from single isotropic-uniform-random or vertical-uniform-random sections (Gundersen and Jensen, 1985). The PSI method with volume-weighted mean particle volume is most commonly used in prognostic studies to assess the relative potential of malignancies to metastasize (Sørensen et al., 1992).

The PSI sampling approach may also be used to estimate neuron number and size from electron microscopy images (Dockery et al., 1997). We applied this approach to the wobbler mouse, a spontaneous model for the investigation of motoneuron diseases, including amyotrophic lateral sclerosis and infantile spinal muscular atrophy. A characteristic feature of this mutant is the development of swollen vacuolated motoneuron cell bodies in the ventral horn of the spinal cord. Using this murine model of motoneuron disease, neuronal cell and nuclear volumes were estimated. These data were combined with volume fraction data obtained from a subsequent electron microscopical study (Treacy et al., 2002) to produce a comprehensive account of the cytoarchitecture of this cell population.

Two groups of mice ($n = 6$ per group) were studied at two ages: young (3 weeks) and old (12 weeks). Mice were anesthetized and perfusion-fixed for electron microscopy (Dockery et al., 1997; Treacy et al., 2002). The spinal cord was cut transversely to its long axis into approximately 1-mm thick slices, which were trimmed under a binocular microscope to remove all but the ventral gray horn. Tissues were then embedded in Epon resin in spherical molds using the isector method (Nyengaard and Gundersen, 1992; Li et al., 2009). The resultant sections were isotropic uniform and random (IUR) in orientation, as required for the application of the stereological probes (Howard and Reed, 2005). Semi-thin sections (0.5 µm thick) were cut for light microscopy and stained with toluidine blue.

The study examined the neurons in the ventral gray horn region using the morphological criteria of Mayhew and Momoh (1974). About 25 microscopic fields from each case were selected in a systematic-random fashion for estimation of perikaryal and nuclear volumes and volume fractions. A systematic series of electron micrographs were collected from thin sections to obtain fractional volumes of subcellular organelles. Volume-weighted mean volume of both nuclei and perikaryon were estimated by the volume-weighted PSI method, which samples particles in proportion to their volume (Gundersen et al., 1988). Briefly, after random placement of a point grid over the area containing the particles of interest (reference area), the volume of each particle intersecting a point on the grid was estimated by measuring the length of the isotropic line l_o passing through the sampled point. The mean weighted particle volume was estimated from a series of measurements according to the following formula:

$$\hat{\bar{V}}_v = \frac{1}{3}\pi \overline{l_o^3},$$

(7.1)

where $\overline{l_o^3}$ is the mean of the cube of the intercept length.

Number-weighted mean nuclear and perikaryal volumes were estimated using the nucleator principle (Gundersen et al., 1988) by sampling neurons using physical disectors (Mayhew, 1992). An unbiased counting frame (Gundersen, 1977) was superimposed on one of the "disector-pairs." Nucleoli that appeared in the reference section but not on the adjacent (look-up) section were counted. The nuclear profiles of the selected nuclei were identified and the position of the nucleolus was noted. A four-way nucleator was then applied to the profile, and the distance was measured from the center of the nucleolus to the nuclear and perikaryal membranes (Gundersen et al., 1988; Tandrup, 1993). Volume was estimated using the following formula:

$$\hat{\bar{V}}_n = \frac{4}{3}\pi \bar{l}_n^3.$$
(7.2)

Number-weighted mean volume and volume-weighted mean volumes are related by the following relationship:

$$\hat{\bar{V}}_v = \hat{\bar{V}}_n(1 + CV_n^2).$$
(7.3)

CV_n^2 is the coefficient of variation (CV) of the number distribution of particle volumes (Gundersen and Jensen, 1985; Cruz-Orive and Hunziker, 1986). These were combined with fractional volumes to provide estimates of organelle volumes.

As shown in Table 7.3, the composition of cells shows the extent of the intracellular vacuolation in the young wobbler group.

The CV of the number distribution of nuclear and perikaryal volumes were calculated (Table 7.4), providing access to the population stucture (Table 7.2). For detailed discussion on the biological implications of these findings, see Dockery et al. (1997).

Length Estimation

Unbiased estimators have been developed to quantify length density (Lv) and total length (L), two useful stereological parameters to estimate the linear dimension of objects within a reference

Table 7.3 Ventral horn cell composition[a,b]

Volume μm³	Young		Old	
	Normal	Wobbler	Normal	Wobbler
Nucleus	1,298	1,337	1,450	768
RER	213	64	171	48
Mitochondria	432	412	528	254
Secretory apparatus	155	102	97	36
Vacuoles	9	2,159	0	598
Cytoplasm	6,437	6,101	8,114	3,702
Cell	8,544	10,175	10,360	5,406

[a]Values represent mean volume for five animals in each group.
[b]Volumes of cell and organelle volumes of ventral horn neurons were obtained by using stereological methods (Dockery et al., 1997; Treacy et al., 2002).

Table 7.4 The percentage coefficient of variation $CV_n\%$ for the number weighted neuronal distributions in the murine ventral horn

Mouse age	$CV_n\%$ nuclei	$CV_n\%$ perikarya
Young normal	48	95
Young wobbler	54	127
Old normal	45	104
Old wobbler	65	96

Source: Adapted from Dockery et al. (1997).

volume. Length is often a parameter of interest for neuroscientists with regard to axons, dendrites, neurites, and blood vessels. Because length estimation is particularly sensitive to orientation, there are a number of solutions to the problem of anisotropy. The orientator or isector methods may be used for isotropic uniform random sections, though these approaches lose tissue landmarks due to random rotation of the tissue prior to sectioning. Nevertheless, this approach has been used to obtain estimates of Lv and total L of myelinated fibers in the white matter of the human brain and accessory sex glands (Chow et al., 1997; Tang and Nyengaard, 1997; Marner and Pakkenberg, 2003). Vertical-uniform-random sections may be used in conjunction with cycloids, where the longer cycloid axis is oriented parallel to the vertical axis and projected through the section depth (Gohkale, 1990; Batra et al., 1995; Stocks et al., 1996; Avendano, 2006). If the entire structure can be visualized via total vertical projections, it is possible to estimate total branch length by counting the number of intersections with projected cycloid arcs on a repeated number of object rotations. This method has been used to examine dendritic length in Golgi-stained neurons (Howard et al., 1992) and in CT angiograms (Dockery and Fraher, 2007). A number of computer-assisted solutions for length estimation include Virtual Isotopic Planes (Larsen et al., 2004) and Virtual Spheres (space balls; Calhoun and Mouton, 2001; Mouton et al., 2002; Calhoun et al., 2004). The advantages of these computerized approaches using virtual probes are that tissue may be sectioned in any convenient orientation, for example, coronal, and length estimation may be carried out on tissue not previously rotated prior to sectioning.

Stereology and imaging technologies provide an important component to enhance our understanding of the functional anatomy of the vascular system (McDonald and Choyke, 2003; Dockery and Fraher, 2007). Despite the fundamental importance of the vascular system to function of the spinal cord, the majority of stereological studies have focused on neuronal and glial composition (Schmitz and Hof, 2005). The following example uses the same wobbler mouse material described earlier where the isector approach was adopted in the production of IUR resin blocks (Dockery et al., 1997; Bane et al., 2002). An unbiased counting frame was applied in a uniform-random pattern using high magnification light microscopy (100× oil immersion) on semi-thin sections to obtain estimates of length density (Lv):

$$L_v = 2N_a. \tag{7.4}$$

Diffusion distance: The radial diffusion distance estimate provides a simple, robust indication of a cylindrical zone of diffusion around a vessel. This can be estimated from the Lv data (Nyengaard and Gundersen, 1992; Dockery and Fraher, 2007) using the following formula:

$$r(diff) = 1/\sqrt{pL_v}. \tag{7.5}$$

A summary of the type of data so obtained is shown in Table 7.5.

The results indicate that diffusion distances is maintained despite the pathologic insult. This pattern between gray and white matter was also noted in the human spinal cord using a similar approach (Dockery and Fraher, 2007).

Axon Number

The axon situated between the cell body and the synaptic terminals is vital in connecting neurons and acting as an instrument for the transmission of information between them. A variety of different types of pathologic insult affect axons. Axonal number is, therefore, often estimated as key indicator of the extent of this insult. The number of axons in a given nerve trunk can vary a great

Table 7.5   Length densities and radial diffusion distances in the ventral horn[a,b]

Mouse age and color	Length density mm^{-1}		Radial diffusion distance μm	
	Normal	Wobbler	Normal	Wobbler
Young white	624	884	23	19
Old white	744	980	21	19
Young gray	1307	1321	15	16
Old gray	1710	1307	16	17

[a]Length densities and radial diffusion distances in the ventral horn of normal and wobbler mice.
[b]Values represent mean six animals in each group (Bane et al., 2002; Dockery et al., 2002).

deal, from tens to over a million, depending on species and location. Since the effort involved in quantification can be considerable, efficient sampling strategies and stereological approaches have made a significant contribution (Mayhew and Sharma, 1984a,b; Mayhew, 1991; Mouton et al., 2002; Perry et al., 2004; Avendano, 2006). These efficient methods include systematic-random sampling using an unbiased counting frame, with results for total axon number calculated by the fractionator method. Unbiased stereological methods have also been used to assess axonal composition (Li et al., 2009; Avandano, 2006). However, many of the questions related to transversely sectioned peripheral nerve trunks or indeed certain central white matter tracts (e.g., the optic nerve) are essentially 2D problems requiring adequate sampling strategies combined with adequate mensuration (Dockery et al., 1996; Avendano, 2006).

As for all stereological approaches, the optimal resolution is the lowest magnification that the structure of interest can be clearly resolved. Design-based sampling is the preferred approach to ensure that morphological variables of biological objects do not influence the probability of each object being sampled. Sampling strategies for enumeration have been well established for both peripheral and central nervous systems (Mayhew and Sharma, 1984a,b; Dockery et al., 1996). For sites other than central and peripheral nerve trunks, the reader should review the approach adopted by Li et al. (2009).

A multicenter study by Kaplin et al. (2010) examined the reliability of two different stereological counting methods by comparing the unbiased counting frame versus the 2D-disector. Both approaches provided efficient and unbiased estimates of fiber numbers, suggesting that in this narrow context, design-based stereological methods and sampling schemes may be considered a priori correct and superior to all other methods. The authors of this report urge caution when handling any quantitative data, even those generated by design-based stereological methods.

Axonal Number and Composition in the Murine Optic Nerve

The following systematic sampling approach illustrates one way in which axon number can be estimated with minimal effort.

This next example presents data from our studies on the wobbler mutant mouse. In this section, data are presented on the old (3 months) wobbler group described earlier (Dockery et al., 2002). The right optic nerve was removed and processed for transmission electron microscopy. Transverse semi-thin sections were cut across the entire nerve trunk and stained with toluidine blue. The transverse area of the endoneurium was estimated by simple point counting (Dockery et al., 1996). Thin sections (60 nm) were also cut and stained for electron microscopy. A systematic series of micrographs were taken across the entire nerve trunk, using an unbiased counting frame (Gundersen, 1977). The number of myelinated and nonmyelinated axons per unit area were estimated in

Table 7.6   Number of fibers in the optic nerve[a,b]

Fiber	Normal	Wobbler
Myelinated	38,584 (31%)	33,352 (22%)
Unmyelinated	5,455 (60%)	16,769 (40%)
Total	44,039 (25%)	48,193 (21%)

[a]Number of fibers in the optic nerve in normal and wobbler mice (Dockery et al., 2002).
[b]Values in parenthesis represent CV% for five animals in each group.

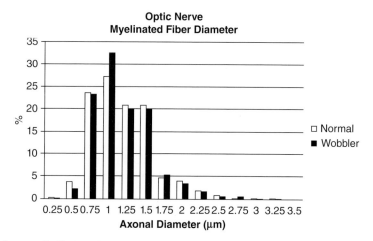

Figure 7.1   Fiber diameter distribution of myelinated axons in the optic nerve of normal and wobbler mice.

this sample to obtain Na (number per unit area). This was then multiplied by the endoneurial area to obtain estimates of total number. This study found no significant difference in the number of axons in normal and wobbler mice; however, the number of unmyelinated axons in the wobbler was significantly greater than the control (Table 7.6).

Axonal and Fiber Size Distributions

The range of size differences of different nerves may reflect anatomical differences between functional groups of axons, as well as regional differences in their target distributions (Dockery et al., 1996).

A commonly measured parameter is the external myelinated nerve fiber diameter, which has been linked to various functional attributes such as nerve conduction velocity (Arbuthnott et al., 1980a) and differences between normal and abnormal populations of nerve fibers (Sharma et al., 1985). Typically, the minimum diameter, or some function of major and minor diameters (Dockery et al., 1996; Tang and Nyengaard, 1997; Yang et al., 2008), is measured by simple light microscopy. Electron microscopy has been used for fibers and umyelinated axons in the CNS, and occasionally PNS-myelinated fibers where the added resolution is needed for quantitative analyses (Dockery, 1992; Dockery et al., 1996).

The data presented in Figure 7.1 shows the diameter (based upon perimeter estimates) of the myelinated axon populations in the normal and wobbler optic nerves (Dockery et al., 2002).

There have been many studies on parametric variations of the various components of the myelinated nerve fibers on saltatory conduction (see Aguayo et al., 1971; Waxman, 1980; Arbuthnott et al., 1980a), including internodal length and relative mylelin sheath thickness (Dockery et al., 1996). Reduction in conduction velocity is observed when axons become atrophic due to compression (Baba et al., 1982) or in nerves proximal to a lesion (Gillespie and Stein, 1983). *In vivo* noncircularity must be considered as a scaling factor for relating fiber caliber to conduction velocity (Arbuthnott et al., 1980b).

It is well established that the axon determines whether or not it is myelinated (Aguayo et al., 1976a,b). Mature nerve fiber populations have demonstrated a positive correlation between axon caliber and myelin sheath thickness and is also evident when quantifying more complex parameters (axonal surface area, internodal length, and sheath volume). During early development, these correlations are often very low or nonsignificant but strengthen as maturation proceeds. For this to occur, the myelinating mechanism are thought to continuously respond to axon size. However, such a system seems unnecessarily complex. The strong correlation between the axon size and myelination for a given myelinated fiber population could be explained by a simpler mechanism such as a single stimulus that switches on during axon growth, persists for a time, and then switches off. Thus, the Schwann cell may form the myelin sheath at a constant rate, that is, in the absence of any quantitative influence exerted by the axon (Fraher et al., 2007).

The Myelin Sheath

Schmidt et al. (1941) observed a periodicity of about 18 nm for fresh peripheral myelin. Central and peripheral myelin sheaths are similar, both formed by the spiral wrapping of glial cell plasma membranes, though important differences exist (Peters et al., 1991). For instance, central myelin has a periodicity about 10% less than peripheral myelin (Inouye and Kirschener et al., 1984). Our rat studies with fixed material (Dockery et al., 1996) found a periodicity of 11.3 nm for optic nerve and 12 nm for sciatic nerve (Dockery et al., 1996). Even lower estimates were obtained in our studies in mice (Table 7.7).

Because the myelin sheath can be affected by fixation, developmental processes, and pathologic insult, care should be taken to confirm similar periodicity between groups by measuring the periodicity on a sample of axons (King and Thomas, 1984). Average periodicity for a nerve may be expressed as the slope of the linear regression line of width of myelin sheath against number of lamellae (Dockery and Sharma, 1991). Table 7.8 shows data on unmyelinated poulations (Dockery et al., 2002).

A systematic series of electron micrographs was taken across the whole nerve and an unbiased counting frame was used to ensure adequate sampling. We estimated a number of parameters such

Table 7.7 Myelinated fibers in the optic nerve[a,b]

	Normal	Wobbler
Axon area μm^2	0.66 (29%)	0.71 (12%)
Fiber area μm^2	1.35 (22%)	1.32 (9%)
Periodicity	9.2 (13%)	10.2 (19%)
g-ratio	0.826	0.832

[a]Parameters of myelinated fibers in the optic nerve of normal and wobbler mice.
[b]Values represent mean and CV% for six animals in each group (Dockery et al., 2002).

Table 7.8 Optic nerve unmyelinated axons[a,b]

	Normal	Wobbler
Axon area μm²	0.147 (25%)	0.183 (17%)
Fiber area μm²	0.149 (46%)	1.557 (8%)
Axon diameter μm	0.432 (15%)	0.496 (8%)

[a]Paramaters of unmyelinated axons in the optic nerve of normal and wobbler mice.
[b]Values represent mean and CV% for six animals in each group (Dockery et al., 2002).

as axon area and axon perimeter using a combined morphometric and stereological approach (Dockery et al., 1996). The width of myelin sheath was estimated using the method similar to that descibed by Li et al. (2009), and number of lamellae was estimated in a subsample of the populations.

Another commonly used descriptor of the axon myelin relationship, the g-ratio, has been discussed as vital for the adequate mensuration of this important parameter (Dockery, 1992; Dockery et al., 1996). Recently Paus and Toro (2009) suggested possible implications of "suboptimal" g-ratio for the emergence of "disconnection" disorders, such as schizophrenia, in late adolescence. The degree of myelination may also influence visualization of anisotropy in techniques such as diffusion tensor magnetic resonance imaging (Rye, 1999). Axer et al. (2011) recently used polarized light microscopy in combination with computer modeling techniques to try and close the gap between large-scale diffusion orientation and microsctuctural histological analysis of connectivity to help understand diffusion tensor mapping of white matter.

The final example in this chapter examines unmyelinated axons in the tibial nerve of genetically diabetic mice C57BL/Ks (db/db) at 6 and 15 months of age. Tibial nerves from five animals in each group were processed for transmission electron microscopy (Sharma et al., 1982). Transverse sections were made, and a systematic series of electron micrgraphs were obtained for morphometric and stereological investigation (Crotty et al., 2002). Neurotubules are a fundamental part of the axonal cytoskeleton involved in axonal transport (Holzbaur and Scherer, 2011). The density and number of this imporant organelle have been examined in a wide variety of nerve types in normal and pathological conditions (Peters et al., 1991).

Numerous techniques exist for the study of spatial patterns (Diggle, 1983; Upton and Fingleton, 1985). In the present study, we used a powerful 2D technique, the Hopkins H_n Statistic (Diggle, 1983). This entailed measuring distances between random points and the nearest neighbor neurotubule and between a randomly chosen neurotubule and the nearest neighbor. The results indicate that the distribution of neurotubules is not random, suggesting that the pathologic insult of diabetes mellitus may affect the pattern-generating process in axons (see Dockery, 1992). This finding and the other structural findings, some of which are presented in Table 7.9, may partially explain the transport disturbances associated with diabetic neuropathy.

Conclusion

This chapter illustrates the type of quantitative first- and second-order information on neural structural that can be obtained using unbiased sampling strategies in combination with simple morphometric and stereological probes. The nervous system presents an elaborate tapestry of interwoven structural and functional elements of wide-ranging size, shape, and orientation. Because they are devised to avoid bias arising from size, shape, and orientation, the methods of design-based stereology have the potential to reveal an enormous amount of quantitative information about structural components of the nervous system under normal and pathological conditions.

Table 7.9 Tibial nerve unmyelinated axons[a,b]

	6-Month control	6-Month diabetic	15-Month control	15-Month diabetic
Axon area μm^2	0.34 (15%)	0.48 (13%)	0.38 (31%)	0.37 (16%)
Neurotubule density	57 (18%)	53 (14%)	63 (13%)	57 (13%)
Vv % Mitochondria	4.5 (25%)	4.5 (15%)	2.0 (64%)	4.8 (26%)
Vv % SER/vesicles	8.7 (24%)	7.9 (3%)	4.7 (26%)	9.9 (8%)
Hopkins test statistic	0.428	0.389	0.370	0.390

[a]Parameters of unmyelinated axons from the tibial nerve of genetically diabetic (db/db) and normal mice.
[b]Values represent mean and CV% for six animals in each group (Dockery, 1992; Crotty et al., 2002).

References

Aguayo, A., Nair, C. P., Midgley, R. 1971. Experimental progressive compression neuropathy in the rabbit. Histologic and electrophysiologic studies. *Arch Neurol* **24** (4): 358–364.

Aguayo, A. J., Charron, L., Bray, G. M. 1976a. Potential of Schwann cells from unmyelinated nerves to produce myelin: a quantitative ultrastructural and radiographic study. *J Neurocytol* **5**: 565–573.

Aguayo, A. J., Epps, J., Charron, L., Bray, G. M. 1976b. Multipotentiality of Schwann cells in cross-anastomosed and grafted myelinated and unmyelinated nerves: quantitative microscopy and radio-autography. *Brain Res* **104**: 1–20.

Arbuthnott, E. R., Boyd, I. A., Kalu, K. U. 1980a. Ultrastructural dimensions of myelinated peripheral nerve fibres in the cat and their relation to conduction velocity. *J Physiol* **308**: 125–157.

Arbuthnott, E. R., Ballard, K. J., Boyd, I. A., Kalu, K. U. 1980b. Quantitative study of the non-circularity of myelinated peripheral nerve fibres in the cat. *J Physiol* **308**: 99–123.

Avendano, C. 2006. Stereology of neural connections: an overview. In *Neuroanatomical Tract-Tracing*, edited by L. Zaborszky, F. G. Wouterlood, and J. L. Lanciego, p. 477. London, UK: Springer.

Axer, M., Grässel, D., Kleiner, M., Dammers, J., Dickscheid, T., Reckfort, J., Hütz, T., Eiben, B., Pietrzyk, U., Zilles, K., Amunts, K. 2011. High-resolution fiber tract reconstruction in the human brain by means of three-dimensional polarized light imaging. *Front Neuroinform* **5**: 34.

Baba, M., Fowler, C. J., Jacobs, J. M., Gilliatt, R. W. 1982. Changes in peripheral nerve fibres distal to a constriction. *J Neurol Sci* **54** (2): 197–208.

Baddeley, A. J., Vedel Jensen, E. B. 2004. *Stereology for Statisticians*. London, UK: Chapman & Hall/CRC.

Bane, V., Tay, D. K. C., Tany, Y., Morais, M., Vacca-Galloway, L. L., Dockery, P. 2002. The vasculature of the spinal cord of the wobbler mutant mouse: a stereological study. *J Anat* **201** (5): 433.

Batra, S., Konig, M. F., Cruz-Orive, L. M. 1995. Unbiased estimation of capillary length from vertical sections. *J Microsc* **178**: 152–159.

Beaulieu, C. 2010. What makes diffusion anisotropic in the nervous system. In *Theory, Methods and Applications*, edited by D. K. Jones. Diffusion MRI. Oxford, UK: Oxford University Press.

Calhoun, M. E., Mouton, P. R. 2001. New developments in neurostereology: length measurement and 3D imagery. *J Chem Neuroanat* **21**: 257–265.

Calhoun, M. E., Mao, Y., Roberts, J. A., Rapp, P. R. 2004. Reduction in hippocampal cholinergic innervation is related to recognition memory impairment in aged rhesus monkeys. *J Comp Neurol* **475**: 238–246.

Chow, P. H., Dockery, P., Cheung, A. 1997. Innervation of accessory sex glands in the adult male golden hamster and quantitative changes of nerve densities with age. *Andrologia* **29** (6): 331–342.

Crotty, S. G., Dockery, P., Sharma, A. K., Thomas, P. K. 2002. Ultrastructural abnormalities of unmyelinated fibres in the peripheral nerves of genetically diabetic (db/db) mutant mice. *J Anat* **200** (2): 207–208.

Cruz-Orive, L. M., Hunziker, E. B. 1986. Stereology for anisotropic cells: application to growth cartilage. *J Microsc* **143** (Pt 1): 47–80.

Diggle, P. 1983. *Statistical Analysis of Spatial Point Patterns*. London and New York.: Academic Press.

Dockery, P. 1992. Peripheral nerve structure in two models of diabetes: a morphometric approach. In *Advances in Physiological Sciences*, edited by S. K. Manchanda, W. Selvamurthy, and V. M. Kumar, pp. 220–229. New Delhi: Macmillan India.

Dockery, P., Fraher, J. 2007. The quantification of vascular beds: a stereological approach. *Exp Mol Pathol* **82** (2): 110–120.

Dockery, P., Sharma, A. K. 1991. Ultrastructural abnormalities of myelinated fibres in the tibial nerve of streptozotocin-diabetic rats. *J Neurol Sci* **98** (2–3): 327–345.

Dockery, P., Chau, W. K. D., So, K. F., Fraher, J. P. 1996. Axon glial interactions: a morphometric approach. In *Morphometry Applications to Medical Sciences*, edited by A. K. Sharma, pp. 93–111. New Delhi: MacMillan India.

Dockery, P., Tang, Y., Morais, M., Vacca-Galloway, L. L. 1997. Neuron volume in the ventral horn in Wobbler mouse motoneuron disease: a light microscope stereological study. *J Anat* **191**: 89–98.

Dockery, P., Tay, D. K. C., Treacy, J., Tang, Y., O'Sullivan, P., Vacca-Galloway, L. L. 2002. Body composition of the wobbler mutant mouse. *J Anat* **200** (2): 214.

Fraher, J. P., Dockery, P., O'Donoghue, O., Riedewald, B., O'Leary, D. 2007. Initial motor axon outgrowth from the developing central nervous system. *J Anat* **211** (5): 600–611.

Gillespie, M. J., Stein, R. B. 1983. The relationship between axon diameter, myelin thickness and conduction velocity during atrophy of mammalian peripheral nerves. *Brain Res* **259** (1): 41–56.

Gohkale, A. M. 1990. Unbiased estimation of curve length in 3D using vertical slices. *J Microsc* **159**: 133–141.

Gundersen, H. J. 1986. Stereology of arbitrary particles: a review of unbiased number and size estimators and the presentation of some new ones, in memory of William R. Thompson. *J Microsc* **143** (Pt 1): 3–45.

Gundersen, H. J., Jensen, E. B. 1985. Stereological estimation of the volume-weighted mean volume of arbitrary particles observed on random sections. *J Microsc* **138** (Pt 2): 127–142.

Gundersen, H. J., Jensen, E. B. 1987. The efficiency of systematic sampling in stereology and its prediction. *J Microsc* **147** (Pt 3): 229–263.

Gundersen, H. J., Bagger, P., Bendtsen, T. F., Evans, S. M., Korbo, L., Marcussen, N., Moller, A., Nielsen, K., Nyengaard, J. R., Pakkenberg, B. 1988. The new stereological tools: disector, fractionator, nucleator and point sampled intercepts and their use in pathological research and diagnosis. *APMIS* **96** (10): 857–881.

Gundersen, H. J. G. 1977. Notes on the estimation of the numerical density of arbitrary particles: the edge effect. *J Microsc* **111**: 219–223.

Hell, S. W. 2007. Far-field optical nanoscopy. *Science* **316** (5828): 1153–1158.

Holzbaur, E. L. F., Scherer, S. S. 2011. Microtubules, axonal transport, and neuropathy. *N Engl J Med* **365**: 2330–2332.

Howard, C. V., Reed, M. G. 1998. *Unbiased Stereology*, London, UK: Springer Scientific.

Howard, C. V., Reed, M. G. 2005. *Unbiased Stereology*, 2nd ed. Oxford: BIOS Scientific Publishers.

Howard, C. V., Cruz-Orive, L. M., Yaegashi, H. 1992. Estimating neuron dendritic length in 3D from total vertical projections and from vertical slices. *Acta Neurol Scand Suppl* **137**: 14–19.

Inouye, H., Kirschner, D. A. 1984. New X-ray spacings from central myelinated tissue. *J Neurocytol* **13** (6): 883–894.

Jensen, E. B. V., Gundersen, H. J. G. 1993. The rotator. *J Microsc* **170**: 35–44.

Kaplin, S., Geuna, S., Ronchi, G., Ulkay, M.B., von Bartheld, C.S. 2010. Calibration of the stereological estimation of the number of myelinated axons in the rat sciatic nerve: a multicenter study. *J Neurosci Methods* **187** (1): 90–99.

King, R. H., Thomas, P. K. 1984. The occurrence and significance of myelin with unusually large periodicity. *Acta Neuropathol* **63** (4): 319–329.

Kristiansen, S. L., Nyengaard, J. R. 2012. Digital stereology in neuropathology. *APMIS* **120** (4): 327–340.

Larsen, J. O., Von Euler, M., Janson, A. M. 2004. Virtual test systems for estimation of orientation-dependent parameters in thick, arbitrarily orientated sections exemplified by length quantification of regenerating axons in spinal cord lesions using isotropic, virtual planes. In *Quantitative Methods in Neuroscience*, edited by S. M. Evans, A. M. Janson, and J. R. Nyengaard, pp. 264–384. Oxford: Oxford University Press.

Li, C., Yang, S., Chen, L., Lu, W., Qiu, X., Gundersen, H. J., Tang, Y. 2009. Stereological methods for estimating the myelin sheaths of the myelinated fibers in white matter. *Anat Rec* **292** (10): 1648–1655.

Marner, L., Pakkenberg, B. 2003. Total length of nerve fibers in prefrontal and global white matter of chronic schizophrenics. *J Psychiatr Res* **37** (6): 539–547.

Mayhew, T. M. 1991. The new stereological methods for interpreting functional morphology from slices of cells and organs. *Exp Physiol* **76**: 639–665.

Mayhew, T. M. 1992. A review of recent advances in stereology for quantifying neural structure. *J Neurocytol* **21**: 313–328.

Mayhew, T. M., Momoh, C. K. 1974. Stereological description of the anterior horn cervical cord of the adult rat: a quantitative study using the optical microscope. *J Comp Neurol* **156**: 107–121.

Mayhew, T. M., Olsen, D. R. 1991. Magnetic resonance imaging (MRI) and model-free estimates of brain volume determined using the Cavalieri principle. *J Anat* **178**: 133–144.

Mayhew, T. M., Sharma, A. K. 1984a. Sampling schemes for estimating nerve fibre size: II. Methods for unifascicular nerve trunks. *J Anat* **139** (Pt 1): 59–66.

Mayhew, T. M., Sharma, A. K. 1984b. Sampling schemes for estimating nerve fibre size: I. Methods for nerve trunks of mixed fascicularity. *J Anat* **139** (Pt 1): 45–58.

McDonald, D. M., Choyke, P. L. 2003. Imaging of angiogenesis: from microscope to clinic. *Nat Med* **9**: 713–725.

Mouton, P. R. 2002. *Principles and Practices of Unbiased Stereology: An Introduction for Bioscientists*. Baltimore, MD: Johns Hopkins University Press.

Mouton, P. R. 2011a. Applications of unbiased stereology to neurodevelopmental toxicology. In *Developmental Neurotoxicology Research: Principles, Models, Techniques, Strategies and Mechanisms*, edited by C. Wang and W. Slikke, pp. 53–77. Hoboken, NJ: John Wiley & Sons.

Mouton, P. R. 2011b. *Unbiased Stereology: A Concise Guide*. Baltimore, MD: The Johns Hopkins University Press.

Mouton, P. R., Gordon, M. 2010. Stereological and image analysis techniques for quantitative assessment of neurotoxicology. In *Neurotoxicology*, 3rd ed., Target Organ Toxicology Series, edited by G. J. Harry and H. A. Tilson, pp. 243–267. London: Taylor & Francis Press.

Mouton, P. R., Martin, L. J., Calhoun, M. E., Dal Forno, G., Troncoso, J. C., Price, D. L. 1998. Cognitive decline strongly correlates with cortical atrophy in Alzheimer's dementia. *Neurobiol Aging* **19**: 371–377.

Mouton, P. R., Gokhale, A. M., Ward, N. L., West, M. J. 2002. Stereological length estimation using spherical probes. *J Microsc* **206**: 54–64.

Nyengaard, J. R., Gundersen, H. J. 1992. The isector: a simple and direct method for generating isotropic, uniform random sections from small specimens. *J Microsc* **165**: 427–431.

Nyengaard, J. R., Gundersen, H. J. 2006. Direct and efficient stereological estimation of total cell quantities using electron microscopy. *J Microsc* **222**: 182–187.

Paus, T., Toro, R. 2009. Could sex differences in white matter be explained by g ratio? *Front Neuroanat* **3**: 14.

Perry, T. A., Weerasuriya, A., Mouton, P. R., Holloway, H. W., Greig, N. H. 2004. Pyridoxine-induced toxicity in rats: a stereological quantification of the sensory neuropathy. *Exp Neurol* **190**: 133–144.

Peters, A., Palay, S. L., Webster, H. D. 1991. *The Fine Structure of the Nervous System: Neurons and Their Supporting Cells.* Oxford, UK: Oxford University Press.

Rye, D. B. 1999. Tracking neural pathways with MRI. *Trends Neurosci* **22** (9): 373–374.

Schmidt, F. O., Bear, R. S., Palmer, K. J. 1941. X-ray diffraction studies on the structure of the nerve myelin sheath. *J Cell Comp Physiol* **18**: 31–41.

Schmitz, C., Hof, P. R. 2005. Design-based stereology in neuroscience. *Neuroscience* **130** (4): 813–831.

Sharma, A. K., Thomas, P. K., Gabriel, G., Stolinski, C., Dockery, P., Hollins, G. W. 1982. Peripheral nerve abnormalities in the diabetic mutant mouse. *Diabetes* **32**: 1152–1161.

Sharma, A. K., Duguid, I. G., Blanchard, D. S., Thomas, P. K. 1985. The effect of insulin treatment on myelinated nerve fibre maturation and integrity and on body growth in streptozotocin-diabetic rats. *J Neurol Sci* **67**: 285–297.

Sørensen, F. B., Biche, P., Jakobsen, A. 1992. DNA level and stereologic estimates of nuclear volume in squamous cell carcinomas of the uterine cervix: a comparative study with analysis of prognostic impact. *Cancer* **69**: 187–199.

Stocks, E. A., McArthur, J. M., Griffin, J. W., Mouton, P. R. 1996. An unbiased method for estimation of total epidermal nerve fiber length. *J Neurocytol* **25**: 11–18.

Subbiah, P., Mouton, P. R., Fedor, H., Mcarthur, J., Glass, J. D. 1996. Stereological analysis of cerebral atrophy in human immunodeficiency virus-associated dementia. *J Neuropath Exp Neurol* **55**: 1032–1037.

Tandrup, T. 1993. A for unbiased and efficient estimation of number and mean volume of specified neuron subtypes in rat dorsal root ganglion. *J Comp Neurol* **329**: 209–279.

Tandrup, T., Gundersen, H. J. G., Vedel-Jensen, B. B. 1997. The optical rotator. *J. Microsc.* **172**: 108–120.

Tang, Y., Nyengaard, J. R. 1997. A stereological method for estimating the total length and size of myelin fibers in human brain white matter. *J Neurosci Methods* **73**: 193–200.

Testa, I., Urban, N. T., Jakobs, S., Eggeling, C., Willig, K. I., Hell, S. W. 2012. Nanoscopy of living brain slices with low light levels. *Neuron* **75** (6): 992–1000.

Treacy, J., Tay, D. K. C., Tang, Y., Morais, M., vacca-Galloway, L. L., Dockery, P. 2002. The ultrastucture of the ventral horn of the wobbler mutant mouse; a stereological study. *J Anat* **200** (2): 214–215.

Tuohy, E., Leahy, C., Dockery, P., Fraher, J., Fitzgerald, E., Galvin, R., Dansie, P. 2004. An anatomical and MRI study of the human thalamus. *J Anat* **205** (6): 527.

Upton, G. J. G., Fingleton, B. 1985. *Spatial Data Analysis by Example: Categorical and Directional Data.* Boston: Wiley.

Waxman, S. G. 1980. Determinants of conduction velocity in myelinated nerve fibers. *Muscle Nerve* **3** (2): 141–150.

Witte, S., Negrean, A., Lodder, J. C., de Kock, C. P., Testa, S. G., Mansvelder, H. D., Louise Groot, M. 2011. Label-free live brain imaging and targeted patching with third-harmonic generation microscopy. *Proc Natl Acad Sci U S A* **108** (15): 5970–5975.

Yang, S., Li, C., Zhang, W., Wang, W., Tang, Y. 2008. Sex differences in the white matter and myelinated nerve fibers of Long-Evans rats. *Brain Res* **1216**: 16–23.

8 Comparative Stereology Studies of Brains from Marine Mammals

Nina Eriksen and Bente Pakkenberg

Research Laboratory for Stereology and Neuroscience, Bispebjerg Hospital, University Hospital of Copenhagen, Copenhagen, Denmark

Background

The number of neurons and their relative abundance in different brain regions is at least partly determined by neural functions and behavior. According to Jerison (1973), phyla with larger brains and more neurons have greater behavioral range and versatility. For this reason, it is assumed that somehow neurons adapt to environmental change, forming the basis for the evolution of intelligence.

The amount of brain mass (encephalization) exceeding that required for a given body mass, the so-called encephalization quotient (EQ), refers to the tendency of a species to evolve larger brains over time. For small mammals, the EQ increases in a nearly linear manner but becomes becomes more nonlinear in the brains of large animals like cetaceans (Jerison, 1973). Smaller cetaceans such as odontocetes (toothed whales) possess above-average EQ levels compared to other mammals, ranking second only to humans (Oelschläger and Oelschläger, 2002; Manger, 2006; Marino, 2008). In contrast, the EQ is low for mysticetes (baleen whales) and large odontocetes such as the sperm whale, the species with the largest brain (about 8 kg) in the Animal Kingdom (Pilleri and Gihr, 1970; Marino et al., 2004. Despite these low EQ values, the large absolute size and high degree of cortical gyrification of these large cetaceans indicate substantial enlargement and elaboration through the course of their evolution (Oelschläger and Oelschläger, 2002).

Information on EQ in pinnipeds and fissipeds is limited but shows values in the range of terrestrial carnivores (EQ 1.25–2; Würsig, 2008). The EQ for sirenians, the lowest for marine mammals, varies in the range 0.25–0.5 (Marino, 2008).

Description of Different Marine Mammalian Brains

The Cetacean Brain

The brains of cetaceans differ in numerous ways from terrestrial mammals and pinnipeds, showing a higher degree of gyrification. Like the rest of the cetacean body, cetaceans possess several adaptations to life in the marine environment. The migration of the blowhole from the front to the top of the head to facilitate breathing at the water's surface occurred in association with changes

---

Neurosterology: Unbiased Stereology of Neural Systems, First Edition. Edited by Peter R. Mouton.
© 2014 John Wiley & Sons, Inc. Published 2014 by John Wiley & Sons, Inc.

in the shape of the brain and the distribution of cranial nerves (Oelschläger and Oelschläger, 2002). Cytoarchitectural organization in the cetacean brain, which does not resemble that of terrestrial mammals, includes far more cellularity in layer I, with more atypical neurons in layer II and very large pyramidal neurons in layer III (Glezer, 2002; Hof et al., 2005). Cortical layer IV is absent or poorly developed, indicating that inputs, outputs, and interneuronal connections differ from other mammals (Glezer et al., 1988; Morgane and Glezer, 1990).

Figure 8.1 shows the cytoarchitectural organization in an odontocete (a) and a mysticete (b). In the cetacean brain, the cortical arrangement of functional areas has changed from terrestrial

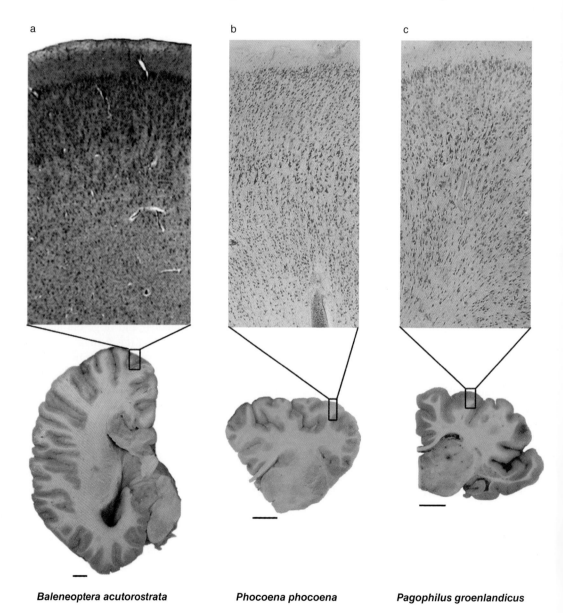

a

b

c

Baleneoptera acutorostrata   **Phocoena phocoena**   **Pagophilus groenlandicus**

Figure 8.1 Cytoarchitectural organization in marine mammals. (a) Odontocetes as represented by the harbor porpoise. (b) Mysticetes as represented by the Minke whale. (c) Pinnipeds as presented by the harp seal. Notice that layer IV in (a) and (b) is not recognizable or absent. Scale bars represent 1 cm, magnification = 65×.

mammals, with the frontal region very poorly developed or even absent (Morgane et al., 1980). Compared to primates, the frontal region in cetaceans displays a unique pattern of differentiation but remains distinctly laminated with several cortical fields as in other lobes (Hof et al., 2005). Electrophysiological mapping studies have placed both the auditory and visual cortices of dolphins and porpoises in the parietal regions (Supin et al., 1978), whereas in pinnipeds and terrestrial mammals, they are located in the temporal (auditory) and occipital (visual) regions. The auditory region is located on the suprasylvian gyrus, which adjoins the visual areas in the lateral gyrus and dorsal parietal regions. There is no intervening cortex between the auditory areas and the visual areas or between the visual-auditory areas and the sensorimotor areas (Glezer et al., 1988). The auditory systems are smaller in mysticetes than in odontocetes, but the mysticete visual system contains more axons (Oelschläger and Oelschläger, 2002). In cetaceans, the olfactory system is essentially absent, a finding more pronounced in odontocetes than mysticetes (Oelschläger and Oelschläger, 2002).

Odontocetes also show specialized hemispheric independency, such as independent eye movements and closure in beluga whales (*Delhinapterus leucas*) and unihemispheric sleep in Amazon river dolphins (*Inia geoffrensis*) (Mukhametov, 1987), beluga whales (Lyamin et al., 2002), and bottlenose dolphins (*Tursiops truncatus*) (Mukhametov et al., 1988; Ridgway et al., 2006).

The Pinniped Brain

Despite the fact that pinnipeds are semiaquatic, the cytoarchitectural organization of the pinniped brain resembles that of terrestrial carnivores (see Figure 8.1c), though larger than their terrestrial relatives (Oelschläger and Oelschläger, 2002). This is probably due to the fact that pinnipeds diverged from terrestrial carnivores during the early Miocene, about 23–16 million years ago, which is much later than cetaceans returned to an aquatic environment about 50 million years ago (Gingerich et al., 1983). Both evolutionary lines have developed large, complex CNS with highly developed neocortices. A thorough comparison between the two helps to illustrate some of the basic mechanisms essential for convergent evolution of these marine mammals.

The auditory and visual cortices of pinnipeds are located in the temporal and occipital lobes, respectively, and are connected with their association cortices. The frontal lobe has maintained an elongated appearance. The olfactory system is small and thin, larger than found in cetaceans, but smaller than in terrestrial mammals (Oelschläger and Oelschläger, 2002). Eared seals, like odontocetes, also exhibit hemispheric independency in the form of unihemispheric sleep (Lyamin et al., 2004, 2008).

The Sirenian Brain

The sirenian brain is unusually small for the animals' size, and structurally simpler than other marine mammals. The hemispheres lack gyrification and are completely smooth (lissencephalic). No actual cell numbers have been reported, but one publication has noted that cell numbers are sparse, and their encephalization numbers are among the lowest of modern mammals (Oelschläger and Oelschläger, 2002).

The Fissiped Brain

Although the polar and sea otter brain share many similarities with the terrestrial carnivore brain (Oelschläger and Oelschläger, 2002), information on these species is very limited.

Parts of the Brain

Cerebellum

Most marine mammals have a well-developed cerebellum. Dolphins have the greatest cerebellar volume, which is lower in pinnipeds and otters and comparatively small in sirenians (Oelschläger and Oelschläger, 2002). This may arise because the cerebellum is responsible for controlling movement and balance, and the rather sedentary sirenians do not require the large, highly developed, cerebellum of other marine mammals.

Within the cerebellum, there is an obvious allometric shift in the size relationship between the vermis and the hemispheres that occurred during the adaptation to aquatic life. The result is a small vermis and large cerebellar hemispheres in fully aquatic cetaceans (Oelschläger and Oelschläger, 2002).

Neocortical Cell Numbers and Cell Size

Table 8.1 gives the estimation of total neocortical neurons and glial cells in different marine mammals. There are both stereological (see Appendix) and nonstereological estimates. The harbor porpoise (*Phoncoena phocoena*) has the largest number of neurons of all animals, an estimated 15×10^9 despite its small body (120–130 cm long) and brain size (~415 g) (Walloe et al., 2010). It is closely followed by the much larger Minke whale (*Balenoptera acutorustrata*) (body size 7–8 m long, brain size ~2700 g) with an average of 13×10^9 neurons (Eriksen and Pakkenberg, 2007). Harp seals (*Pagophilus groenlandicus*) have 6×10^9 neocortical neurons with brain weight just half that of the harbor porpoise.

Glia/Neuron Ratio

The Minke whale has the highest number of neocortical glial cells in any mammal studied to date (Eriksen and Pakkenberg, 2007). The ratio of neocortical glial cells to neocortical neurons is species specific and therefore varies among the mammalian groups and during ontogenesis due to changes in neuron density (Oelschläger and Oelschläger, 2002; Nishiyama et al., 2005). The glia/neuron ratio is 7.7:1 in Minke whales, 2.3:1 in harbor porpoises, 2.8:1 in harp seals, and only 1.4:1 in humans. Ratios have not been reported for many other cetaceans, with the exceptions of *Tursiops* (~3:1) and fin whales (~5:1) (Oelschläger and Oelschläger, 2002), but these numbers have not been estimated using modern stereology. Still, these data demonstrate a tendency for glia/neuron ratio to increase with greater brain mass. Consequently, the glia/neuron ratio signals the importance of glia for facilitating neuron growth, and thus for neocortical function, and they probably play a crucial role in cetaceans with high glial ratios. Since the neocortical neurons in the brains of Minke whales appear relatively large, it is also possible that large neurons require more glia than smaller neurons.

The harbor porpoise is the marine mammal with the largest number of neurons estimated to date (~15 billion) (Walloe et al., 2010), approaching the number (~20 billion neocortical neurons) estimated for humans (Pakkenberg and Gundersen, 1997), with comparable size to the human brain. This indicates that (at least for Minke whales) cetaceans have a substantially larger number of neocortical neurons and glial cells than other nonhuman mammals, even larger than lower primates such as the rhesus monkey. This may be an adaptation to the maintenance and control of large body size, a consequence of complex social systems, or an adaptation to the aquatic environment, as suggested for odontocetes by Marino and coauthors (Marino et al., 2005).

Brain Cell Density

The densities of neocortical neurons in cetaceans (Table 8.1) are lower than in other mammals, leading to the previous hypothesis that neuron density declines with increasing brain size (Tower, 1954; Haug, 1987). However, this relationship does not apply to the cetacean brain. Minke whales have larger brains but lower neuron densities than odontocetes. Also, within odontocetes, there seems to be no relationship between brain size and neuron density.

The neuron density in Minke whales is about the same as in fin whales, which are twice as large. Therefore, it is possible that there might be a lower limit for neuron density at around $60-85 \times 10^6/cm^3$, at least for larger cetaceans. Glial cell density, however, was originally thought to be independent of brain volume (Haug, 1987), but it seems to be fairly stable around $60-80 \times 10^6/cm^3$ for different mammalian species (Eriksen and Pakkenberg, 2007).

Functional Cortices

Poth and coworkers have estimated neuron numbers in different functional cortices (sensomotory, auditory, and visual) in six species of odontocetes, but they were not calculated as total numbers, merely as neuron number per neocortical unit (the number of perikarya below a defined area of the cortical surface). They found that common dolphins (*Delphinus delphinus*) have many more neurons per cortex unit in the auditory (506 vs. average 219) and visual (419 vs. average 212) cortices than other delphinid species (see Table 8.2). The authors did not find any difference in neuron number per standard cortical unit for the three sensory systems studied (Poth et al., 2005), even though these animals use sounds as their primary communication channel and also heavily rely on sound reception for hunting. The opposite was the case in investigations of harbor porpoises and Minke whales, where the auditory cortices contained more cells and had larger volumes than the visual cortices (Table 8.2). In the Minke whale, the auditory cortex had the highest glia/neuron ratio. This is not surprising since cetaceans are much more dependent on sound than on vision in an aquatic environment with poor visibility. Likely because Minke whales do not echolocate, their auditory cortex is less developed than expected for echolocating odontocetes. Mysticetes do use their vision to a greater extent than odontocetes (Oelschläger and Oelschläger, 2002), suggesting that they may have a more complex visual system. However, Poth et al. (2005) reported decreasing neuron numbers per neocortical unit with increasing brain mass in sensory neocortices of delphinids that seem to be equally reliant on audition. More knowledge on visual and auditory structures is needed to further clarify the relationship between neuron density and brain function.

A recent study by Kern et al. (2011) used an optical fractionator and Cavalieri methods to investigate the quantitative morphology of the neocortex (gray matter) in two odontocetes: the harbor porpoise and the bottlenose dolphin. Rather than estimate total neuron numbers, the authors assessed cell densities in layers III and V in four primary projection areas (motor, somatosensory, auditory, and visual fields), as shown in Table 8.2. Along cortical areas M1, S1, A1, and V1 in Tursiops, neuron density was higher in layer III than in layer V, whereas the data in Phocoena were variable. Moreover, neuron density in layer III was generally around 1.5 times higher in Tursiops than in Phocoena. Thus, layer III in the bottlenose dolphin could have greater intrinsic connectivity. The authors concluded that the neuron density of standard cortical units may be correlated with specific adaptations to their respective habitats.

Neuronal Perikaryon Volume

Some studies have measured the perikaryon volume of neurons, and two performed stereological assessments (see Appendix for method used to estimate perikaryon volume). Haug measured

Table 8.1 Neocortex data for both hemispheres

Species	Common name	Mean brain weight, g	Neocortical volume, cm³	Surface area, cm²	Neuron number, 10⁹	Neuron density, 10⁶/cm³	Avg. neuron size, μm³	Glial number, 10⁹	Glial density, 10⁶/cm³	Sample size	Method used	Reference
Mysticetes												
Baleoptera physalus	Fin whale	6,800				6.9				2	Count in 1 mm², convert to cm³	Tower (1954)
Megaptera novaeangliae	Humpback whale	6,500				8.3				1	Not stated	Oelschläger and Oelschläger (2002)
Baleoptera acutorostrata	Minke whale	2,750	★1,622	★5,912	★12.8	★8.02	†4,880	★98.2	★6.26	5	★Optical fractionator, Cavalieri †Rotator method	★Eriksen and Pakkenberg (2007) †Unpublished data by Eriksen, Pakkenberg, and Pakkenberg
Odontocetes												
Orcinus orca	Killer whale	5,439		13,800						2	Stereology, grid plate technique	Ridgway and Bronson (1984)
Pseudorca crassidens	False killer whale	3,650	~900	8,000		9				1	Cavalieri, fractionator	Haug (1987)
Globicephala macrorryncha	Pilot whale	2,760	⊛~1,000	⊛5,000, ★6,200		⊛10	⊛2,900		⊛47.6	⊛1, ★1	⊛Cavalieri, fractionator ★Stereology, grid plate technique,	⊛Haug (1987) ★Ridgway and Bronson (1984)
Grampus griseus	Risso's dolphin	2,500		5,800						2	Stereology, grid plate technique	Ridgway and Bronson (1984)
Ziphius caviostris	Cuvier's beaked whale	2,000		4,000						1	Stereology, grid plate technique	Ridgway and Bronson (1984)

Species	Common name									Method	References
Tursiops truncatus	Bottlenose dolphin	1,461	❀~500	3,745✱	❀18	❀3,100		❀52	✱13, ❀1, ✥8	✱Stereology, grid plate technique ❀Cavalieri, fractionator	✱Ridgway and Bronson (1984) ❀Haug (1987)
Delphinus delphinus	Common dolphin	802	❀~250	2,136✱	❀20	❀2,600		❀65	✱9, ❀1	✱Stereology, grid plate technique ❀Cavalieri, fractionator	✱Ridgway and Bronson (1984) ❀Haug (1987)
Stenella spp.	Saddleback and Spinner dolphins	646		1474					11	Stereology, grid plate technique	Ridgway and Bronson (1984)
Phocoena phocoena	Harbor porpoise	413	✥166	✥14.9	✥92	✥5,100	✥34.8	✥210	✥5, ❀1	✥Optical fractionator, Cavalieri ❀Cavalieri, fractionator	✥Walloe et al. (2010), ❀Haug (1987)
Pinnipeds											
Pagophilus groenlandicus	Harp seal	228	93.1	6.1	70		17.5	105	5	Optical fractionator, Cavalieri	Walloe et al. (2010)

Symbols before data refer to specific references in final column.

Table 8.2 Results for functional neocortical subregions (both hemispheres)

Species	Common name	Mean brain weight, g	Volume of auditory cortex	Auditory neuron number	Auditory glial number	Volume of visual cortex	Visual neuron number	Visual glial number	Somatosensory neuron number	Sample size	Method used	Reference
Mysticetes												
Baleoptera acutorostrata	Minke whale	2750	56.9 cm³	0.58 × 109	6.9 8 × 109	24.51 cm³	0.46 × 109	7.11 × 109		5	Optical fractionator, Cavalieri	Eriksen and Pakkenberg (2007)
Odontocetes												
Orcinus orca	Killer whale	6052		135/neocortical unit			168/neocortical unit		91/neocortical unit	1	Number of perikarya below a defined area of the cortex surface	Poth et al. (2005)
Pseudorca crassidens	False killer whale	4307		208/neocortical unit			160/neocortical unit		177/neocortical unit	1	Number of perikarya below a defined area of the cortex surface	Poth et al. (2005)
Kogia breviceps	Pygmy sperm whale	3680		235/neocortical unit			188/neocortical unit		195/neocortical unit	1	Number of perikarya below a defined area of the cortex surface	Poth et al. (2005)
Globicephala macrorryncha	Pilot whale	2733		257/neocortical unit			220/neocortical unit		205/neocortical unit	1	Number of perikarya below a defined area of the cortex surface	Poth et al. (2005)
Tursiops truncatus	Bottlenose dolphin	1563		✗276/neocortical unit ✓layer III: 4.79 × 106 layer V: 0.97 × 106			✗300/neocortical unit ✓layer III: 4.42 × 106 layer V: 0.94 × 106		✗268/neocortical unit ✓layer III: 3.49 × 106 layer V: 0.75 × 106	1	✗Neuron number per cortical unit. ✓Optical fractionator, Cavalieri only in cortical layers III and V	✗Poth et al. (2005) ✓Kern et al. (2011)
Delphinus delphinus	Common dolphin	834		506/neocortical unit			419/neocortical unit		338/neocortical unit	1	Number of perikarya below a defined area of the cortex surface	Poth et al. (2005)
Phocoena phocoena	Harbor porpoise	461	✲16cm³	✲1.56 × 109 ✓layer III: 2.95 × 106 layer V: 0.61 × 106	✲3.52 × 109	✲7.25 cm³	✲0.68 × 109 ✓layer III: 2.97 × 106 layer V: 0.47 × 106	✲1.56 × 109	✓layer III: 2.15 × 106 layer V: 0.70 × 106	5	✲Optical fractionator, Cavalieri ✓Optical fractionator, Cavalieri only in cortical layers III and V	✲Walloe et al. (2010) ✓Kern et al. (2011)
Pinnipeds												
Pagophilus groenlandicus	Harp seal	228	1.76cm³	0.1 × 109	0.29 × 109	2.33 cm³	0.15 × 109	0.38 × 109		5	Optical fractionator, Cavalieri	Walloe et al. (2010)

Note: Symbols before data refer to specific references in final column.

neuronal perikaryon in the harbor porpoise (Haug, 1987), and the perikaryon volume of the Minke whale is presented here for the first time (Table 8.1). The perikaryon volume in harbor porpoises and Minke whales are about the same size ($5100 \mu m^3$ and $4880 \mu m^3$, respectively). However, a sexual difference was observed in Minke whale—females have larger perikarya ($5422 \mu m^3$) than males ($3977 \mu m^3$) ($p = 0.035$, Student's t-test). Other cetaceans (common dolphins, bottlenose dolphins, and pilot whales) have perikaryon volumes from $2600–3100 \mu m^3$, but these were measured on single animals using semiquantitative (nonstereology) methods. All of these perikarya volumes are larger than cortical neuron volumes in humans, which are $1430 \mu m^3$ on average (Stark et al., 2007).

Intelligence and Neuron Number

A common question refers to the functional relevance of possessing many neurons. Is the large number of neurons in certain marine mammals a sign of relative intelligence or, as Manger suggests, does the brain of certain marine mammals merely reflect an efficient thermogenetic organ that effectively counteracts heat loss to the water (Manger, 2006)? Manger's alternative hypothesis is supported, at least in part, by quantitative findings: the large number of glial cells in mysticetes supports the idea that an unusually high number of glial cells, together with unihemispheric sleep phenomenology, makes the cetacean brain an efficient thermogenetic organ. However, the Minke corpus callosum area is rather large, much larger than investigated in other odontocete species (see below), suggesting that mysticetes lack the specialized hemispheric independency observed in several odontocetes. But the theory of unihemispheric sleep evolved to counteract heat loss may only apply to deep diving species, which are all odontocetes (sperm whales, beaked whales) without high EQs. Dolphins, the marine mammals with high EQs that approach those in humans, have very complex social and behavioral patterns, whereas fissipeds and pinnipeds with more moderate EQ have behavior patterns that more closely resemble terrestrial mammals (Würsig, 2008). It should be mentioned that humpback whales (*Megaptera novaeangliae*) have the most complex vocalizations in the Animal Kingdom (Payne and McVay, 1971), and they, like the rest of the mysticetes, do not possess high EQs. A further area for future research is the relationship between high EQ relates and high numbers of neuron. With the highest EQ (around 7), humans have the largest number of neurons (~15–35 billion) (Pakkenberg and Gundersen, 1997). The harbor porpoise EQ is 3.15 (Marino et al., 2004), and their brains contain approximately 15 billion neurons. The EQ of the Minke whale is unknown, but most mysticetes lie around 0.2 (Marino, 2008) despite a high number of neocortical neurons (13 billion). These findings indicate that for certain mammals, for example, harbor porpoises and humans, EQ is a rather good measure for neuronal number, but this relationship does not account for high neuronal numbers in the Minke whale brain. However, as mentioned earlier, due to nonlinearity, EQ may not be a good measure of intelligence for relatively large animals (Jerison, 1973).

Corpus Callosum

The corpus callosum is generally small in cetaceans (Tarpley and Ridgway, 1994; Pakkenberg and Gundersen, 1997; Oelschläger and Oelschläger, 2002; Keogh and Ridgway, 2008; Ratner et al., 2010) and sirenians compared to terrestrial mammals, but it is well developed in pinnipeds (Oelschläger and Oelschläger, 2002). This observation gave rise to speculation that small corpus callosi are a full aquatic trait, as both cetaceans and sirenians are the only full aquatic members of the marine mammal groups. Table 8.3 shows the corpus callosal area and most common fiber diameter in four cetacean species. The mysticete callosal area, as studied in the Minke whale (Ratner et al., 2010), is larger than that in the odontocete (Tarpley and Ridgway, 1994; Pakkenberg and

Table 8.3   Corpus callosum

Species	Common name	Mean brain weight, g	Corpus callosal fiber diameter, μm^3	CC area, mm^2	Sample size	Method used	Reference
Mysticetes							
Baleoptera acutorostrata	Minke whale	2750	0.82–1.14	675	5	Optical fractionator, Cavalieri	Ratner et al. (2010)
Odontocetes							
Orcinus orca	Killer whale	5439	1.0–2.99	535	1	All fibers counted	Keogh and Ridgway (2008)
Tursiops truncatus	Bottlenose dolphin	1461	1.0 2.99	233	8	All fibers counted	Keogh and Ridgway (2008)
Inia geoffrensis	Amazon river dolphin	630	1.0–2.99	139	1	All fibers counted	Keogh and Ridgway (2008)

Gundersen, 1997; Keogh and Ridgway, 2008). Ratner et al. (2010) speculated that the specialized hemispheric independency observed in some odontocete species is probably nonexistent in mysticetes. The most common fiber diameter of the corpus callosum was smaller in the Minke whales compared to delphinids (see Appendix).

Surface Area and Gyrification

The surface area of the odontocete cerebral cortex is directly related to brain size (Ridgway and Bronson, 1984), as clearly indicated by the data in Table 8.1. Prothero and Sundsten (1984) hypothesized that there is an upper limit for brain mass, and as brain mass increases so does the cortical surface area, resulting is an increase in gyrification ("gyral-window hypothesis"). Hence, increased brain mass and cortical surface is only possible by increasing the number of cortical fissures and thickening the neocortex. All cetaceans and pinnipeds have highly gyrified neocortices with large surfaces. If volume grows and cortical thickness remains stable, the cortical surface must increase in area. Therefore, as brain volume increases, so does neocortical volume, with increased surface area and more cortical fissures in the large cetacean brain (Table 8.1). This observation was also made by Poth and colleagues (Poth et al., 2005). The level of gyrification is similar in all cetaceans, with the greatest level in dolphins, but all cetaceans have higher levels than observed in humans (Figure 8.2). That part of the gyral-window hypothesis holds for the cetacean brain; nevertheless, it might be an aquatic trait rather than a "large brain" trait, especially considering the level of gyrification in the harp seal.

In summary, adaptation to marine life required three-dimensional locomotion and deep diving, which resulted in four major adaptations in the marine mammal brain: (1) increased brain size due to enlarged special functional areas for the auditory and motor systems, (2) increased neocortical volume, (3) increased neocortical surface and gyrification, and (4) strong reduction or loss of the olfactory system. Other specified adaptations include a greater number of neurons and glial cells and larger neurons, although more research in greater numbers of species is needed to determine whether or not these findings represent general traits of marine mammals.

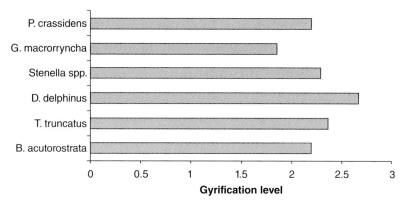

Figure 8.2 Gyrification in different cetaceans. Note that gyrification is higher in delphinid species: common dolphin (*Delphinus delphinus*), bottlenose dolphin (*Tursiops truncatus*), false killer whale (*Pseudorca crassidens*), saddleback and spinner dolphins (*Stenella* spp.).

References

Baddeley, A. J., Gundersen, H. J., Cruz-Orive, L. M. 1986. Estimation of surface area from vertical sections. *J Microsc* **142**: 259–276.

Eriksen, N., Pakkenberg, B. 2007. Total neocortical cell number in the mysticete brain. *Anat Rec (Hoboken)* **290**: 83–95.

Gingerich, P. D., Wells, N. A., Russell, D. E., Shah, S. M. 1983. Origin of whales in epicontinental remnant seas: new evidence from the early Eocene of Pakistan. *Science* **220**: 403–406.

Glezer, I. 2002. Neural morphology. In *Marine Mammal Biology (An Evolutionary Approach)*, edited by R. Hoezel. Oxford, UK: Blackwell Publishing.

Glezer, I. I., Jacobs, M. S., Morgane, P. J. 1988. Implications of the "initial brain" concept for brain evolution in Cetacea. *Behavioral and Brain Sciences.* **11**: 75–89.

Gundersen, H. J., Bendtsen, T. F., Korbo, L., Marcussen, N., Moller, A., Nielsen, K., Nyengaard, J. R., Pakkenberg, B., Sorensen, F. B., Vesterby, A. et al. 1988. Some new, simple and efficient stereological methods and their use in pathological research and diagnosis. *APMIS* **96**: 379–394.

Haug, H. 1987. Brain sizes, surfaces, and neuronal sizes of the cortex cerebri: a stereological investigation of man and his variability and a comparison with some mammals (primates, whales, marsupials, insectivores, and one elephant). *Am J Anat* **180**: 126–142.

Hof, P. R., Chanis, R., Marino, L. 2005. Cortical complexity in cetacean brains. *Anat Rec A Discov Mol Cell Evol Biol* **287**: 1142–1152.

Jensen, E. B. V., Gundersen, H. J. G. 1993. The rotator. *J Microsc* **170**: 35–44.

Jerison, H. J. 1973. *Evolution of the Brain and Intelligence.* New York: Academic Press.

Keogh, M. J., Ridgway, S. H. 2008. Neuronal fiber composition of the corpus callosum within some odontocetes. *Anat Rec (Hoboken)* **291**: 781–789.

Kern, A., Siebert, U., Cozzi, B., Hof, P. R., Oelschläger, H. H. 2011. Stereology of the neocortex in Odontocetes: qualitative, quantitative, and functional implications. *Brain Behav Evol* **77**: 79–90.

Lyamin, O. I., Mukhametov, L. M., Siegel, J. M., Nazarenko, E. A., Polyakova, I. G., Shpak, O. V. 2002. Unihemispheric slow wave sleep and the state of the eyes in a white whale. *Behav Brain Res* **129**: 125–129.

Lyamin, O. I., Mukhametov, L. M., Siegel, J. M. 2004. Relationship between sleep and eye state in Cetaceans and Pinnipeds. *Arch Ital Biol* **142**: 557–568.

Lyamin, O. I., Lapierre, J. L., Kosenko, P. O., Mukhametov, L. M., Siegel, J. M. 2008. Electroencephalogram asymmetry and spectral power during sleep in the northern fur seal. *J Sleep Res* **17**: 154–165.

Manger, P. R. 2006. An examination of cetacean brain structure with a novel hypothesis correlating thermogenesis to the evolution of a big brain. *Biol Rev Camb Philos Soc* **81**: 293–338.

Marino, L. 2008. Brain evolution. In *Encyclopedia of Marine Mammals*, edited by W. F. Perrin, B. Würsig, and J. G. M. Thewissen, pp. 149–152. San Diego, CA: Academic Press.

Marino, L., McShea, D. W., Uhen, M. D. 2004. Origin and evolution of large brains in toothed whales. *Anat Rec A Discov Mol Cell Evol Biol* **281**: 1247–1255.

Marino, L., Uhen, M. D., McShea, D. W. 2005. Encephalization in odontocetes: what's being aquatic got to do with it? In Fourth Triennial Convention on the Evolution on Aquatic Tetrapods, p. 50, Akron, OH, May 16–20.

Morgane, P. J., Glezer, I. I. 1990. Sensory neocortex in dolphin brain. In *Sensory Abilities of Cetaceans. Laboratory and Field Evidence*, edited by J. A. Thomas and R. A. Kastelein, pp. 101–137. New York: Plenum Press.

Morgane, P. J., Jacobs, M. S., McFarland, W. L. 1980. The anatomy of the brain of the bottlenose dolphin (*Tursiops truncates*): surface configurations of the telencephalon of the bottlenose dolphin with comparative anatomical observation sin four other cetacean species. *Brain Res Bull* **5**: 1–107.

Mukhametov, L. M. 1987. Unihemispheric slow-wave sleep in the Amazonian dolphin, *Inia geoffrensis*. *Neurosci Lett* **79**: 128–132.

Mukhametov, L. M., Oleksenko, A. I., Poliakova, I. G. 1988. [Quantitative characteristics of the electrocorticographic sleep stages in bottle-nosed dolphins]. *Neirofiziologiia* **20**: 532–538.

Nishiyama, A., Yang, Z., Butt, A. 2005. Astrocytes and NG2-glia: what's in a name? *J Anat* **207**: 687–693.

Oelschläger, H. H. A., Oelschläger, J. S. 2002. Brain. In *Encyclopedia of Marine Mammals*, edited by W. F. Perrin, B. Würsig, and J. G. M. Thewissen, pp. 133–158. San Diego, CA: Academic Press.

Pakkenberg, B., Gundersen, H. J. 1997. Neocortical neuron number in humans: effect of sex and age. *J Comp Neurol* **384**: 312–320.

Payne, R. S., McVay, S. 1971. Songs of Humpback Whales. *Science* **173**: 585–597.

Pilleri, G., Gihr, M. 1970. The central nervous system of the mysticete and odontocete whales. *Investigations Cetacea* **2**: 89–135.

Poth, C., Fung, C., Gunturkun, O., Ridgway, S. H., Oelschlager, H. H. 2005. Neuron numbers in sensory cortices of five delphinids compared to a physeterid, the pygmy sperm whale. *Brain Res Bull* **66**: 357–360.

Prothero, J. W., Sundsten, J. W. 1984. Folding of the cerebral cortex in mammals: a scaling model. *Brain Behav Evol* **24** (2–3): 152–167.

Ratner, C., Riise, J., Eriksen, N., Pakkenberg, B. 2010. A postmortem study of the corpus callosum in the common Minke whale (*Balaenoptera acutorostrata*). *Marine Mammal Science*. **27**: 688–700.

Ridgway, S., Houser, D., Finneran, J., Carder, D., Keogh, M., Van Bonn, W., Smith, C., Scadeng, M., Dubowitz, D., Mattrey, R., Hoh, C. 2006. Functional imaging of dolphin brain metabolism and blood flow. *J Exp Biol* **209**: 2902–2910.

Ridgway, S. H., Bronson, R. H. 1984. Relative brain size and cortical surface areas in odontocetes. *Acta Zool. Fennica.* **172**: 149–152.

Stark, A. K., Toft, M. H., Pakkenberg, H., Fabricius, K., Eriksen, N., Pelvig, D. P., Moller, M., Pakkenberg, B. 2007. The effect of age and gender on the volume and size distribution of neocortical neurons. *Neuroscience* **150**: 121–130.

Supin, A. Y., Mukhametov, L. M., Ladygina, T. F., Popov, V. V., Mass, A. M., Polyakova, I. G. 1978. *Electrophysiological Studies of the Dolphin's Brain*, edited by V. E. Solokov, pp. 7–85. Moscow: Izdatel'stvo Nauka.

Tarpley, R. J., Ridgway, S. H. 1994. Corpus callosum size in delphinid cetaceans. *Brain Behav Evol* **44**: 156–165.

Tower, D. B. 1954. Structural and functional organization of mammalian cerebral cortex; the correlation of neurone density with brain size; cortical neurone density in the fin whale (*Balaenoptera physalus* L.) with a note on the cortical neurone density in the Indian elephant. *J Comp Neurol* **101**: 19–51.

Walloe, S., Eriksen, N., Dabelsteen, T., Pakkenberg, B. 2010. A neurological comparative study of the harp seal (*Pagophilus groenlandicus*) and harbor porpoise (*Phocoena phocoena*) brain. *Anat Rec (Hoboken)* **293**: 2129–2135.

West, M. J., Slomianka, L., Gundersen, H. J. 1991. Unbiased stereological estimation of the total number of neurons in the subdivisions of the rat hippocampus using the optical fractionator. *Anat Rec* **231**: 482–497.

Würsig, B. 2008. Intelligence and cognition. In *Encyclopedia of Marine Mammals*, edited by W. F. Perrin, B. Würsig, and J. G. M. Thewissen, pp. 638–637. San Diego, CA: Academic Press.

Appendix: Cited Stereological Approaches

Total Neocortical Cell Number

The optical fractionator is a combination of two stereological principles: the optical disector and fractionator sampling design (West et al., 1991). The optical fractionator method involves counting particles with optical disectors in a systematic, uniform, random sample that constitutes a known fraction of the neocortex. This is achieved by counting cells in a known fraction of sections (ssf), under a known fraction of the sectional area of the region (asf) in a known fraction of the thickness of a section (hsf). The total neocortical cell number is determined by multiplying the total number of counted particles, $\sum Q\text{-}$, by the reciprocal sampling fractions, adding a multiplication factor of 2 for bilateral number:

$$N_{total} = \frac{1}{ssf} \cdot \frac{1}{asf} \cdot \frac{1}{hsf} \cdot \sum Q^{-} \cdot 2 \qquad (8.1)$$

Minke whale neurons were counted at 1900× magnification (paraffin embedding), harbor porpoise and harp seal neurons at 2000× (plastic embedding), and 3400× magnification (paraffin embedding).

Neuronal Size Estimation

The rotator method estimates cell volume and requires isotropy (Jensen and Gundersen, 1993). The isotropic test planes can be fulfilled with the use of isotropic random sections or a vertical design that can be selected arbitrarily, but all sections must be made parallel to the vertical axis after random rotation, and all subsequent measurements must be made with respect to the axis, which must therefore be identifiable in all sections (Baddeley et al., 1986). A vertical axis is aligned parallel to the y-axis on the computer screen, and the nucleolus is set as the center point. The top and bottom are indicated, and systematic random test lines are created perpendicular to the vertical axis. Intersections with the cell boundary and test lines are marked, for example, in a total of six places, and an estimate of cell volume is calculated using the formula

$$V = \sum l_i^2 \cdot t \cdot \frac{\pi}{2}, \qquad (8.2)$$

where l_i is the distance between the intersections and the vertical axis, and t is the distance between the test lines, defined by $t = h/3$, where h is the height of the profile projected on the vertical axis.

Minke whale neuronal perikarya were estimated at 2330× magnification in plastic embedded samples, which were used to prevent severe neuronal shrinkage.

Corpus Callosum Fiber Estimation

The total number of fibers was estimated using the fractionator principle. It involves taking out a predetermined number of uniform, systematic, random samples, which constitute a known fraction of the corpus callosum (Gundersen et al., 1988). This is achieved by counting fibers on a known fraction of corpus callosal strips: the strip-sampling fraction (f1), and in a known fraction of the area: the area-fraction sampling (f2). f2 is defined as the ratio between the area of the counting frames Aframes and the area associated with each step in the x and y directions ($x \cdot y$):

$$f_2 = \frac{\left(\dfrac{A_{frame}}{Mag^2} \right)}{x \cdot y}. \qquad (8.3)$$

The total number of callosal fibers is found with the equation

$$N = \sum Q \cdot \frac{1}{f_1} \cdot \frac{1}{f_2},$$ (8.4)

where $\sum Q$ is the total number of counted fibers, and $1/f_1$ and $1/f_2$ are the inverse sampling fractions (Gundersen et al., 1988).

Corpus callosum fiber estimation in Minke whales was done at 3100× magnification (plastic embedding, epoxy-epon). Plastic embedding was chosen to prevent severe tissue shrinkage.

Surface Estimation

Surface estimation was performed in combination with volume estimation and Cavalieri's principle. Surface areas are estimated from the following equation, when the neocortical volume is known:

$$S = \left(\frac{2 \cdot \sum I}{l(p) \cdot \sum P} \right) \cdot V_{neocortex},$$ (8.5)

where S is total surface area of the structure, $V_{neocortex}$ is the reference volume of neocortex, 2 is a constant, $\sum I$ is the total number of intersections of a test line and the pial surface of neocortex, $l(p)$ is the test line length per point, and $\sum P$ is the total number of the points contacting the neocortex.

Minke whale neocortex surface area was estimated at 20× magnification (paraffin embedding). Tissue shrinkage (both volume and surface area) should always be taken into account when using paraffin embedding.

9 Quantitative Assessment of Hippocampus Architecture Using the Optical Disector

Shozo Jinno

Department of Developmental Molecular Anatomy, Graduate School of Medical Sciences, Kyushu University, Fukuoka, Japan

Background

The optical disector, one of the most commonly used design-based stereological techniques, enables accurate counting of total number of objects (neurons, synapses) using thick 2D sections through the reference space of interest (Braendgaard et al., 1990). Because numerical density (number of cells per unit area or volume) is affected by volume changes such as shrinkage of target areas, uncorrected densities of neurons and synapses in specific brain areas do not make sense for assessment of the possible structural alterations related to development, aging, stress, trauma, and so on (for reviews, see West, 1999; Mouton, 2011a,b). However, for studies where the objective is to assess the anatomical differences along the longitudinal axis of a brain structure, densities of various cellular elements provide the preferred method. In our studies, numerical density estimates provide the parameter of choice to assess regional differences within the hippocampus that cannot be deduced from the total number of neurons in the entire structure.

The optical disector applied to thick immunostained sections requires attention to several technical issues. First is a potential bias from incomplete penetration of antibodies. Because some antibodies do not enter deeply into 40- to 50-μm-thick sections, the optical disector height and location should be adjusted carefully prior to every experiment. Comparison of the numbers of labeled cells at the surface and the middle of the immunostained sections provides an indication of antibody penetration. If the numbers of labeled cells at the middle of the section appear significantly fewer than those at the surface of the section, changes may be required of tissue processing protocols, for example, longer time in primary antibody, to ensure complete penetration of the antibody through the full thickness of the preparation. If complete penetration is not possible, counting with optical disectors should be limited to regions with complete penetration, for example, just beneath the section surface, rather than through the entire thickness of the section.

As mentioned above, differential shrinkage of tissue presents a major problem for accurate density estimation by the optical disector. To address this issue, we have developed an approach to correct density data using shrinkage correction factors. To determine the extent of shrinkage by the immunostaining procedure, morphological alterations in the area and thickness of sections were measured (Jinno et al., 1998, 1999). The planer images of individual sections were captured with a light microscope before immunoprocessing and after mounting in Vectashield and the thickness of each selected section measured using the differential interference contrast (DIC) microscopy with a water immersion objective in the free-floating condition. After immunostaining and mounting on glass slides, these measurements were repeated using an oil immersion objective. The differences before and after tissue processing allowed the areal and thickness shrinkage factors to be calculated for each section.

The Hippocampus

Dorsoventral Differentiation of the Hippocampus

The hippocampus, a major limbic structure, and its contribution to learning and memory have consistently attracted the interest of neuroscientists. Although many studies emphasize the hippocampal as a network, at least in part the hippocampus also functions in a lamellar fashion (Andersen et al., 2000) with copious intrinsic connections that extend in both the dorsoventral and transverse directions (Hampson et al., 1999; Zappone and Sloviter, 2004). Thus, the hippocampus is composed of complicated 3D networks of neural connections.

In the rodent hippocampus, the longitudinal alignment, also referred to as the dorsoventral axis, appears grossly as an elongated structure extending in a C-shaped fashion from the septal nuclei of the basal forebrain to the temporal lobe. The extrinsic and intrinsic connections differ between dorsal and ventral hippocampus (Amaral and Witter, 1989). The dorsal CA1 region gives rise to extrinsic connections to the subicular, retrosplenial, perirhinal, and entorhinal cortices, as well as to the lateral septum. The ventral CA1 region projects to the subicular, entorhinal, and infraradiata cortices, amygdale, and hypothalamus (van Groen and Wyss, 1990). The dorsal CA3 region innervates the medial and dorsal areas of the medial septum, while the ventral CA3 region projects to the lateral and ventral areas of the medial septum (Gaykema et al., 1991). The dorsal dentate gyrus (DG) receives afferents from both the lateral and medial areas of the entorhinal cortex, whereas the ventral DG receives projections from the medial areas of the entorhinal cortex (Witter et al., 1989; van Groen et al., 2003).

Lesion and electrophysiological studies substantiate the functional differentiation of the hippocampus along the dorsoventral axis (Bannerman et al., 2004). Lesions on the dorsal hippocampus impair spatial learning and memory in rats (Moser et al., 1993) where receptors for N-methyl-D-aspartate (NMDA) are associated with spatial working memory performance (McHugh et al., 2008). Lesions to the ventral hippocampus affect anxiety-related behavior, with little to no effect on spatial learning in rats (Kjelstrup et al., 2002). Similarly, electrophysiological studies show that distinct spatial firing patterns differentiate dorsal and ventral hippocampus in rats (Jung et al., 1994). Modern genomic analyses also report significant discrepancies in molecular profiles between dorsal and ventral hippocampus (Leonardo et al., 2006; Thompson et al., 2008).

To address the anatomical differentiation, we divided the hippocampus into dorsal, middle, and ventral parts perpendicular to the longitudinal axis (Figure 9.1a). Each brain block was cut transversely into 40- to 50-μm-thick serial sections on a vibrating microtome. Our preliminary studies indicated that densities and cell sizes of glutamic acid decarboxylase 67 (GAD67)-positive neurons and nitric oxide synthase (NOS)-positive neurons in the middle part were intermediate between the dorsal and ventral parts of the hippocampus (Jinno et al., 1998, 1999). We considered the anatomical characteristics of the middle part of the hippocampus to be intermediate between dorsal and ventral parts. For the sake of concentrating our studies on the dorsal and ventral aspects of the hippocampus, our subsequent studies excluded the middle part of the hippocampus.

Density and Numbers of Glutamatergic Principal Neurons in the Hippocampus

To estimate possible differences along the transverse axis, the mouse hippocampus was divided into six subfields (Figure 9.1b,c). Each of the CA1 and CA3 regions was divided into the distal

a

1. Divide the hipocampus into dorsal, middle, and ventral parts with a razor blade.

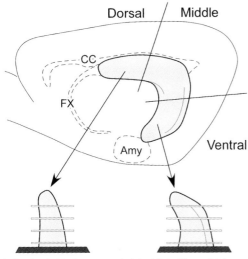

2. Cut brain block transversly into 40- to 50-μm-thick serial sections.

3. Select 4-8 sections in a random manner.

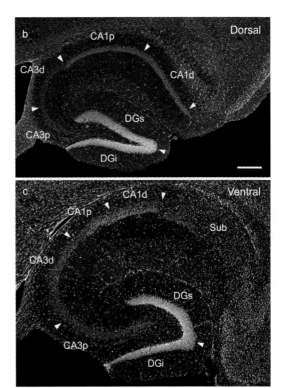

Figure 9.1   Estimation of anatomical differentiation of the mouse hippocampus along the dorsoventral and transverse axes. (a) Procedure for preparation of serial transverse sections for immunostaining. (b,c) Digital photomicrograph of DAPI-stained section of the dorsal (b) and ventral (c) hippocampus. The borders of subfields are indicated by arrowheads. Amy, amygdala; CA1d, distal portion of the CA1 region; CA1p, proximal portion of the CA1 region; CA3d, distal portion of the CA3 region; CA3p, proximal portion of the CA3 region; CC, corpus callosum; DGi, inferior blade of the dentate gyrus; DGs, superior blade of the dentate gyrus; FX, fornix; Sub, subiculum. Scale bar in panel b = 200 μm (applies to b,c). Modified and reproduced from Jinno and Kosaka (2010), with permission of the publisher.

and proximal portions at the midpoint, and the DG was divided into the superior and inferior blades at the crescent.

Densities of glutamatergic principal neurons (ND, neuron number per unit volume) were estimated using the optical disector (Table 9.1). The results show pyramidal neurons in the entire CA1 region with significantly higher density in the dorsal ($447.5 \times 10^3/mm^3$) than in the ventral ($180.5 \times 10^3/mm^3$) aspect of the hippocampus. The proximal and distal portions of the CA1 region showed similar dorsoventral gradients. We also examined possible differences in the densities along the transverse axis, and found that the densities of CA1 pyramidal neurons in the dorsal and ventral hippocampus were significantly higher in the proximal portion than in the distal portion. The densities of CA3 pyramidal neurons were generally low (156.8 to $187.6 \times 10^3/mm^3$), with no significant differences along the dorsoventral and transverse axes. The DG cells showed the highest densities among all hippocampal regions, ranging from about $760 \times 10^3/mm^3$ to about $940 \times 10^3/mm^3$ neurons. In the entire DG, the densities of granule cells were significantly higher in the dorsal part ($916.3 \times 10^3/mm^3$) than in the ventral part ($788.9 \times 10^3/mm^3$). Although there were no statistically significant differences in the densities of granule cells along the transverse axis, the inferior and superior blades of the DG showed different dorsoventral gradients: the densities in the superior blade were significantly higher in the dorsal part than in the ventral part, while those in the inferior blade showed no significant difference.

Table 9.1 Density ($\times 10^3$/mm^3) of glutamatergic principal neurons and GABAergic nonprincipal neurons in the mouse hippocampus

Glutamatergic principal neurons			GABAergic nonprincipal neurons		
Region	Dorsal	Ventral	Region	Dorsal	Ventral
CA1	447.5 ± 33.3	180.5 ± 11.5**	CA1	7.0 ± 0.3	8.3 ± 0.9
CA3	165.2 ± 10.6	172.4 ± 21.6	CA3	5.7 ± 0.7	7.1 ± 0.7*
DG	916.7 ± 48.8	788.9 ± 56.3**	DG	4.0 ± 0.4	6.5 ± 0.2**
Total	377.5 ± 25.5	217.8 ± 12.0**	Total	5.7 ± 0.2	7.3 ± 0.4**
Layer			Layer		
CA1			CA1		
so	–	–	so	6.5 ± 0.5	10.5 ± 0.6**
sp (distal)	407.5 ± 28.7	150.5 ± 15.6**	sp (total)	13.5 ± 0.9	10.1 ± 1.6*
(proximal)	505.7 ± 47.8††	216.4 ± 12.6**††	–	–	–
sr	–	–	sr	3.2 ± 0.8	4.3 ± 0.5
slm	–	–	slm	8.4 ± 0.9	8.8 ± 1.1
CA3			CA3		
so	–	–	so	3.2 ± 1.0	5.5 ± 1.3*
sp (distal)	160.1 ± 27.4	156.8 ± 19.4	sp (total)	7.6 ± 0.7	10.5 ± 1.4*
(proximal)	168.6 ± 11.6	187.6 ± 23.8	–	–	–
sl	–	–	sl	2.6 ± 0.8	4.6 ± 0.7**
sr	–	–	sr	7.9 ± 0.7	6.6 ± 0.6*
slm	–	–	slm	5.8 ± 1.4	7.2 ± 1.0
DG			DG		
hilus	–	–	hilus	7.0 ± 0.5	11.3 ± 1.0**
gl (infra)	891.3 ± 33.3	823.1 ± 86.7	gl (total)	7.7 ± 1.0	11.9 ± 1.8**
(supra)	936.5 ± 70.3	756.3 ± 31.3**	–	–	–
ml	–	–	ml	1.7 ± 0.2	3.4 ± 0.5**

DG, dentate gyrus; gl, granule cell layer; ml, molecular layer; sl, stratum lucidum; slm, stratum lacunosum-moleculare; so, stratum oriens; sp, stratum pyramidale; sr, stratum radiatum.
The statistical difference is determined by Welch's t-test. The significance is described as follows: Difference along the dorsoventral axis (*$p < 0.05$, **$p < 0.01$) and along the transverse axis (††$p < 0.01$). Modified and Reproduced from Jinno and Kosaka (2006, 2010).

The majority of axons originating from glutamatergic principal neurons are oriented parallel to each other and course in a transverse manner to the dorsoventral axis of the hippocampus (Andersen et al., 1971; Witter and Amaral, 2004). The principal cells are activated in a strip-like manner with impulses conveyed sequentially in a near-transverse band called lamellae. The quantitative data of glutamatergic principal cells provide a basic anatomical foundation for understanding the information processing mechanisms of the hippocampus.

Expression Ratios of Calbindin D28K (CB) in Glutamatergic Principal Neurons

In the hippocampus, calcium-binding protein, calbindin D28K (CB), is present in most dentate granule cells and a subset of CA1 pyramidal neurons, but absent in CA3 pyramidal neurons (Baimbridge and Miller, 1982). Among the functions for CB is a role in neuroprotection against seizure-induced damage (Sloviter, 1989). In addition, recent studies have shown that CB sharpens Ca^{2+} microdomains in space and time, and regulates paired-pulse facilitation in the hippocampus (Müller et al., 2005). Another function for CB is regulation of synaptic plasticity (Schmidt, 2012).

The expression ratios of CB in pyramidal neurons were estimated in the CA1 region of the hippocampus (Jinno and Kosaka, 2010). In the total area of CA1 region, the expression rates were about 45%, without significant dorsoventral differences. However, the distal and proximal portions of the CA1 region showed the reciprocal dorsoventral gradients with CB expression in the distal portion were significantly higher in the ventral part (58%) than in the dorsal part (38%), and those in the proximal portions were higher in the dorsal part (50%) than in the ventral part (34%). The three-dimensional organization of projections from the CA3 to CA1 region should be emphasized. For instance, the proximal CA3 cells project to both dorsal and ventral but tend to send axons more dorsally to distal portion of the CA1 region (Ishizuka et al., 1990). Thus, topographically organized connections between the CA3 and CA1 regions may be specifically modulated by neuronal CB.

General Distributions of GABAergic Neurons in the Hippocampus

Rhythmic activity in the cortical circuits critically relies on GABAergic neurons regulating the balance between excitation and inhibition (Mann and Paulsen, 2007). GABAergic neurons are usually identified immunocytochemically using either GAD (Ribak et al., 1978) or GABA-like (Ottersen and Storm-Mathisen, 1984) antibodies. We found almost identical labeling patterns for GAD and GABA in the mouse hippocampus without colchicine (Jinno et al., 1998). Furthermore, the penetration into thick sections by antibodies against GAD was much better than for GABA antibodies. Thus, we used GAD immunostaining to identify GABAergic neurons in a series of studies using the optical disector method.

GAD67-positive cells were scattered throughout all regions of the mouse hippocampus (Figure 9.2a,b), with clusters of GAD67-positive axon terminals scattered among the fine elements in the stratum pyramidale and dentate granule cell layer and mossy fibers in the bands in the stratum lucidum and in the dentate hilus. No discriminative differences were observed in the patterns of distributions of GAD67-positive neurons between dorsal and ventral hippocampus.

The densities of GAD67-positive neurons were estimated by the optical disector, and their dorsoventral differences were statistically analyzed (Figure 9.2c; Table 9.1). Because of the complexity, the statistical analysis of interlaminar differences was omitted. However, there was a trend for higher densities of GAD67-positive neurons in the ventral part as compared to the dorsal part, with the exception of two layers, that is, the stratum pyramidale of the CA1 region and the stratum radiatum of the CA3 region. In addition, the densities of GAD67-positive neurons were relatively higher in the principal cell layers than in the dendritic layers.

Neurochemical Diversities of GABAergic Nonprincipal Neurons in the Hippocampus

Since Ramón y Cajal (1911) described the morphological difference of neurons, many studies reported the diversities of GABAergic neurons in the cortex from morphological, neurochemical, and electrophysiological viewpoints (Freund and Buzsáki, 1996; Markram et al., 2004). The diversity of GABAergic interneurons appears to support numerous brain functions, including regulation of synchronized oscillation and synaptic plasticity (Whittington et al., 1995; Bacci and Huguenard, 2006). Furthermore, recent reports demonstrated that distinct classes of GABAergic neurons coordinate the activity of pyramidal neurons in a temporally different and brain-state-dependent manner (Klausberger et al., 2003, 2004).

Klausberger and Somogyi (2008) classified hippocampal GABAergic interneurons into >21 classes based primarily on the differences in distributions of inputs and outputs. By contrast, Rudy et al., (2011) suggest that three neurochemical markers account for nearly 100% of GABAergic neurons in the somatosensory cortex. In the absence of a classification scheme for GABAergic, international efforts are under way to develop functional terms for descriptions of GABAergic neurons (Ascoli et al., 2008).

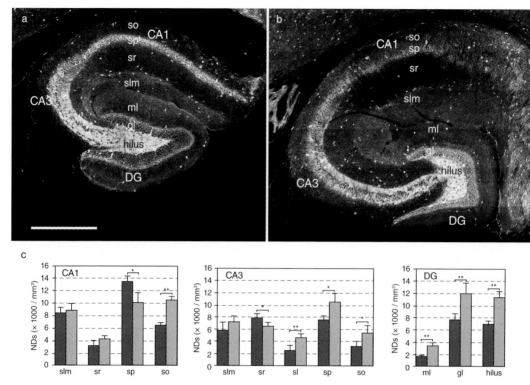

Figure 9.2 Spatial distributions of GAD67-positive neurons in the hippocampus. (a,b) Montage images of the dorsal (a) and ventral (b) hippocampus showing immunofluorescence for GAD67. (c) Comparisons of the densities of GAD67-positive neurons in the CA1 and CA3 regions and dentate gyrus (DG). Dark columns represent the dorsal part and bright columns represent the ventral part. Scale bar in panel a = 500 μm (applies to a and b). $*p < 0.05$ and $**p < 0.01$. gl, granule cell layer; ml, molecular layer; sl, stratum lucidum; slm, stratum lacunosum-moleculare; so, stratum oriens; sp, stratum pyramidale; sr, stratum radiatum. Reproduced from Jinno and Kosaka (2006), with permission of the publisher.

Earlier studies indicated the specific relationship between morphological characteristics and electrophysiological activities of chemically defined GABAergic neurons in the hippocampus and neocortex (Kawaguchi et al., 1987; Wang et al., 2002). However, the most practical and widely used classification is based upon the neurochemical markers (Maccaferri et al., 2000). Though some neurochemical markers are coexpressed in single GABAergic neurons (Dun et al., 1994; Jinno and Kosaka, 2000, 2002a), neurochemical markers enable precise estimation of the densities of GABAergic neurons via obtaining a mass of labeled cells, which helps to understand pathological changes in diseases such as ischemia, (Arabadzisz and Freund, 1999) and epilepsy (Cossart et al., 2001). Here we review the spatial distributions and provide density estimates from optical disector counts of eight classes of GABAergic neurons in the hippocampus defined by the following neurochemical markers: three calcium-binding proteins (parvalbumin [PV], calretinin [CR], and calbindin D28K [CB]); four neuropeptides (neuropeptide Y [NPY], somatostatin [SOM], cholecystokinin [CCK], and vasoactive intestinal protein [VIP]); and neuronal NOS.

Distribution of Eight Classes of GABAergic Nonprincipal Neurons Defined by Neurochemical Markers

The majority of PV-positive GABAergic neurons are considered basket (axo-axonic) cells that mediate perisomatic inhibition (Kosaka et al., 1987; Katsumaru et al., 1988). Recent studies showed that PV was also expressed in dendritic inhibitory cells, for example, oriens/alveus inter-neurons with lacunosum-moleculare axon arborizations (O-LM cells; Jinno and Kosaka, 2000; Ferraguti et al., 2004) and bistratified cells (Pawelzik et al., 2002). In addition, some of the weakly PV-positive cells projected to the medial septum (Jinno and Kosaka, 2002b). The majority of PV-positive cells were considered to be fast-spiking cells in the hippocampus (Kawaguchi et al., 1987), but some of them were bust firing (Pawelzik et al., 2002). Recent *in vivo* studies using optogenetic techniques have indicated that activity of PV-positive neurons is essential for driving cortical gamma oscillations in mice (Cardin et al., 2009; Sohal et al., 2009). Clinically, several studies have shown that bipolar disorder and schizophrenia are accompanied by decreased density of PV-positive interneurons in the parahippocampal region (Wang et al., 2011). It has also been suggested that schizophrenia may be associated with dysfunctions of PV-positive basket cells (Lewis et al., 2012).

Because CR-positive GABAergic neurons are thought to innervate other GABAergic neurons, they are referred to as interneuron specific cells (Gulyás et al., 1996). In addition, CR was expressed in hilar mossy cells in the ventral hippocampus of mice (Liu et al., 1996; Blasco-Ibanez and Freund, 1997). Previous studies indicate that CR-positive cells belong to regular firing cells or to burst firing cells (Kawaguchi and Kondo, 2002). Recently, Caputi et al., (2009) reported that CR-positive bipolar cells exhibit burst-firing pattern, while CR-positive multipolar cells show regular firing pattern. The presence of CR-positive dystrophic neurites was reported in Alzheimer's disease (AD) hippocampus (Brion and Resibois, 1994). It has been hypothesized that CR-positive GABAergic neurons are early targets of extracellular amyloid-β pathology of AD (Baglietto-Vargas et al., 2010).

The majority of CB-positive GABAergic neurons are considered to innervate the distal dendrite of glutamatergic principal cells and control the efficacy of afferent inputs, for example, Schaffer collateral associated cells (Vida et al., 1998). A subset of CB-positive GABAergic neurons pro-jected to the medial septum (T th and Freund, 1992; Jinno and Kosaka, 2002b). In addition, CB was expressed in dentate granule cells and a subset of CA1 pyramidal neurons. Postmortem ste-reological analysis has shown a selective increase in the density of CB-positive neurons in the DG of individuals with autism (Lawrence et al., 2010).

SOM-positive GABAergic neurons mainly belong to dendritic inhibitory cells, for example, O-LM cells (Sik et al., 1995) and hilar perforant path-associated neurons (HIPP cells; Han et al., 1993). More than 90% of hippocampal GABAergic neurons project to the medial septum and express SOM (Jinno and Kosaka, 2002b), which are different from dendritic inhibitory cells (Gulyás et al., 2003). Some of the SOM-positive cells also project to the subiculum and retrosple-nial cortex (Jinno et al., 2007). A recent study reported that hippocampal SOM-positive neurons project to GABAergic interneurons in the medial entorhinal cortex, which may modulate rhythmic theta activity of postsynaptic neurons in the target areas (Melzer et al., 2012). Alterations in SOM expression occur in pathological conditions. Sloviter (1987) noted a highly selective loss of SOM-positive neurons in the dentate hilus after repeated seizures in rats. Shortly thereafter, the specific loss of SOM-positive neurons and upregulation of SOM binding sites was confirmed in humans with temporal lobe epilepsy (de Lanerolle et al., 1989; Robbins et al., 1991). Age-dependent reduction of SOM has been hypothesized as a trigger for accumulation of amyloid β-protein in the hippocampus (Burgos-Ramos et al., 2008).

The distributions of NPY-positive GABAergic neurons were rather similar to those of SOM-positive neurons (Deller and Leranth, 1990). A recent study demonstrated NPY expression in bistratified cells (Klausberger et al., 2004). Interestingly, maternally separated rats in a model of depression-related behavior exhibited lower levels of NPY in the hippocampus in adulthood (Jiménez-Vasquez et al., 2001). Recent studies have suggested that NPY may be involved in depression-like disorders and stress responses (Morales-Medina et al., 2010).

CCK-positive GABAergic neurons are morphologically classified into several distinct subtypes, for example, basket cells, Schaffer collateral-associated cells, perforant path-associated cells, bistratified cells, trilaminar cells, and quadrilaminar cells (Cope et al., 2002; Pawelzik et al., 2002). CCK was also found in some subsets of non-GABAergic neurons in the mouse hippocampus (Jinno and Kosaka, 2003). Electrophysiologically, the vast majority of CCK-positive GABAergic neurons were regular spiking (Pawelzik et al., 2002). In the hippocampus, CCK-positive neurons and PV-positive neurons are considered to play complementary roles in network oscillations (Klausberger et al., 2005). It has been suggested that CCK-positive neurons carry information from subcortical pathways about the emotional, motivational, and general physiological state of the animal (Freund, 2003).

VIP-positive GABAergic neurons are also heterogeneous (Acsády et al., 1996a,b; Hájos et al., 1996), with some specifically innervating other GABAergic neurons. Recent pharmacological studies have raised the possibility that VIP in the hippocampus may critically modulate learning and memory processes (Ivanova et al., 2008). An intercellular messenger, nitric oxide (NO), is synthesized from L-arginine by NOS. In the hippocampus, relatively large numbers of GABAergic neurons express NOS (Valtschanoff et al., 1993; Megías et al., 1997; Jinno et al., 1999). A recent study has shown that NO is a homeostatic regulator, tuning neuronal excitability to the recent history of excitatory synaptic inputs over intervals of minutes to hours (Steinert et al., 2011).

Densities of Eight Classes of Chemically Defined GABAergic Nonprincipal Neurons in the Hippocampus

The densities of eight classes of GABAergic neurons in the mouse hippocampus were estimated using the optical disector principle (Figure 9.3). The densities in the entire hippocampus and the CA1 stratum oriens were generally higher in the ventral part than in the dorsal part in all classes of GABAergic neurons, including neurons immunopositive for NPY, PV, CR, CB, SOM, CCK, and VIP and NOS. In contrast, the majority of GABAergic neurons in the CA1 stratum pyramidale exhibit higher densities in the dorsal part than in the ventral part, with statistically significant increases in PV-positive neurons, CR-positive neurons, NPY-positive neurons, and NOS-positive neurons. In the CA1 strata radiatum and lacunosum-moleculare, the dorsoventral discrepancies were not prominent in most classes of GABAergic neurons.

The densities of GABAergic neurons in each layer of the CA3 area were generally higher in the ventral part than in the dorsal part. One exception is that SOM-positive neurons in the stratum lucidum and NPY-positive neurons in the stratum lacunosum-moleculare showed significantly higher densities in the dorsal part than in the ventral part.

In the DG, the majority of eight classes of GABAergic neurons showed higher densities in the ventral part than in the dorsal part while the densities of NPY-positive neurons in the molecular layer were significantly higher in the dorsal subregion than in the ventral subregion.

Numbers of Eight Classes of Chemically Defined GABAergic Nonprincipal Neurons in a 300-µm-thick Virtual Slice

Because modern multidisciplinary analyses often use slice preparations, we estimated the absolute numbers of eight classes of GABAergic neurons contained in a 300-µm-thick virtual transverse slice of the mouse hippocampus (Table 9.2). For this purpose, volume of the virtual slice of the mouse hippocampus was estimated from 50-µm-thick immunostained sections. Then, the numbers

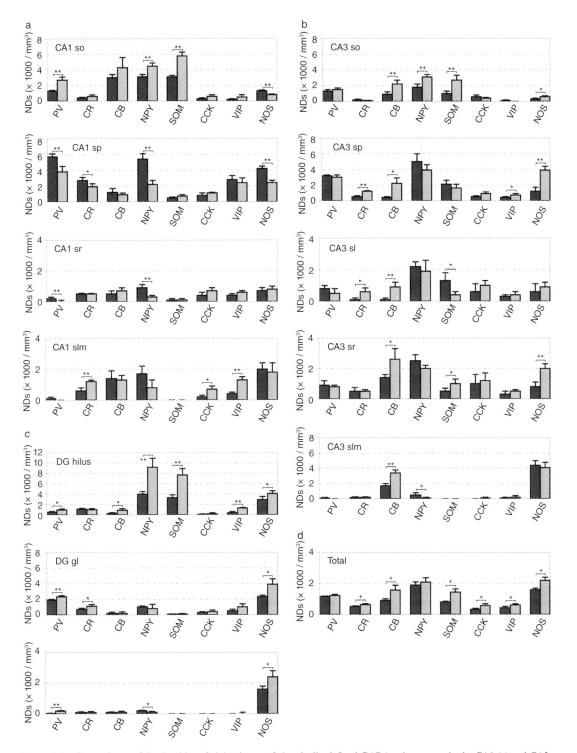

Figure 9.3 Comparisons of the densities of eight classes of chemically defined GABAergic neurons in the CA1 (a) and CA3 (b) regions, and dentate gyrus (DG; c), and the entire area (d). Dark columns represent the dorsal part and bright columns represent the ventral part. $*p < 0.05$ and $**p < 0.01$. Reproduced from Jinno and Kosaka (2006), with permission of the publisher.

Table 9.2   Numbers of eight classes of chemically defined GABAergic nonprincipal neurons contained in a 300-μm-thick virtual slice

	Dorsal								Ventral							
Region	PV	CR	CB	NPY	SOM	CCK	VIP	NOS	PV	CR	CB	NPY	SOM	CCK	VIP	NOS
CA1	145	79	160	247	106	40	74	166	178	124	198	204	180	91	139	175
CA3	92	19	45	150	65	33	14	73	261	97	441	471	274	138	65	387
DG	48	27	13	71	27	8	19	175	88	52	33	226	166	16	56	413
Total	286	128	224	468	197	81	105	413	526	274	672	893	615	244	262	975
Layer																
CA1																
so	42	11	93	97	97	9	8	37	73	16	118	121	158	15	12	21
sp	101	47	21	94	8	13	49	70	111	56	27	62	19	31	69	61
sr	9	19	20	35	3	16	15	22	2	20	29	11	4	27	23	47
slm	1	14	31	37	1	4	10	40	0	36	41	25	0	20	40	46
CA3																
so	20	3	14	27	15	9	2	6	94	6	132	190	162	25	2	27
sp	55	8	7	86	36	9	7	27	116	45	85	150	61	33	28	144
sl	6	1	0	18	11	5	3	7	7	9	15	32	6	17	7	10
sr	8	5	13	23	5	9	3	11	39	26	134	102	50	62	23	98
slm	0	1	12	3	0	0	1	25	0	5	79	2	1	3	5	110
DG																
hilus	4	9	2	31	26	1	3	27	18	19	18	175	146	4	24	97
gl	48	18	4	25	1	6	14	72	61	30	5	20	3	10	26	140
ml	2	3	6	12	0	2	2	75	14	7	8	7	1	1	3	177

of eight classes of chemically defined GABAergic neurons were calculated by multiplying the densities by the volume of individual layers and regions.

The numbers of eight classes of GABAergic neurons in a 300-μm-thick virtual slice revealed some previously overlooked facts. For instance, only a few CCK-positive neurons ($n = 13$) were present in the stratum pyramidale of the dorsal CA1 area, with a larger number of PV-positive neurons (101). Emerging thought during the past decade indicates a complementary role for PV-positive neurons and CCK-positive neurons in the hippocampus (Klausberger et al., 2005; Glickfeld and Scanziani, 2006). The present data may help to understand the role for PV and CCK in the inhibitory control in the hippocampus.

Balance between Glutamatergic Excitation and GABAergic Inhibition in the Hippocampus

The balance between excitation and inhibition (E/I balance) in the neuronal circuits is critical for proper brain function (Zhang and Sun, 2011). Disturbed E/I balance occurs in numerous neuropsychological disorders, such as autism, epilepsy, and schizophrenia (Yizhar et al., 2011). To understand the potential dorsoventral differences in E/I balance of the hippocampus, we examined the ratio of the number of glutamatergic neurons to the number of GABAergic neurons using virtual slices (Figure 9.4).

The total numbers of glutamatergic neurons in the entire hippocampus were comparable between dorsal (333,334) and ventral (313,222) slices. In the CA1 region, the numbers of pyramidal neurons were significantly larger in the dorsal slice (7608) than in the ventral slice (4692). By contrast, in the CA3 region, the numbers were larger in the ventral slice (6549) than in the dorsal slice (2808). The numbers of dentate granule cells were larger in the dorsal slices (22,918) than in the ventral slice (20,081). In the entire hippocampus, the numbers of GAD67-positive neurons in the ventral slice (3124) were more than twice the dorsal slice (1404). The same dorsoventral

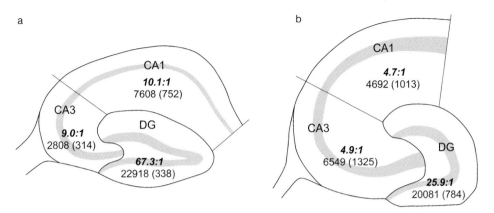

Figure 9.4 Schematic representations of the E/I ratios and neuron numbers in 300-μm-thick virtual slices of the dorsal (a) and the ventral (b) hippocampus. The bold italic numerals represent the ratios of the numbers of excitatory glutamatergic to the number of inhibitory GABAergic neurons. The plain numerals represent the numbers of glutamatergic neurons and those in parenthesis represent the GABAergic neurons. Modified and reproduced from Jinno and Kosaka (2010), with permission of the publisher.

gradient was seen in the CA1 and CA3 regions and the DG. The dorsoventral difference was the most prominent in the CA3 region (dorsal = 314, ventral = 1326).

In the CA1 and CA3 regions, the ratios of the number of glutamatergic neurons to the number of GABAergic neurons in the dorsal slice (CA1, 10.1:1; CA3, 9.0:1) were over twice as high as those in the ventral slice (CA1, 4.7:1; CA3, 4.9:1). Those in the DG were almost three times higher in the dorsal slice (67.3:1) than in the ventral slice (25.9:1). Together, we propose that excitability of the neuronal circuit is higher in the dorsal slice than in the ventral slice. Such dorsoventral difference in the E/I balance may underlie the functional differentiation of the hippocampus. It should also be noted that these findings may be especially important for the interpretation of physiological experiments using hippocampal slices *in vitro*.

Conclusion

Solid quantitative data about structural organization of central nervous system remains scarce. Although many challenges remain, the present stereological data on the neural architecture of the hippocampus may serve as a foundation for future research.

References

Acsády, L., Arabadzisz, D., Freund, T. F. 1996a. Correlated morphological and neurochemical features identify different subsets of vasoactive intestinal polypeptide-immunoreactive interneurons in rat hippocampus. *Neuroscience* **73** (2): 299–315.

Acsády, L., Gorcs, T. J., Freund, T. F. 1996b. Different populations of vasoactive intestinal polypeptide-immunoreactive inter- neurons are specialized to control pyramidal cells or interneurons in the hippocampus. *Neuroscience* **73** (2): 317–334.

Amaral, D. G., Witter, M. P. 1989. The three-dimensional organization of the hippocampal formation: a review of anatomical data. *Neuroscience* **31**: 571–591.

Andersen, P., Bliss, T. V., Skrede, K. K. 1971. Lamellar organization of hippocampal pathways. *Exp Brain Res* **13**: 222–238.

Andersen, P., Soleng, A. F., Raastad, M. 2000. The hippocampal lamella hypothesis revisited. *Brain Res* **886**: 165–171.

Arabadzisz, D., Freund, T. F. 1999. Changes in excitatory and inhibitory circuits of the rat hippocampus 12–14 months after complete forebrain ischemia. *Neuroscience* **92** (1): 27–45.

Ascoli, G. A., Alonso-Nanclares, L., Anderson, S. A., Barrionuevo, G., Benavides-Piccione, R., Burkhalter, A., Buzsáki, G., Cauli, B., Defelipe, J., Fairén, A. et al., 2008. Petilla terminology: nomenclature of features of GABAergic interneurons of the cerebral cortex. *Nat Rev Neurosci* **9**: 557–568.

Bacci, A., Huguenard, J. R. 2006. Enhancement of spike-timing precision by autaptic transmission in neocortical inhibitory interneurons. *Neuron* **49** (1): 119–130.

Baglietto-Vargas, D., Moreno-Gonzalez, I., Sanchez-Varo, R., Jimenez, S., Trujillo-Estrada, L., Sanchez-Mejias, E., Torres, M., Romero-Acebal, M., Ruano, D., Vizuete, M., et al., 2010. Calretinin interneurons are early targets of extracellular amyloid-beta pathology in PS1/AbetaPP Alzheimer mice hippocampus. *J Alzheimers Dis* **21** (1): 119–132.

Baimbridge, K. G., Miller, J. J. 1982. Immunohistochemical localization of calcium-binding protein in the cerebellum, hippocampal formation and olfactory bulb of the rat. *Brain Res* **245**: 223–229.

Bannerman, D. M., Rawlins, J. N., McHugh, S. B., Deacon, R. M., Yee, B. K., Bast, T., Zhang, W. N., Pothuizen, H. H., Feldon, J. 2004. Regional dissociations within the hippocampus—memory and anxiety. *Neurosci Biobehav Rev* **28**: 273–283.

Blasco-Ibanez, J. M., Freund, T. F. 1997. Distribution, ultrastructure, and connectivity of calretinin-immunoreactive mossy cells of the mouse dentate gyrus. *Hippocampus* **7** (3): 307–320.

Braendgaard, H., Evans, S. M., Howard, C. V., Gundersen, H. J. 1990. The total number of neurons in the human neocortex unbiasedly estimated using optical disectors. *J Microsc* **157** (Pt 3): 285–304.

Brion, J. P., Resibois, A. 1994. A subset of calretinin-positive neurons are abnormal in Alzheimer's disease. *Acta Neuropathol (Berl)* **88**: 33–43.

Burgos-Ramos, E., Hervás-Aguilar, A., Aguado-Llera, D., Puebla-Jiménez, L., Hernández-Pinto, A. M., Barrios, V., Arilla-Ferreiro, E. 2008. Somatostatin and Alzheimer's disease. *Mol Cell Endocrinol* **286** (1–2): 104–111.

Cajal, R. y. 1911. *Histologie du System Nerveux de l'Homme et des Vertebres* (translated by L. Azoulay). Maloine, .

Caputi, A., Rozov, A., Blatow, M., Monyer, H. 2009. Two calretinin-positive GABAergic cell types in layer 2/3 of the mouse neocortex provide different forms of inhibition. *Cereb Cortex* **19** (6): 1345–1359.

Cardin, J. A., Carlén, M., Meletis, K., Knoblich, U., Zhang, F., Deisseroth, K., Tsai, L. H., Moore, C. I. 2009. Driving fast-spiking cells induces gamma rhythm and controls sensory responses. *Nature* **459** (7247): 663–667.

Cope, D. W., Maccaferri, G., Marton, L. F., Roberts, J. D., Cobden, P. M., Somogyi, P. 2002. Cholecystokinin-immunopositive basket and Schaffer collateral-associated interneurones target different domains of pyramidal cells in the CA1 area of the rat hippocampus. *Neuroscience* **109** (1): 63–80.

Cossart, R., Dinocourt, C., Hirsch, J. C., Merchan-Perez, A., De Felipe, J., Ben-Ari, Y., Esclapez, M., Bernard, C. 2001. Dendritic but not somatic GABAergic inhibition is decreased in experimental epilepsy. *Nat Neurosci* **4** (1): 52–62.

de Lanerolle, N. C., Kim, J. H., Robbins, R. J., Spencer, D. D. 1989. Hippocampal interneuron loss and plasticity in human temporal lobe epilepsy. *Brain Res* **495** (2): 387–395.

Deller, T., Leranth, C. 1990. Synaptic connections of neuropeptide Y (NPY) immunoreactive neurons in the hilar area of the rat hippocampus. *J Comp Neurol* **300** (3): 433–447.

Dun, N. J., Dun, S. L., Wong, R. K., Forstermann, U. 1994. Colocalization of nitric oxide synthase and somatostatin immunoreactivity in rat dentate hilar neurons. *Proc Natl Acad Sci U S A* **91** (8): 2955–2959.

Ferraguti, F., Cobden, P., Pollard, M., Cope, D., Shigemoto, R., Watanabe, M., Somogyi, P. 2004. Immunolocalization of metabotropic glutamate receptor 1alpha (mGluR1alpha) in distinct classes of interneuron in the CA1 region of the rat hippocampus. *Hippocampus* **14** (2): 193–215.

Freund, T. F. 2003. Interneuron diversity series: rhythm and mood in perisomatic inhibition. *Trends Neurosci* **26** (9): 489–495.

Freund, T. F., Buzsáki, G. 1996. Interneurons of the hippocampus. *Hippocampus* **6** (4): 347–470.

Gaykema, R. P., van der Kuil, J., Hersh, L. B., Luiten, P. G. 1991. Patterns of direct projections from the hippocampus to the medial septum-diagonal band complex: anterograde tracing with *Phaseolus vulgaris* leucoagglutinin combined with immunohistochemistry of choline acetyltransferase. *Neuroscience* **43**: 349–360.

Glickfeld, L. L., Scanziani, M. 2006. Distinct timing in the activity of cannabinoid-sensitive and cannabinoid-insensitive basket cells. *Nat Neurosci* **9** (6): 807–815.

Gulyás, A. I., Hajos, N., Freund, T. F. 1996. Interneurons containing calretinin are specialized to control other interneurons in the rat hippocampus. *J Neurosci* **16** (10): 3397–3411.

Gulyás, A. I., Hájos, N., Katona, I., Freund, T. F. 2003. Interneurons are the local targets of hippocampal inhibitory cells which project to the medial septum. *Eur J Neurosci* **17** (9): 1861–1872.

Hájos, N., Acsády, L., Freund, T. F. 1996. Target selectivity and neurochemical characteristics of VIP-immunoreactive interneurons in the rat dentate gyrus. *Eur J Neurosci* **8** (7): 1415–1431.

Hampson, R. E., Simeral, J. D., Deadwyler, S. A. 1999. Distribution of spatial and nonspatial information in dorsal hippocampus. *Nature* **402**: 610–614.

Han, Z. S., Buhl, E. H., Lorinczi, Z., Somogyi, P. 1993. A high degree of spatial selectivity in the axonal and dendritic domains of physiologically identified local-circuit neurons in the dentate gyrus of the rat hippocampus. *Eur J Neurosci* **5** (5): 395–410.

Ishizuka, N., Weber, J., Amaral, D. G. 1990. Organization of intrahippocampal projections originating from CA3 pyramidal cells in the rat. *J Comp Neurol* **295**: 580–623.

Ivanova, M., Ternianov, A., Belcheva, S., Tashev, R., Negrev, N., Belcheva, I. 2008. Hippocampal asymmetry in exploratory behavior to vasoactive intestinal polypeptide. *Peptides* **29** (6): 940–947.

Jiménez-Vasquez, P. A., Mathé, A. A., Thomas, J. D., Riley, E. P., Ehlers, C. L. 2001. Early maternal separation alters neuropeptide Y concentrations in selected brain regions in adult rats. *Brain Res Dev Brain Res* **131** (1–2): 149–152.

Jinno, S., Kosaka, T. 2000. Colocalization of parvalbumin and somatostatin-like immunoreactivity in the mouse hippocampus: quantitative analysis with optical disector. *J Comp Neurol* **428** (3): 377–388.

Jinno, S., Kosaka, T. 2002a. Patterns of expression of calcium-binding proteins and neuronal nitric oxide synthase in different populations of hippocampal GABAergic neurons in mice. *J Comp Neurol* **449** (1): 1–25.

Jinno, S., Kosaka, T. 2002b. Immunocytochemical characterization of hippocamposeptal projecting GABAergic nonprincipal neurons in the mouse brain: a retrograde labeling study. *Brain Res* **945** (2): 219–231.

Jinno, S., Kosaka, T. 2003. Heterogeneous expression of the cholecystokinin-like immunoreactivity in the mouse hippocampus, with special reference to the dorsoventral difference. *Neuroscience* **122** (4): 869–884.

Jinno, S., Kosaka, T. 2006. Cellular architecture of the mouse hippocampus: a quantitative aspect of chemically defined GABAergic neurons with stereology. *Neurosci Res* **56**: 229–245.

Jinno, S., Kosaka, T. 2010. Stereological estimation of numerical densities of glutamatergic principal neurons in the mouse hippocampus. *Hippocampus* **20** (7): 829–840.

Jinno, S., Aika, Y., Fukuda, T., Kosaka, T. 1998. Quantitative analysis of GABAergic neurons in the mouse hippocampus, with optical disector using confocal laser scanning microscope. *Brain Res* **814** (1–2): 55–70.

Jinno, S., Aika, Y., Fukuda, T., Kosaka, T. 1999. Quantitative analysis of neuronal nitric oxide synthase-immunoreactive neurons in the mouse hippocampus with optical disector. *J Comp Neurol* **410** (3): 398–412.

Jinno, S., Klausberger, T., Marton, L. F., Dalezios, Y., Roberts, J. D., Fuentealba, P., Bushong, E. A., Henze, D., Buzsáki, G., Somogyi, P. 2007. Neuronal diversity in GABAergic long-range projections from the hippocampus. *J Neurosci* **27** (33): 8790–8804.

Jung, M. W., Wiener, S. I., McNaughton, B. L. 1994. Comparison of spatial firing characteristics of units in dorsal and ventral hippocampus of the rat. *J Neurosci* **14**: 7347–7356.

Katsumaru, H., Kosaka, T., Heizmann, C. W., Hama, K. 1988. Immunocytochemical study of GABAergic neurons containing the calcium-binding protein parvalbumin in the rat hippocampus. *Exp Brain Res* **72** (2): 347–362.

Kawaguchi, Y., Kondo, S. 2002. Parvalbumin, somatostatin and cholecystokinin as chemical markers for specific GABAergic interneuron types in the rat frontal cortex. *J Neurocytol* **31** (3–5): 277–287.

Kawaguchi, Y., Katsumaru, H., Kosaka, T., Heizmann, C. W., Hama, K. 1987. Fast spiking cells in rat hippocampus (CA1 region) contain the calcium-binding protein parvalbumin. *Brain Res* **416** (2): 369–374.

Kjelstrup, K. G., Tuvnes, F. A., Steffenach, H. A., Murison, R., Moser, E. I., Moser, M. B. 2002. Reduced fear expression after lesions of the ventral hippocampus. *Proc Natl Acad Sci U S A* **99** (16): 10825–10830.

Klausberger, T., Somogyi, P. 2008. Neuronal diversity and temporal dynamics: the unity of hippocampal circuit operations. *Science* **321**: 53–57.

Klausberger, T., Magill, P. J., Marton, L. F., Roberts, J. D., Cobden, P. M., Buzsaki, G., Somogyi, P. 2003. Brain-state- and cell-type-specific firing of hippocampal interneurons in vivo. *Nature* **421** (6925): 844–848.

Klausberger, T., Marton, L. F., Baude, A., Roberts, J. D., Magill, P. J., Somogyi, P. 2004. Spike timing of dendrite-targeting bistratified cells during hippocampal network oscillations in vivo. *Nat Neurosci* **7** (1): 41–47.

Klausberger, T., Marton, L. F., O'Neill, J., Huck, J. H., Dalezios, Y., Fuentealba, P., Suen, W. Y., Papp, E., Kaneko, T., Watanabe, M., et al. 2005. Complementary roles of cholecystokinin- and parvalbumin-expressing GABAergic neurons in hippocampal network oscillations. *J Neurosci* **25** (42): 9782–9793.

Kosaka, T., Katsumaru, H., Hama, K., Wu, J. Y., Heizmann, C. W. 1987. GABAergic neurons containing the Ca2+-binding protein parvalbumin in the rat hippocampus and dentate gyrus. *Brain Res* **419** (1–2): 119–130.

Lawrence, Y. A., Kemper, T. L., Bauman, M. L., Blatt, G. J. 2010. Parvalbumin-, calbindin-, and calretinin-immunoreactive hippocampal interneuron density in autism. *Acta Neurol Scand* **121** (2): 99–108.

Leonardo, E. D., Richardson-Jones, J. W., Sibille, E., Kottman, A., Hen, R. 2006. Molecular heterogeneity along the dorsal-ventral axis of the murine hippocampal CA1 field: a microarray analysis of gene expression. *Neuroscience* **137**: 177–186.

Lewis, D. A., Curley, A. A., Glausier, J. R., Volk, D. W. 2012. Cortical parvalbumin interneurons and cognitive dysfunction in schizophrenia. *Trends Neurosci* **35** (1): 57–67.

Liu, Y., Fujise, N., Kosaka, T. 1996. Distribution of calretinin immunoreactivity in the mouse dentate gyrus. I. General description. *Exp Brain Res* **108** (3): 389–403.

Maccaferri, G., Roberts, J. D., Szucs, P., Cottingham, C. A., Somogyi, P. 2000. Cell surface domain specific postsynaptic currents evoked by identified GABAergic neurones in rat hippocampus in vitro. *J Physiol* **524** (Pt 1): 91–116.

Mann, E. O., Paulsen, O. 2007. Role of GABAergic inhibition in hippocampal network oscillations. *Trends Neurosci* **30** (7): 343–349.

Markram, H., Toledo-Rodriguez, M., Wang, Y., Gupta, A., Silberberg, G., Wu, C. 2004. Interneurons of the neocortical inhibitory system. *Nat Rev Neurosci* **5** (10): 793–807.

McHugh, S. B., Niewoehner, B., Rawlins, J. N., Bannerman, D. M. 2008. Dorsal hippocampal N-methyl-D-aspartate receptors underlie spatial working memory performance during non-matching to place testing on the T-maze. *Behav Brain Res* **186**: 41–47.

Megías, M., Verduga, R., Fernandez-Viadero, C., Crespo, D. 1997. Neurons co-localizing calretinin immunoreactivity and reduced nicotinamide adenine dinucleotide phosphate diaphorase (NADPH-d) activity in the hippocampus and dentate gyrus of the rat. *Brain Res* **744** (1): 112–120.

Melzer, S., Michael, M., Caputi, A., Eliava, M., Fuchs, E. C., Whittington, M. A., Monyer, H. 2012. Long-range-projecting GABAergic neurons modulate inhibition in hippocampus and entorhinal cortex. *Science* **335** (6075): 1506–1510.

Morales-Medina, J. C., Dumont, Y., Quirion, R. 2010. A possible role of neuropeptide Y in depression and stress. *Brain Res* **1314**: 194–205.

Moser, E., Moser, M. B., Andersen, P. 1993. Spatial learning impairment parallels the magnitude of dorsal hippocampal lesions, but is hardly present following ventral lesions. *J Neurosci* **13**: 3916–3925.

Mouton, P. R. 2011a. Applications of unbiased stereology to neurodevelopmental toxicology. In *Developmental Neurotoxicology Research: Principles, Models, Techniques, Strategies and Mechanisms*, edited by C. Wang and W. Slikke, pp. 53–77. Hoboken, NJ: John Wiley & Sons.

Mouton, P. R. 2011b. *Unbiased Stereology: A Concise Guide*. Baltimore, MD: The Johns Hopkins University Press.

Müller, A., Kukley, M., Stausberg, P., Beck, H., Müller, W., Dietrich, D. 2005. Endogenous Ca2+ buffer concentration and Ca2+ microdomains in hippocampal neurons. *J Neurosci* **25** (3): 558–565.

Ottersen, O. P., Storm-Mathisen, J. 1984. Glutamate- and GABA-containing neurons in the mouse and rat brain, as demonstrated with a new immunocytochemical technique. *J Comp Neurol* **229** (3): 374–392.

Pawelzik, H., Hughes, D. I., Thomson, A. M. 2002. Physiological and morphological diversity of immunocytochemically defined parvalbumin- and cholecystokinin-positive interneurones in CA1 of the adult rat hippocampus. *J Comp Neurol* **443** (4): 346–367.

Ribak, C. E., Vaughn, J. E., Saito, K. 1978. Immunocytochemical localization of glutamic acid decarboxylase in neuronal somata following colchicine inhibition of axonal transport. *Brain Res* **140** (2): 315–332.

Robbins, R. J., Brines, M. L., Kim, J. H., Adrian, T., de Lanerolle, N., Welsh, S., Spencer, D. D. 1991. A selective loss of somatostatin in the hippocampus of patients with temporal lobe epilepsy. *Ann Neurol* **29** (3): 325–332.

Rudy, B., Fishell, G., Lee, S., Hjerling-Leffler, J. 2011. Three groups of interneurons account for nearly 100% of neocortical GABAergic neurons. *Dev Neurobiol* **71** (1): 45–61.

Schmidt, H. 2012. Three functional facets of calbindin D-28k. *Front Mol Neurosci* **5**: 25.

Sik, A., Penttonen, M., Ylinen, A., Buzsaki, G. 1995. Hippocampal CA1 interneurons: an in vivo intracellular labeling study. *J Neurosci* **15** (10): 6651–6665.

Sloviter, R. S. 1987. Decreased hippocampal inhibition and a selective loss of interneurons in experimental epilepsy. *Science* **235** (4784): 73–76.

Sloviter, R. S. 1989. Calcium-binding protein (calbindin-D28k) and parvalbumin immunocytochemistry: localization in the rat hippocampus with specific reference to the selective vulnerability of hippocampal neurons to seizure activity. *J Comp Neurol* **280** (2): 183–196.

Sohal, V. S., Zhang, F., Yizhar, O., Deisseroth, K. 2009. Parvalbumin neurons and gamma rhythms enhance cortical circuit performance. *Nature* **459** (7247): 698–702.

Steinert, J. R., Robinson, S. W., Tong, H., Haustein, M. D., Kopp-Scheinpflug, C., Forsythe, I. D. 2011. Nitric oxide is an activity-dependent regulator of target neuron intrinsic excitability. *Neuron* **71** (2): 291–305.

T th, K., Freund, T. F. 1992. Calbindin D28k-containing nonpyramidal cells in the rat hippocampus: their immunoreactivity for GABA and projection to the medial septum. *Neuroscience* **49** (4): 793–805.

Thompson, C. L., Pathak, S. D., Jeromin, A., Ng, L. L., MacPherson, C. R., Mortrud, M. T., Cusick, A., Riley, Z. L., Sunkin, S. M., Bernard, A., et al. 2008. Genomic anatomy of the hippocampus. *Neuron* **60**: 1010–1021.

van Groen, T., Wyss, J. M. 1990. Extrinsic projections from area CA1 of the rat hippocampus: olfactory, cortical, subcortical, and bilateral hippocampal formation projections. *J Comp Neurol* **302**: 515–528.

van Groen, T., Miettinen, P., Kadish, I. 2003. The entorhinal cortex of the mouse: organization of the projection to the hippocampal formation. *Hippocampus* **13**: 133–149.

Valtschanoff, J. G., Weinberg, R. J., Kharazia, V. N., Nakane, M., Schmidt, H. H. 1993. Neurons in rat hippocampus that synthesize nitric oxide. *J Comp Neurol* **331** (1): 111–121.

Vida, I., Halasy, K., Szinyei, C., Somogyi, P., Buhl, E. H. 1998. Unitary IPSPs evoked by interneurons at the stratum radiatum-stratum lacunosum-moleculare border in the CA1 area of the rat hippocampus in vitro. *J Physiol* **506** (Pt 3): 755–773.

Wang, A. Y., Lohmann, K. M., Yang, C. K., Zimmerman, E. I., Pantazopoulos, H., Herring, N., Berretta, S., Heckers, S., Konradi, C. 2011. Bipolar disorder type 1 and schizophrenia are accompanied by decreased density of parvalbumin- and somatostatin-positive interneurons in the parahippocampal region. *Acta Neuropathol (Berl)* **122** (5): 615–626.

Wang, Y., Gupta, A., Toledo-Rodriguez, M., Wu, C. Z., Markram, H. 2002. Anatomical, physiological, molecular and circuit properties of nest basket cells in the developing somatosensory cortex. *Cereb Cortex* **12** (4): 395–410.

West, M. J. 1999. Stereological methods for estimating the total number of neurons and synapses: issues of precision and bias. *Trends Neurosci* **22**: 51–61.

Whittington, M. A., Traub, R. D., Jefferys, J. G. 1995. Synchronized oscillations in interneuron networks driven by metabotropic glutamate receptor activation. *Nature* **373** (6515): 612–615.

Witter, M. P., Amaral, D. G. 2004. The hippocampal region. In *The Rat Brain*, edited by G. Paxinos. San Diego, CA: Elsevier Academic Press.

Witter, M. P., Van Hoesen, G. W., Amaral, D. G. 1989. Topographical organization of the entorhinal projection to the dentate gyrus of the monkey. *J Neurosci* **9**: 216–228.

Yizhar, O., Fenno, L. E., Prigge, M., Schneider, F., Davidson, T. J., O'Shea, D. J., Sohal, V. S., Goshen, I., Finkelstein, J., Paz, J. T., et al., 2011. Neocortical excitation/inhibition balance in information processing and social dysfunction. *Nature* **477** (7363): 171–178.

Zappone, C. A., Sloviter, R. S. 2004. Translamellar disinhibition in the rat hippocampal dentate gyrus after seizure-induced degeneration of vulnerable hilar neurons. *J Neurosci* **24**: 853–864.

Zhang, Z., Sun, Q. Q. 2011. The balance between excitation and inhibition and functional sensory processing in the somatosensory cortex. *Int Rev Neurobiol* **97**: 305–333.

10   The Possible Applications (and Pitfalls!) of Stereological Analysis in Postmortem Brain Research

Ahmad A. Khundakar and Alan J. Thomas

Institute for Ageing and Health, Newcastle University Campus for Ageing and Vitality, Newcastle upon Tyne, UK

Background

Analysis of human postmortem tissue has significantly advanced our understanding of the structural and molecular abnormalities associated with neurodegenerative and psychiatric disorders. Such developments have been entirely reliant upon the ultimate act of generosity from the patient and families through the gift of brain donation. In order to reciprocate the faith shown by the donor in the scientific value of brain research, it is imperative that the donated tissue is used in the most effective way possible. However, despite increases in the number of brain tissue banks and demand for tissue samples for research purposes (Dedova et al., 2009), disparate, nonstandardized processing and sampling protocols exist across institutions.

As detailed throughout this book, stereological analysis represents the "gold standard" for the unbiased assessment of the structural components comprising the brain; it is also an all-encompassing discipline that affects not only how these structures are examined but further how tissue is collected and sampled. The strict protocol that stereological analysis requires is thus often misaligned with the "realpolitik" of the brain bank environment, where a balance must be met between diagnostic and research requirements. Before embarking on a morphometric study with neuronal postmortem human tissue, one must therefore be aware of the substantial confounding factors that may affect the outcome and reliability of the resultant data and conclusions. Through identifying these inherent issues and integrating stereological methodology, a more uniform and coordinated approach may be applied to the investigation of brain disorders worldwide.

The Legacy of Two-Dimensional (2D) Analysis

During the 1990s, debate arose on the relative merits of stereological tools, for example, the use of the optical disector for cell counting in three-dimensional (3D), in the quantitative morphology of brain structures against prevailing 2D analysis (for competing views, see Benes and Lange, 2001; West and Slomanka, 2001; Schmitz and Hof, 2005). 2D analysis requires a far less rigorous sampling regime than stereology approaches. Typically, a small number of thin (5–10 μm-thick) sections from a predefined region of a paraffin-embedded block are histochemically stained and mounted for microscopic examination. Disector grids (2D frames) are projected over the image at low or high

Neurostereology: Unbiased Stereology of Neural Systems, First Edition. Edited by Peter R. Mouton.
© 2014 John Wiley & Sons, Inc. Published 2014 by John Wiley & Sons, Inc.

magnification and the number of cell profiles touching or within the grid counted. The properties of other parameters, for example, volume and surface area, are also estimated using equivalent probes such as a point-grid or line probes, respectively. Problems arising from 2D analysis, including issues surrounding "reducing fraction" and "correction" formulae, such as that devised by Abercrombie, have been well documented (Clarke, 1992; Hedreen, 1998). However, the shadow of 2D analysis looms large on the brain bank, with an archive of brains cut, stored, and sampled with these older protocols in mind. This fairly ad hoc method has made it considerably more difficult to use these sampled predefined blocks for the purposes of stereology. A particularly frustrating consequence of older sampling regimes is the inability to calculate the volume of a structure due to incomplete sampling of the reference area in question. Without knowledge of the volume of the structure, absolute values for first-order stereological parameters, for example, total cell number, cannot be estimated in a reliable manner, forcing researchers faced with this situation to rely on the use of assumption-based parameters, such as cell density, with all their inherent problems.

Density: A Necessary Evil

Herbert Haug's seminal study highlights the perils of using a ratio estimator, such as density, as an indicator of the total number of neurons in defined brain regions (Haug et al., 1984). This work reported that the process of fixation for tissue preservation causes shrinkage in neural tissue that is more severe in neural tissue from younger subjects. Ignoring differential shrinkage, while relying on the ratio between the numerator (the number of cells or profiles counted) and the denominator (the area or volume of tissue or "neuropil"), leaves open the possibility of a bias known as the "reference trap" (Braendgaard and Gundersen, 1986; Dorph-Petersen and Lewis, 2011); that is, the assumption that neuron density acts as a proxy for total neuron number within a reference volume, requiring the further assumption that the reference volume of the structure remains constant across groups.

The less rigorous cutting and sampling regime described above for typical 2D morphometric approaches may initially represent an avoidable situation, but also one that could be resolved by modifying the procedure for brain banking. There are, however, several technical and anatomical restrictions inherent to analysis of postmortem brain tissue that complicate the estimation of absolute parameters, such as total cell number. In certain brain regions, such as the neocortex, cytoarchitectural borders are often indistinct, making the precise volume of the studied regions difficult to identify. Exceptions to this rule may be applied where the cortical area contains a distinct cytoarchitectural feature, for example, myelinated layer (4) in the primary visual cortex, or can be reliably identified by surrounding features, for example, Brodmann area 24 of the anterior cingulate cortex, the gyrus located anteriorly to the corpus callosum. Technical issues may also prohibit estimation of total parameters using stereological approaches. For instance, the use of virtual probes in 3D, such as the optical disector for estimation of total number (Sterio, 1984) or "space balls" for estimation of total object length (Calhoun and Mouton, 2001; Mouton et al., 2002), requires relatively thick sections, typically 30–100 µm in the z-axis after tissue processing. Consistent immunohistochemical particle labeling, that is, complete antibody penetration through the depth of thick sections may also create difficulties depending on antibody used. As a result, the degree of penetration may vary between diagnostic groups, thus creating bias.

"Come on, Feel the Noise": Recognizing Confounding Factors

Unlike laboratory-bred animal tissue, where variables related to tissue processing may be easily controlled by experimental design, postmortem human tissue is subject to a range of uncontrolled and potentially confounding factors. The inability to account and control the noise arising from such factors, and the subsequent effects of these factors on the research findings, played a major role in the initial skepticism toward research on postmortem human tissue (Plum, 1972). Such uncertainties are pertinent in the consideration of neurochemical studies but may also weaken the impact morphometric analysis.

Postmortem interval (PMI), the delay between death and fixation or freezing, has been widely reported as a major confounding factor in tissue viability; however, its impact has also been questioned (Everall and Harrison, 2002). Autolysis of the brain is believed to commence at death, but its effect on mRNA, proteins and morphometric measures may not be realized until sometime afterward (24–72 hours) (Ross et al., 1992; Barton et al., 1993; Bahn et al., 2001). Autolysis may be enhanced by factors that manifest in the period between life and death. In subjects with a prolonged agonal state, signified by, for example, shallow infrequent breaths after cardiogenic shock or septicemia, a lower tissue pH is frequently seen in respective postmortem brain tissue (McCullumsmith and Meador-Woodruff, 2011). Tissue pH has been shown to affect tissue shrinkage and is thus an empirical predictor of neuronal and glial cell density. Tissue acidosis may also impact protein status (Harrison et al., 1995), and thus neuronal density, though this remains controversial (Stan et al., 2006).

Paraffin or celloidin embedding is the most commonly used embedding method for stereological analysis of postmortem tissue. Frozen tissue acquired by rapid cooling in liquid nitrogen, followed by storage at −70°C, has been employed in human brain stereological studies (Stockmeier et al., 2004); however, the probability of tissue fracture, ice crystal formation (Vonsattel et al., 2008) and z-axis collapse during processing (Dorph-Petersen et al., 2001) reduces its applicability. For light microscopy stereology, brains are usually fixed in 10% phosphate-buffered formaldehyde or 4% paraformaldehyde in 0.1 M phosphate buffer; for electron microscopy studies a glutaraldehyde solution is generally employed. The goal of fixation is to preserve the structure of tissue components, with a minimum alteration from living state regarding volume, morphology, and spatial relationships. However, this process inevitably changes the intrinsic properties of the tissue and introduces artifacts. Maintaining the properties of the fixative solution in all sampled tissue is vital as deviation may lead to hidden confounding factors that may introduce bias to a stereological study. Ionic composition, pH, osmolarity, temperature, length of fixation, and method of application (Hyatt, 1989) have all been cited as determinants of tissue integrity. The primary method of human brain fixation by immersion, which is largely borne out of convenience, demands less time and expertise than intra-arterial perfusion. In contrast to perfusion fixation, immersion has been reported to cause uneven staining in certain antigens through the z-axis of a tissue block, with immunohistochemical staining restricted to the outermost 1–2 mm (Beach et al., 1987).

"I Am Not a Number": The Importance of Sound Patient Clinical History

If conducted blindly, that is, without knowledge of treatment group, a stereology rater will receive slides or blocks of postmortem tissue removed from the postmortem brain, typically with a patient number and a few supplementary details, such as the section thickness and sample number. Further knowledge, including the stratification into disease groups, is best carried out by a third party in possession of the key demographic and premortem information relating to the individual. Studies of postmortem tissue rely on accurate and consistent medical diagnoses through comprehensive clinical information, especially in studies involving psychiatric disorders without gross histopathological hallmarks. Antemortem diagnostic assessment is thus a vital component in the characterization of subject groups, as well as for establishing a rigid and reliable inclusion and exclusion criteria among patient cohorts. The addition of prospective characterization of subjects for post-mortem research typically adds cost, time, and may reduce the sample sizes. Assessment of clinical history by retrospective examination of patient records may substantially increase tissue yield, but introduces a new complication: the lack of standardized guidelines for recording and validation of clinical information, with well-defined inclusion and exclusion criteria, which may limit the generalizability of the study findings. To help make accurate group assignments for each subject, medical records may also be supplemented with information gleaned from surviving relatives, friends, and health-care professionals, the so called "psychological autopsy."

Knowledge of prior exposure to medication (prescribed and illicit) is fundamental to any post-mortem brain tissue study. Subjects with chronic neurological or psychiatric illness are often treated with a wide range of psychoactive compounds that affect numerous neurotransmitter receptors and activate a multitude of postreceptor cascades. The symptomatic use of prescribed psychotropic drugs is linked with clinical diagnoses; it is thus very rare to find a "naïve" test subject not taking medication for the symptoms relating to their primary illness. Whether such drugs alter the structural coordinates relating to the underlying pathology associated with the disease may depend on the drug's mode of action. For example, antidepressant drugs were initially thought to provide symptomatic relief through the direct effects on serotonin and noradrenaline transmission; however, the latency period between enhanced extracellular monoamine levels and therapeutic effect suggests numerous serotonin and noradrenaline receptor-linked targets underlie their action. A commonly identified target of antidepressant drugs, brain-derived neurotrophic factor, is thought to modulate synaptic function and induce neuroplastic events in the hippocampus (D'Sa and Duman, 2002; Monteggia et al., 2004). Conversely, components of brain affective circuitry including the hippocampus, amygdala, and frontal cortex are particularly sensitive to high levels of adrenal stress hormones. The hippocampus contains a high concentration of both mineralocorticoid and glucocorticoid receptors (Lowenberg et al., 2008), and the chronic administration of corticosteroids has long been predicted to produce atrophic changes in neurons within the hippocampal formation (Arbel et al., 1994; Sousa et al., 2000). Thus, stereologic studies of postmortem tissue require full consideration of each patient's full pharmacological profile and their possible impact on brain structure.

Lessons Learned from Stereology: Toward a More Unified Approach to Brain Banking and Postmortem Tissue Research (and Beyond!)

The relative paucity in studies that use stereological methods reflects the potential pitfalls associated with scientifically sound and meaningful analyses using human postmortem brain tissue. Published studies of this type vary in quality in terms of the degree of adherence to stereological protocol, as well as the ability to account for the potential confounds, such as histopathological factors and the quality of clinical assessment. Nevertheless, such studies have yielded vital information on potential neuroanatomical deficits in psychiatric disorders, such as schizophrenia (Stark et al., 2004; Kreczmanski et al., 2007; Dorph-Petersen et al., 2009; Schmitt et al., 2009), major depression (Rajkowska et al., 1999, 2005; Khundakar et al., 2009, 2011), and bipolar disorder (Rajkowska, 2002), alcohol abuse (Miguel-Hidalgo et al., 2002, 2006; Andersen, 2004; Underwood et al., 2007), and neurodegenerative disorders such as Alzheimer's (Mouton et al., 1998; Gemmell et al., 2012) and Parkinson's disease (Joelving et al., 2006). The fact that *in vivo* neuroimaging techniques currently do not provide sufficient temporal, spatial, and neurochemical resolution highlights the need for expansion of high quality, scientifically robust studies using well-documented postmortem tissue. One should therefore not be discouraged from what may seem insurmountable issues when planning a stereological study using brain bank material. Rather, as stated in an excellent review of stereological approaches in neuropathology (Dorph-Petersen and Lewis, 2011), thorough documentation of methodological details and references will allow readers to judge the rigor of each study, as well as to perform replication experiments. As summarized in he following section, lessons learned from prior stereological analysis in the brain bank setting ensure that brains donated for scientific research receive proper processing for systematic and unbiased analysis.

Obtain the Full Reference Volume or "Make Do and Mend"

As described earlier, optimal analysis of brain tissue using design-based stereology requires proper tissue sampling at dissection. An important first step is sampling through the entire extent of tissue to support total volume estimation for the maximal number of subregions. In the past two decades, pioneers in the stereology field have published excellent examples of applications to postmortem tissue obtained from human brains, including teams led by Gundersen (Tang et al., 1997), Pakkenberg (Pedersen et al., 2005), West (Korbo and West, 2000), Mouton (Mouton et al., 1998), and Dorph-Petersen and Lewis (Dorph-Petersen et al., 2009). These studies show the advantages of collecting tissue with the express purpose of carrying out high-quality stereological studies. Studies in a typical brain bank setting, however, must depend on a library of predefined blocks, with little or no influence over tissue dissection or sampling at brain cutting. As tissue from certain disease groups is often precious, and many stereology parameters, such as total cell number, require thicker sections (>10 um after processing), the responsibility falls to individual researchers to justify, either to staff members, fund-holders or lay members of a committee, requests for comparatively large tissue samples than that for 2D analysis. One obvious approach is to convince brain bank staff of the merits of standardizing stereological protocols into brain banking procedure. The involvement of a dedicated stereology expert, or neuropathology technician with knowledge of stereological theory and practice, allows for a more systematic approach to dissection and sampling of brains and tissue blocks. Such protocols facilitate routine analyses of numerous small and large anatomical regions from the each brain, including the hippocampus, striatum, amygdala, and neocortex, as well as nonstructural estimates such as volume of brain ventricles volumes and cerebral infarct volumes.

As a first step, the entire brain may be cut into blocks at precisely defined intervals (from 5 mm to 1 cm) using a cutting guide (Fabricius et al., 2007; Pelvig et al., 2008), or alternatively dissected to allow for neuropathological assessment, with the structures of interest removed and subdissected into blocks of known thickness (for an excellent summary of this protocol see Perl et al. (2000). Second, random positioning of a point grid with known area per point may be used to estimate the reference area for volume estimation of defined brain regions. Finally, these methods allow for estimation of total volume for defined anatomical regions using Cavalieri's formulae:

$$V = T \cdot a(p) \cdot \sum P, \tag{10.1}$$

where T is the slab thickness or intersectional distance, $a(p)$ is the area per point, and $\sum P$ is the sum of points hitting the reference area.

Alternatively, one section may be removed from the face of tissue blocks (slabs) sampled in a systematic-random manner, stained, and regional volume(s) estimated by the point counting-Cavalieri method with assistance from a computerized stereology system. Volume estimation for brain regions of interest provides the basis for analyzing other parameters or damage such as neuron and glial cell number, vessel length, white matter infarct volume, and so on, according to stereological principles.

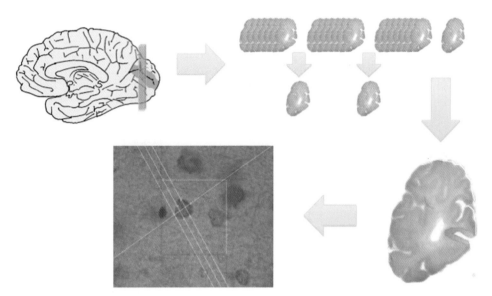

Figure 10.1 Calculation of neuronal density using an adapted optical disector approach. A number of serial sections are cut from the front of a block and sampled in a uniform random manner (e.g., 3 taken from 21). Reference area (e.g., calcarine fissure of the primary visual cortex) drawn at low magnification. Counts and particle volume measured at high magnification using the "optical disector" and "rotator" probes.

The ideal scenario outlined above follows implementation of stereological protocol at an early stage. However, many established brain banks have large libraries of blocks cut prior to the recognition of proper tissue processing and sampling for stereology. If only a single block, or other amount of tissue representing an unknown fraction of the total reference volume is available, then sampling can be performed from a number of serial sections taken from an anatomically defined structure present in all specimens, as shown in Figure 10.1. Though tissue samples may differ in length from the frontal pole, this strategy allows for representative sampling through a consistent volume of tissue, that is, from the frontal pole through a distance available for sampling in all specimens for the study. When a consistent volume of tissue can be sampled from an anatomically defined point in this manner, total parameters such as total cell number, total capillary length, and so on, may be estimated for comparison purposes.

Turn Down the "Noise"

Questions remain about the extent of molecular damage that occurs in the interval between death and tissue preservation. Nevertheless, shorter PMIs effectively reduce tissue damage that begins immediately after death. For this reason, the most favorable tissue preparation results when brain removal occurs as soon as possible after death, that is, with minimal PMI, such as through an "on-call" service 24 hours a day, 7 days a week. In addition to the PMI for each brain, detailed recording of all possible mortality-related variables should be part of the brain bank's operating procedure since several factors, such as agonal state, refrigeration of the body, and method of brain removal (Lewis, 2002), as well as the specific fixative solution and the duration of brain storage in fixative could affect the degree of tissue preservation, and thus may confound subsequent comparison of stereology parameters between groups. As stated earlier, numerous factors can affect tissue shrinkage and antigenicity of certain proteins, and as such should be controlled and monitored. By standardizing the properties and duration of the fixation process, one can minimize potential hidden sources of bias that may affect the final outcome of any stereological study. If using immunohistochemical procedures, a pilot calibration study is critical to ensure the penetration of z-axis labeling of antigens in the reference volume. If full penetration is not readily apparent, then methodological adjustments may be taken, for example, modification in antigen retrieval method, longer primary antibody incubation. Failing this, stereological approaches applicable to thin sections, such as the physical disector method, could be implemented.

"Check the Information, Expand the Knowledge"

The depth of knowledge of the donor's clinical profile determines the value of the tissue sample to the researcher. For the application of stringent inclusion and exclusion criteria, standardized clinical information for each case, including detailed clinical information collected during life by qualified physicians and psychologists using strict diagnostic criteria, provides the most accurate and reliable data. Though retrospective "psychological autopsies" are still frequently used to define specific patient groups, the robustness of this approach has been questioned. In one study, 30% of chart-based retrospective diagnoses were not confirmed after clinical reassessment of patients (Haroutunian and Davis, 2002). Thus, the strength of conclusions depends on the quality of the information collected on a case-by-case basis. Ideally, the database will contain all information describing and characterizing the clinical and postmortem features of the brain tissue, as well as antemortem or postmortem neuroimaging data and any other light microscopic and ultrastructural analyses carried out on each case. Such a readily accessible database of key information provides valuable support for stereological studies of human postmortem brains. A final but important step is database management to include regular updates of analysis carried out on postmortem tissue, for example, volume estimates from the Cavalieri method.

Show Your Work!

Though design-based stereology is based on the fundamental principles of stochastic geometry and probability theory, the applications of these concepts to each study requires careful attention on the part of individual investigators to identify, avoid, and/or minimize the introduction of nonverifiable assumptions and sources of systematic error (bias). To help disseminate accurate conclusions to the neuroscience community, the more information disclosed to the reader regarding study design, the greater their ability to judge its strength and to identify potential weaknesses. We recommend the following as the basic information for research papers involving the applications of stereological protocols to human postmortem tissue:

- *Dissection procedure.* How the brain was removed and cut.
- *Cutting process.* Whether the sampled sections were taken from serial sectioning or at intervals throughout the reference volume.
- *Staining method.* The histochemical or immunohistochemical procedure, whether on free-floating or slide-mounted sections, counterstaining, and calibration study done to identify optimal antibody concentration for full penetration.
- *Tissue sampling design.* How sections were sampled from the reference volume, for example, systematic-random sampling, with fraction of sections sampled from the total number of sections through the reference volume (section sampling fraction).
- *Instrumentation.* Cryostat/microtome, microscope, objectives, stage, microcator, software package, and so on.

- *Analytical procedure.* Specific probe(s), for example, disector, area and height, distance between sprobe, guard zones, tissue thickness.
- *Sampling error information.* Pilot information revealing optimal study design, method for calculation of the coefficient of error (CE), comparison of CE with biological variation (BV).

Conclusion

The gift of brain donation affords scientists the opportunity to examine the most complex tissue known to man. It is thus vitally important that the most appropriate analytical methods are used to ensure that the gift is worthwhile. The revolution of stereological research in the past five decades offers the powerful opportunity to better understand the human postmortem tissue collected in the brain bank setting.

Acknowledgments

We sincerely thank Chris Morris, Johannes Attems, Arthur Oakley, and the technical staff at the Newcastle Brain Tissue Resource for their expert advice and comments.

References

Andersen, B. B. 2004. Reduction of Purkinje cell volume in cerebellum of alcoholics. *Brain Res* **1007**: 10–18.

Arbel, I., Kadar, T., Silbermann, M., Levy, A. 1994. The effects of long-term corticosterone administration on hippocampal morphology and cognitive performance of middle-aged rats. *Brain Res* **657**: 227–235.

Bahn, S., Augood, S. J., Ryan, M., Standaert, D. G., Starkey, M., Emson, P. C. 2001. Gene expression profiling in the post-mortem human brain—no cause for dismay. *J Chem Neuroanat* **22**: 79–94.

Barton, A. J., Pearson, R. C., Najlerahim, A., Harrison, P. J. 1993. Pre- and post-mortem influences on brain RNA. *J Neurochem* **61**: 1–11.

Beach, T. G., Tago, H., Nagai, T., Kimura, H., McGeer, P. L., McGeer, E. G. 1987. Perfusion-fixation of the human brain for immunohistochemistry: comparison with immersion-fixation. *J Neurosci Methods* **19**: 183–192.

Benes, F. M., Lange, N. 2001. Two-dimensional versus three-dimensional cell counting: a practical perspective. *Trends Neurosci* **24**: 11–17.

Braendgaard, H., Gundersen, H. J. 1986. The impact of recent stereological advances on quantitative studies of the nervous system. *J Neurosci Methods* **18**: 39–78.

Calhoun, M. E., Mouton, P. R. 2001. Length measurement: new developments in neurostereology and 3D imagery. *J Chem Neuroanat* **21**: 257–265.

Clarke, P. G. 1992. How inaccurate is the Abercrombie correction factor for cell counts? *Trends Neurosci* **15**: 211–212.

Dedova, I., Harding, A., Sheedy, D., Garrick, T., Sundqvist, N., Hunt, C., Gillies, J., Harper, C. G. 2009. The importance of brain banks for molecular neuropathological research: the New South wales tissue resource centre experience. *Int J Mol Sci* **10**: 366–384.

Dorph-Petersen, K. A., Lewis, D. A. 2011. Stereological approaches to identifying neuropathology in psychosis. *Biol Psychiatry* **69**: 113–126.

Dorph-Petersen, K. A., Nyengaard, J. R., Gundersen, H. J. 2001. Tissue shrinkage and unbiased stereological estimation of particle number and size. *J Microsc* **204**: 232–246.

Dorph-Petersen, K. A., Caric, D., Saghafi, R., Zhang, W., Sampson, A. R., Lewis, D. A. 2009. Volume and neuron number of the lateral geniculate nucleus in schizophrenia and mood disorders. *Acta Neuropathol* **117**: 369–384.

D'Sa, C., Duman, R. S. 2002. Antidepressants and neuroplasticity. *Bipolar Disord* **4**: 183–194.

Everall, I., Harrison, P. J. 2002. Methodological and stereological considerations in post-mortem psychiatric research. In *The Post-mortem Brain in Psychiatric Research*, edited by G. Agam, I. Everall, and R. Belmaker, pp. 21–36. Boston: Kluwer Academic.

Fabricius, K., Pakkenberg, H., Pakkenberg, B. 2007. No changes in neocortical cell volumes or glial cell numbers in chronic alcoholic subjects compared to control subjects. *Alcohol* **42**: 400–406.

Gemmell, E., Bosomworth, H., Allan, L., Hall, R., Khundakar, A., Oakley, A. E., Deramecourt, V., Polvikoski, T. M., O'Brien, J. T., Kalaria, R. N. 2012. Hippocampal neuronal atrophy and cognitive function in delayed poststroke and aging-related dementias. *Stroke* **43**: 808–814.

Haroutunian, V., Davis, K. L. 2002. Issues and perspectives on brain tissue banking. *Curr Psychiatry Rep* **4**: 233–234.

Harrison, P. J., Heath, P. R., Eastwood, S. L., Burnet, P. W., McDonald, B., Pearson, R. C. 1995. The relative importance of premortem acidosis and post-mortem interval for human brain gene expression studies: selective mRNA vulnerability and comparison with their encoded proteins. *Neurosci Lett* **200**: 151–154.

Haug, H., Kuhl, S., Mecke, E., Sass, N. L., Wasner, K. 1984. The significance of morphometric procedures in the investigation of age changes in cytoarchitectonic structures of human brain. *J Hirnforsch* **25**: 353–374.

Hedreen, J. C. 1998. What was wrong with the Abercrombie and empirical cell counting methods? *A review. Anat Rec* **250**: 373–380.

Hyatt, M. A. 1989. *Priciples and Techniques of Electron Microscopy*, 3rd ed. Gaithersburg, MD: Macmillan Press.

Joelving, F. C., Billeskov, R., Christensen, J. R., West, M., Pakkenberg, B. 2006. Hippocampal neuron and glial cell numbers in Parkinson's disease—a stereological study. *Hippocampus* **16**: 826–833.

Khundakar, A., Morris, C., Oakley, A., Thomas, A. J. 2011. Morphometric analysis of neuronal and glial cell pathology in the caudate nucleus in late-life depression. *Am J Geriatr Psychiatry* **19**: 132–141.

Khundakar, A. A., Morris, C. M., Oakley, A. E., McMeekin, W., Thomas, A. J. 2009. Morphometric analysis of neuronal and glial cell pathology in the dorsolateral prefrontal cortex in late-life depression. *Br J Psychiatry* **195**: 163–169.

Korbo, L., West, M. 2000. No loss of hippocampal neurons in AIDS patients. *Acta Neuropathol* **99**: 529–533.

Kreczmanski, P., Heinsen, H., Mantua, V., Woltersdorf, F., Masson, T., Ulfig, N., Schmidt-Kastner, R., Korr, H., Steinbusch, H. W., Hof, P. R., Schmitz, C. 2007. Volume, neuron density and total neuron number in five subcortical regions in schizophrenia. *Brain* **130**: 678–692.

Lewis, D. A. 2002. The human brain revisited: opportunities and challenges in post-mortem studies of psychiatric disorders. *Neuropsychopharmacology* **26**: 143–154.

Lowenberg, M., Stahn, C., Hommes, D. W., Buttgereit, F. 2008. Novel insights into mechanisms of glucocorticoid action and the development of new glucocorticoid receptor ligands. *Steroids* **73**: 1025–1029.

McCullumsmith, R. E., Meador-Woodruff, J. H. 2011. Novel approaches to the study of post-mortem brain in psychiatric illness: old limitations and new challenges. *Biol Psychiatry* **69**: 127–133.

Miguel-Hidalgo, J. J., Overholser, J. C., Meltzer, H. Y., Stockmeier, C. A., Rajkowska, G. 2002. Glia pathology in the prefrontal cortex in alcohol dependence with and without depressive symptoms. *Biol Psychiatry* **52**: 1121–1133.

Miguel-Hidalgo, J. J., Wei, J., Andrew, M., Overholser, J. C., Jurjus, G., Stockmeier, C. A., Rajkowska, G. 2006. Reduced glial and neuronal packing density in the orbitofrontal cortex in alcohol dependence and its relationship with suicide and duration of alcohol dependence. *Alcohol Clin Exp Res* **30**: 1845–1855.

Monteggia, L. M., Barrot, M., Powell, C. M., Berton, O., Galanis, V., Gemelli, T., Meuth, S., Nagy, A., Greene, R. W., Nestler, E. J. 2004. Essential role of brain-derived neurotrophic factor in adult hippocampal function. *Proc Natl Acad Sci U S A* **101**: 10827–10832.

Mouton, P. R., Martin, L. J., Calhoun, M. E., Dal Forno, G., Price, D. L. 1998. Cognitive decline strongly correlates with cortical atrophy in Alzheimer's dementia. *Neurobiol Aging* **19**: 371–377.

Mouton, P. R., Gokhale, A. M., Ward, N. L., West, M. J. 2002. Stereological length estimation using spherical probes. *J Microsc* **206**: 54–64.

Pedersen, K. M., Marner, L., Pakkenberg, H., Pakkenberg, B. 2005. No global loss of neocortical neurons in Parkinson's disease: a quantitative stereological study. *Mov Disord* **20**: 164–171.

Pelvig, D. P., Pakkenberg, H., Stark, A. K., Pakkenberg, B. 2008. Neocortical glial cell numbers in human brains. *Neurobiol Aging* **29**: 1754–1762.

Perl, D. P., Good, P. F., Bussiere, T., Morrison, J. H., Erwin, J. M., Hof, P. R. 2000. Practical approaches to stereology in the setting of aging- and disease-related brain banks. *J Chem Neuroanat* **20**: 7–19.

Plum, F. 1972. Neuropathological findings. In *Prospects for Research in Scizophrenia*, edited by S. S. Kety and S. M. Malthysse, pp. 385–388. Cambridge, MA: MIT Press.

Rajkowska, G. 2002. Cell pathology in bipolar disorder. *Bipolar Disord* **4**: 105–116.

Rajkowska, G., Miguel-Hidalgo, J. J., Wei, J., Dilley, G., Pittman, S. D., Meltzer, H. Y., Overholser, J. C., Roth, B. L., Stockmeier, C. A. 1999. Morphometric evidence for neuronal and glial prefrontal cell pathology in major depression. *Biol Psychiatry* **45**: 1085–1098.

Rajkowska, G., Miguel-Hidalgo, J. J., Dubey, P., Stockmeier, C. A., Krishnan, K. R. 2005. Prominent reduction in pyramidal neurons density in the orbitofrontal cortex of elderly depressed patients. *Biol Psychiatry* **58**: 297–306.

Ross, B. M., Knowler, J. T., McCulloch, J. 1992. On the stability of messenger RNA and ribosomal RNA in the brains of control human subjects and patients with Alzheimer's disease. *J Neurochem* **58**: 1810–1819.

Schmitt, A., Steyskal, C., Bernstein, H. G., Schneider-Axmann, T., Parlapani, E., Schaeffer, E. L., Gattaz, W. F., Bogerts, B., Schmitz, C., Falkai, P. 2009. Stereologic investigation of the posterior part of the hippocampus in schizophrenia. *Acta Neuropathol* **117**: 395–407.

Schmitz, C., Hof, P. R. 2005. Design-based stereology in neuroscience. *Neuroscience* **130**: 813–831.

Sousa, N., Lukoyanov, N. V., Madeira, M. D., Almeida, O. F., Paula-Barbosa, M. M. 2000. Reorganization of the morphology of hippocampal neurites and synapses after stress-induced damage correlates with behavioral improvement. *Neuroscience* **97**: 253–266.

Stan, A. D., Ghose, S., Gao, X. M., Roberts, R. C., Lewis-Amezcua, K., Hatanpaa, K. J., Tamminga, C. A. 2006. Human post-mortem tissue: what quality markers matter? *Brain Res* **1123**: 1–11.

Stark, A. K., Uylings, H. B., Sanz-Arigita, E., Pakkenberg, B. 2004. Glial cell loss in the anterior cingulate cortex, a subregion of the prefrontal cortex, in subjects with schizophrenia. *Am J Psychiatry* **161**: 882–888.

Sterio, D. C. 1984. The unbiased estimation of number and sizes of arbitrary particles using the disector. *J Microsc* **134**: 127–136.

Stockmeier, C. A., Mahajan, G. J., Konick, L. C., Overholser, J. C., Jurjus, G. J., Meltzer, H. Y., Uylings, H. B., Friedman, L., Rajkowska, G. 2004. Cellular changes in the post-mortem hippocampus in major depression. *Biol Psychiatry* **56**: 640–650.

Tang, Y., Nyengaard, J. R., Pakkenberg, B., Gundersen, H. J. 1997. Age-induced white matter changes in the human brain: a stereological investigation. *Neurobiol Aging* **18**: 609–615.

Underwood, M. D., Mann, J. J., Arango, V. 2007. Morphometry of dorsal raphe nucleus serotonergic neurons in alcoholism. *Alcohol Clin Exp Res* **31**: 837–845.

Vonsattel, J. P., Del Amaya, M. P., Keller, C. E. 2008. Twenty-first century brain banking. Processing brains for research: the Columbia University methods. *Acta Neuropathol* **115**: 509–532.

West, M. J., Slomanka, L. 2001. 2-D versus 3-D cell counting—a debate. What is an optical disector? *Trends Neurosci* **24**: 374; author reply 378–380.

11 Visualization of Blood Vessels in Two-Dimensional and Three-Dimensional Environments for Vascular Stereology in the Brain

Zerina Lokmic

Department of Plastic and Maxillofacial Surgery and Department of Nursing Research, Murdoch Children's Research Institute and the Royal Children's Hospital, Parkville, Victoria, Australia

Background

The survival and function of the central nervous system (CNS) critically depend on blood flow for oxygen and nutrients and removal of carbon dioxide and other metabolic waste. In addition to this extreme reliance on a continuous blood supply, the CNS maintains spatial separation between the systemic blood circulation and the brain/spinal cord via two structural entities: the blood–brain barrier (BBB) at the level of CNS microvasculature and blood–cerebrospinal fluid barrier at the epithelial cells of the choroid plexus (Engelhardt and Sorokin, 2009).

The fully differentiated BBB includes a variety of structures such as highly specialized endothelial cells (ECs), their underlying basement membrane (BM) with numerous pericytes in direct communication with the ECs, perivascular antigen presenting cells, and astrocyte end-feet with their associated parenchymal BM (Zlokovic, 2008; Engelhardt and Sorokin, 2009). In contrast to the peripheral vascular system, the blood vessels in CNS lack fenestrations in their ECs, and show extremely low pinocytic activity and junctional complexes in the form of tight junctions and adherens junctions (both act to restrict EC permeability) and recently identified gap junctions likely to mediate intercellular communication (Nagasawa et al., 2006; Zlokovic, 2008). The BBB combined with neurons and non-neuronal cells form a functional unit also known as the neurovascular unit (Figure 11.1a) (Lo et al., 2003).

Loss or impairment of BBB integrity in pathological conditions alters the cellular chemical milieu of neurons, which in turn impairs neuronal function and may result in permanent neuronal damage. Understanding the role of blood vessels in these pathological processes, such as in the mouse model of experimental autoimmune encephalomyelitis (EAE) (Sixt et al., 2001) or in Alzheimer's disease (Bailey et al., 2004), helps to better understand disease pathophysiology and facilitates the delivery of potential therapeutic agents.

Vascular Stereology of Tissue Sections

Our approach to vascular stereology of visualized blood vessels is based on methodology described in excellent reference books by stereology experts, including Cruz-Orive and Weibel (1990), Dockery and Fraher (2007), Howard and Reed (2005), and Mouton (2011). Selection of the best

Neurostereology: Unbiased Stereology of Neural Systems, First Edition. Edited by Peter R. Mouton.
© 2014 John Wiley & Sons, Inc. Published 2014 by John Wiley & Sons, Inc.

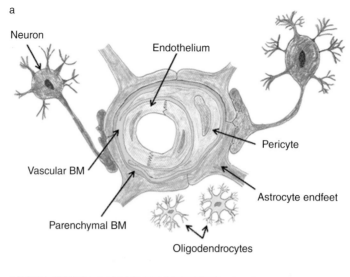

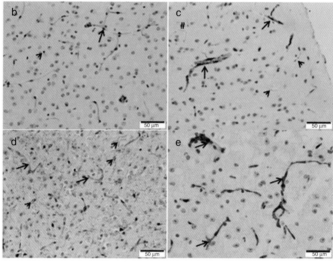

Figure 11.1 (a) Schematic representation of the neurovascular unit (see Zlokovic, 2008 and Engelhardt and Sorokin, 2009) whose vascular components can be individually visualized for the purpose of vascular morphometry. ECs and pericytes are encased in vascular BM. Parenchymal BM surrounds the vascular components and separates the blood vessel from the brain tissue cells such as neurons and oligodendrocytes. (b) CD31 antibody effectively labels all blood vessels within the mouse brain tissue (arrow) using diaminobenzidine chromogen. Note that careful evaluation is required particularly where CD31 labels only the smallest visible parts of the vessel (due to section plane). (c) The von Willebrand factor also labels most of the blood vessels (arrows); however, on some occasions, depending on the section, the staining is granular (small arrow) and hardly noticeable due to the absence of defined EC structure. Also note that some vessels do not label at all (#) which will affect the vascular morphometry results. This emphasizes the need to test multiple markers for optimal vascular identification to ensure accurate morphometric counts. (d) Tomato lectin is often used to visualize blood vessels (arrow); however, its interpretation in thin brain sections is hindered by lectin labeling of microglial cells (short arrow) which may be an issue when the user is not familiar with the vascular structures. (e) α-SMA antibody is used here in combination with Fast Red chromogen to identify individual blood vessels containing smooth muscle cells (arrows).

vascular parameters to investigate and the particular methodology is made during the earliest stages of the experimental design, that is, when the research question is posed and hypothesis defined. Our laboratory focuses on the biology of atrioventricular malformations (AVMs) and angiogenesis. As a result, the most frequently assessed vascular stereological parameters analyzed involve vascular volume/volume density, surface/surface density, length/length density, and number/numerical density. Other parameters available for specific study designs include number of brain segments in three dimensional (3D), segment length, vessel diameter and cross-sectional area, diffusion distance, vessel wall thickness, and vessel network branching (Weibel, 1973, 1975; Parsons-Wingerter et al., 1998; Howard and Reed, 2005; Lee et al., 2005; Dockery and Fraher, 2007; Hyde et al., 2007).

The value of performing design-based stereology is in the statistical (random) sampling combined with geometric probes to generate 3D data where no assumptions exist regarding tissue or target size, shape, distribution, or orientation of the target analyzed (Howard and Reed, 2005). However, the stereological data generated, particularly in regard to tissue volume, are affected by biological and technical factors such as tissue collection, fixation, tissue processing into frozen or paraffin blocks, storage, defining region of interest, targets to count, and reference space and sources of random and systemic errors (Howard and Reed, 2005; Dockery and Fraher, 2007; Mouton, 2011). Subsequently, every attempt is made to minimize the influence of these factors. Once the decision is made on parameters to count, the choice is made on the best vascular marker and visualization method to delineate as many blood vessels as possible and the tissue is prepared accordingly. A word of caution: not every vascular marker will identify every blood vessel in the tissue. Therefore, failure to critically evaluate vessel staining will detrimentally affect the accuracy of vascular stereology.

Tissue Processing

In our laboratory, the brain tissue is collected by dissection of unfixed brain tissue from the skull, followed by weight and volume displacement measurement using an electronic balance with the water displacement method (Hughes, 2005). Tissue is sliced vertically with 2 mm between slices before embedding into O.C.T. freezing media (4583, Tissue-Tek®, Sekura Finetek, Torrance, CA). The tissue is frozen by simply gently lowering the tissue onto the surface of liquid nitrogen until the O.C.T. turns white, then transferring the specimen onto dry ice for a further 10 minutes before storage at −80°C for 24 h prior to sectioning. The brain sections (ranging from 5- to 100-μm thickness) are always stored at −80°C (for a maximum of 6 months) and are fixed prior to immunostaining. Various fixatives (fixation duration maximum is 2 minutes for thin sections and 10 minutes for 100-μm-thick sections) are employed in pursuit of optimal immunohistochemical staining and minimal tissue shrinkage.

Quantitative analysis of vascular parameters with unbiased stereology avoids or minimizes the introduction of systematic error (bias) while reducing random errors (biological and error variance) to an acceptable level (Cruz-Orive and Weibel, 1990; Howard and Reed, 2005; Dockery and Fraher, 2007; Mouton, 2011).

Defining the Reference Volume

The volume of reference space is the tissue region of interest based on anatomical boundaries. This reference volume may be the entire region containing the target of interest, for example, stained vessels. Systematic-random sampling ensures that each section through the reference volume has an equal probability of being selected for analysis.

Choosing the Appropriate Stereological Probe

To estimate various vascular parameters, a range of different probes (grids) of zero dimension (0D) to 3D are placed at systematic-random locations through the reference space. Since design-based stereology provides information on valid 3D structural data, the sum of the dimension probe and feature analyzed must sum to 3 (Howard and Reed, 2005; Mouton, 2011). For example, to estimate vessel volume (a 3D feature), a 0D probe (point grid) is used (3 + 0 = 3); to estimate vessel length, a plane (two-dimensional [2D] probe) with a one-dimensional feature (2 + 1 = 3) is used. With the aid of computerized microscope stage and stereology software, the grid is randomly applied to the tissue section and the intersection between the test probe and the object of interest is counted in order to estimate the parameter of interest.

Visualization of Brain Blood Vessels

Unequivocal identification of blood vessels in any tissue is possible when vascular components are clearly delineated from the surrounding tissue. In morphological terms, the layers of arteries, veins, and capillaries include three layers from luminal to abluminal surfaces: tunica intima, tunica media, and tunica adventitia. Tunica intima ("inner coat") is composed of ECs and abluminal endothelial BM. In arteries, the internal elastic lamina is easily identifiable as a part of the tunica intima situated deep to the EC layer and associated BM. The tunica media ("middle coat") of arteries and veins contain vascular smooth muscle cells (vSMCs), while tunica media of capillaries consists of pericytes. The tunica adventitia or tunica externa ("outer coat") is composed of connective tissue embedded with small nerves and vasa vasorum, the feeding vessels for the blood vessel itself. The ECs, vSMCs, pericytes, and the BM components can be identified with antibodies targeting cell-specific markers, as well as major and minor building blocks of the BM, a thin sheath-like structure whose primary function is to physically separate tunica intima from tunica media and separate the blood vessel from the surrounding tissue structures (Lokmic et al., 2008).

For examining cellular components that may participate in the disease process, researchers often use multiple vascular cell markers in combination with markers for nonvascular components. For example, studies of the transmigration of leukocytes in brain blood vessels, transmigrating leukocytes, and vascular and astrocyte BMs are simultaneously visualized as reported in the murine EAE model (Sixt et al., 2001). From a histological and morphometric viewpoint, vascular structures can be examined by visualizing blood vessels in 5- to 7-μm-thick tissue sections (2D) or in 3D, such as vascular resin casts of the whole organ, or alternatively in thick tissue sections (30–100 μm) perfused intraluminaly with space-occupying compounds, such as fluorescently labeled dextran or 1,1′-dioctadecyl-3,3,3′,3′-tetramethylindocarbocyanine perchlorate (DiI) (Lokmic and Mitchell, 2011). The following section will review cellular markers currently in use to identify blood vascular ECs, vSMCs, and pericytes and components of BMs in brain tissue sections (2D), followed by current approaches to label blood vessels in 3D environments (whole organ perfusion).

Visualization of Blood Vessels in 2D

EC Identification

Because vascular ECs are highly heterogenous in chemical structure (Garlanda and Dejana, 1997), the optimal choice of antibody for quantification depends on a broad specificity to visualize as many vessels as possible. Quantification for stereology involves a two-step process, starting with scanning the tissue section under low power objectives (10×, 40×) for an overall view of tissue staining and vascular distribution, followed by quantification using high power objectives (60×, 100×). The requirement for data collection at higher magnification permits users to clearly distinguish blood vessels from other tissue components, for example, stromal cells with CD34 immunoprobes and lymphocytes with CD31 immunoprobes (Lokmic and Mitchell, 2011).

Cluster of Differentiation (CD) 31

Platelet EC adhesion molecule 1 (PECAM-1), also known as CD31, is a 130 kDa glycoprotein and a member of the immunoglobulin (Ig) superfamily of cell adhesion molecules (Jackson, 2003). Under normal circumstances, CD31 stains vascular ECs as well as leukocytes, including neutrophils and macrophages, platelets (Newman and Albelda, 1992), and lymphatic ECs (Baluk and McDonald, 2008). Because the murine CNS does not contain lymphatic vessels (Alitalo et al., 2005) and leukocytes may be easily distinguished from blood vessels on the basis of morphology, CD31 is a popular choice for identification of brain blood vessels (Figure 11.1b). Endothelial CD31, which is expressed at the lateral junctions of ECs (Jackson, 2003), is thought to participate in a number of important vascular functions including angiogenesis (DeLisser et al., 1997), maintenance of vascular barrier function and BBB integrity, leukocyte diapedesis (Privratsky et al., 2010), control of EC apoptotic events (Ilan and Madri, 2003), and a protective effect against excessive inflammation, as observed in mouse inducible EAE (Graesser et al., 2002).

CD34

CD34 is a 110 kDa membrane-bound sialomycin (Simmons et al., 1992) expressed widely on small vessel vascular endothelium in all murine organs, including CNS vessels in gray and white matter (Baumhueter et al., 1994; Allen et al., 1996), human nerve sheath tumors, and unidentified cell types within the endoneurium of normal nerves (Chaubal et al., 1994). The function of endothelial CD34 in the brain vascular endothelium and maintenance of the BBB remains unclear, although one proposed function *in vivo* is L-selectin mediated neutrophil rolling in lymphoid tissues during inflammation (Baumhueter et al., 1994), which is likely to also occur in neutrophil extravasation in brain inflammation. In addition to vascular endothelium, CD34 is also expressed by hemopoietic stem and progenitor cells, endothelial progenitor cells (Baumhueter et al., 1994; Young et al., 1995), murine mesenchymal stem cells (Copland et al., 2008), activated fibroblasts, and stromal cells of some tumors (Kutzner, 1993).

The degree of CD34 expression by vascular ECs remains unclear because different monoclonal CD34 antibody clones directed against different epitopes on the human CD34 antigen give variable results. In a study by Fina et al. (1990), seven monoclonal antibodies raised to human CD34 antigen and tested in human tissues revealed only a small percentage of vascular capillaries in CNS, suggesting that CD34 is not an optimal vascular marker for CNS tissue. This is in contrast to numerous reports describing strong expression of CD34 in human arterioles, capillaries, and venules of nonpathological CNS, as well as in studies examining vascular changes in Alzheimer's disease, multiple sclerosis, and CNS tumors.

CD105

CD105, also known as endoglin, is a homodimeric 180 kDa membrane glycoprotein expressed by arteries, veins, and capillaries (McAllister et al., 1994) and in the adventitia of normal brain arteries (Matsubara et al., 2000). CD105 constitutes a part of the transforming growth factor (TGF) beta 1 and beta 3 receptor complex. Mutation in the CD105 gene results in hereditary hemorrhagic telengiectasia type 1, a vascular anomaly associated with AVMs (Shovlin et al., 1997). However, analysis of sporadic cerebral AVMs did not find a correlation between endoglin expression and AVM presentation (Matsubara et al., 2000). Endoglin also labels pericytes (Crisan et al., 2008), vSMCs, bone marrow stromal fibroblasts, and progenitor B cells (Dallas et al., 2008), which may hinder the correct interpretation of vascular parameters in the presence of significant inflammation and tissue repair.

CD146

CD146, also known as Mel-CAM, MUC18, A32 antigen, and S-Endo1 antigen, is a 113- to 119-kDa transmembrane glycoprotein receptor and a member of the Ig superfamily first described as a marker of melanoma progression and metastasis (Johnson et al., 1993). Despite being implicated in pathological processes associated with cancer progression and metastasis and chronic disease development and progression, in nonpathological tissues, CD146 is expressed on vascular ECs, vSMCs and pericytes (Bardin et al., 2001), endothelial progenitor cells (Duda et al., 2006), mesenchymal stem cells (Sorrentino et al., 2008), a subpopulation of activated T lymphocytes (Pickl et al., 1997), and bone marrow fibroblasts (Tormin et al., 2011).

CD146 is predominantly expressed on inter-EC junctions outside of adherens junctions and is coupled to the actin cytoskeleton (Bardin et al., 2001). In the context of EC biology, CD146 plays a role in neovascularization and cation-independent cell adhesion through unknown mechanisms likely to involve an outside-in signaling cascade (Johnson et al., 1997). CD146 is expressed on both brain ECs and pericytes, with stronger expression reported for *in vitro* cultured brain ECs (Tigges et al., 2012), a characteristic useful for flow cytometry-based cell sorting of brain ECs and pericytes.

Vascular Endothelial (VE) Cadherin

Vascular endothelial (VE) cadherin, also known as CD144 and cadherin type 5, is the highly expressed endothelium-specific transmembrane component of the adherens junctions in all endothelia including BBB (Vestweber et al., 2010). During embryological development, VE cadherin plays a significant role in vessel morphogenesis; however, in adult mouse, VE cadherin is an integral regulator of paracellular EC permeability, vascular leukocyte extravasation into inflamed tissue, EC polarity, EC proliferation, and vascular stability (Dejana and Giampietro, 2012). It is thought that VE cadherin mediated downregulation of claudin-5 expression may contribute to impaired BBB integrity (Gavard and Gutkind, 2008).

von Willebrand Factor (vWF)

von Willebrand factor (vWF) (Figure 11.1c) is synthesized by megakaryocytes and ECs, stored in Weibel–Palade bodies, and released to participate in platelet adhesion in response to vessel wall injury and thrombus formation (Ruggeri, 2003). Although intrinsic to ECs, the interpretation of vWF staining may be greatly hindered in the hemorrhagic and traumatized tissues due to release of vWF by both platelets and ECs in an attempt to form a hemostatic plug (Miettinen et al., 1994). Brain tissue contains high concentrations of vWF messenger RNA (mRNA) and vWF antigen (Yamamoto et al., 1998).

Glucose Transporter 1 (GLUT-1)

The transport of glucose across the BBB is mainly regulated by the 55 kDa isoform of GLUT-1 protein (Maher et al., 1994). Electron microscopy studies with immunogold suggest that GLUT-1 is predominantly found on the abluminal membrane (brain side) and not the luminal (blood side) of the endothelial lining in the BBB (Gerhart et al., 1989; Farrell et al., 1992).

Identification of compromised BBB, as well as identification of newly formed BBB in the angiogenic vessels, is facilitated by the combination of GLUT-1 localization with identification of tight junction molecules such as occludin, claudin-3, zona occludens-1, zona occludens-2 and alpha-catenin, and adherens junction molecules such as VE-cadherin and caveolin-1 (Zlokovic, 2008). A 45-kDa GLUT-1 isoform is present in brain glia (Morgello et al., 1995), which should be taken into consideration when purchasing GLUT-1 antibody and interpreting immunohistochemical results.

VSMC and Pericyte Identification

In vivo pericytes and vSMCs, commonly known as "mural cells," located abluminally to ECs are encased in a BM shared with the apposing endothelium. The exact lineage of pericytes, which in the mature form occur in capillaries, precapillary arterioles, collecting venules, and postcapillary venules (Hall, 2006), is unknown. Despite their contractile and vSMC-like phenotype, pericytes act as progenitor cells to osteogenic, chondrogenic, and adipocyte cells (Dellavalle et al., 2007). To date, there have been no reports of a single pericyte-specific marker that would help distinguish pericytes from vSMC *in vivo* or *in vitro*. Instead, the usual approach is to stain with cell markers that detect both pericytes and vSMCs, such as angiopoietin 1, angiopoietin 2, nerve/glial antigen 2 (NG-2), platelet-derived growth factor receptor beta (PDGFR-β), CD 146, alpha smooth muscle actin (α-SMA), and desmin. For staining with multiple immunohistochemical probes, these markers are often used in combination with morphology and EC-specific markers such as CD31 and CD34.

Flow cytometry allows for a more specific distinction of pericytes. Vascular pericytes express mesenchymal stem cell markers CD44, CD73, CD90, CD105 (Crisan et al., 2008), NG-2 proteoglycan, PDGFR-β, the regulator of G-protein signaling (RGS5) (Lamagna and Bergers, 2006), 3G5 anglioside antigen (Sundberg et al., 2002), CD13 (Paradis et al., 2002), and endosialin (CD248), a marker expressed by pericytes in CNS during mouse embryogenesis (Virgintino et al., 2007). In contrast, vSMCs express calponin and caldesmon but lack NG-2 proteoglycan (Hughes and Chan-Ling, 2004). Since α-SMA, desmin, and NG-2 are the most frequently used markers for identification of pericytes and vSMCs, the following section will examine the biology of these molecules.

Alpha Smooth Muscle Actin (α-SMA)

With the NH2 terminal as the major antigenic region, alpha actin is found only in differentiated muscle cells, including vSMCs, microfilamentous bundles of pericytes, and myofibroblasts (Skalli et al., 1989). For the purposes of identifying blood vessels, α-SMA is used alone (Figure 11.1e). Due to the absence of vSMCs on capillaries, not all vessels label with α-SMA. More often, α-SMA is used in combination with CD31, CD34, or lectins since α-SMA also labels activated fibroblasts, which may hinder result interpretation in research models with prominent fibroblasts, that is, tissue repair and regeneration.

It should be emphasized that not all pericytes express α-SMA. In the presence of EC-released TGF-β, pericytes will express α-SMA, whereas in the absence of EC-released TGF-β, the pericytes will express NG-2 and desmin (Song et al., 2005). Interestingly, immunohistochemical analysis of α-SMA distribution in the brain microvasculature of patients with Alzheimer's disease shows reduced α-SMA expression (Ervin et al., 2004), and is inversely related to arteriolar β-amyloid volume (Stopa et al., 2008). The precise mechanism underlying this relationship requires further research.

Desmin

Desmin is a 52-kDa type III intermediate filament found in Z-disk of striated muscle (skeletal and cardiac) and in the dense bodies of smooth muscle cells, including vSMCs (Lazarides and Hubbard, 1976; Hubbard and Lazarides, 1979) and pericytes (Fujimoto and Singer, 1987). Desmin is thought to be essential for the integrity of myofibrils and maintenance of muscle tensile strength since desmin knockout mice develop postnatal defects in skeletal, cardiac, and smooth muscle characterized by cycles of degeneration of myofibers and aberrant regeneration in weight bearing muscles and the diaphragm (Li et al., 1997). Similarly, desmin is likely to play a role in pericyte-regulated capillary blood flow regulation and BBB integrity and permeability (Winkler et al., 2011).

Nerve/Glial Antigen 2 (NG-2)

Transmembrane chondroitin sulfate proteoglycan nerve/glial antigen 2 (NG-2) is a 300-kDa glycoprotein identified in CNS oligodendrocyte progenitors, mural cells of microvasculature, and tumors such as glioblastoma (Stallcup, 2002). In addition to acting as a cell surface receptor for collagen VI (Stallcup et al., 1990), NG-2 also binds directly to basic fibroblast growth factors and platelet-derived growth factor AA (Goretzki et al., 1999), plasminogen, and angiostatin (Goretzki et al., 2000), and plays a role in tumor growth and metastasis (Chekenya et al., 2002).

The brain contains a population of macroglial cells that specifically express NG-2, thus called NG-2 glia, and give rise to oligodendrocytes (Nishiyama et al., 2005). The difficulty of using NG-2 as a marker of pericytes in brain microvasculature is compounded by the presence of NG-2 in immature oligodendrocyte progenitors in the developing brain (Stallcup and Beasley, 1987) and its upregulation in the reactive glia of an injured brain (Levine, 1994). For this reason, a combination of vessel morphology, NG-2, and EC markers is required to identify brain blood vessels with confidence.

Vascular BM Identification

In tissues, two distinct extracellular matrices (ECMs) exist: the interstitial loose connective tissue ECM and thin sheet-like BM matrix. The interstitial ECM is composed of fibrillar-containing collagens and noncollagenous glycoproteins such as tenascin, fibronectin, and various proteoglycans, whereas BM is composed of highly interconnected glycoprotein networks containing collagen IV interconnected to laminin via heparin sulfate proteoglycans, perlecan, and nidogens, as well as some minor components such as agrin and fibulins (Lokmic et al., 2008).

The role of BMs is to separate specific tissue structures such as blood vessels from the surrounding tissues, that is, brain. Structurally, collagen IV remains a part of all BMs, although the laminin composition differs greatly in different BMs. Laminins are cross-shaped heterotrimeric glycoproteins composed of α, β, and γ chains. With five types of α chains, four β, and three γ chains, various combinations have resulted in reports of 15–16 different laminin isoforms to date (Lokmic et al., 2008). Vascular BMs in mouse brain are composed of laminin $\alpha4\beta1\gamma1$ and $\alpha5\beta1\gamma1$ chains, whereas astrocyte BM is composed of $\alpha1\beta1\gamma1$ and $\alpha2\beta1\gamma1$ laminin chains (Figure 11.2c) (Sixt et al., 2001).

Blood vessel endothelium, pericytes, and vSMCs synthesize the components of the BM including laminins. In practice, collagen IV (Figure 11.2a) and pan-laminin antibody (Figure 11.2b,e) that detects $\alpha1$ and $\beta1$ chains are most frequently used to identify BMs in the tissue. Combined with EC markers (Figure 11.2b) and vessel morphology, these antibodies are powerful tools in

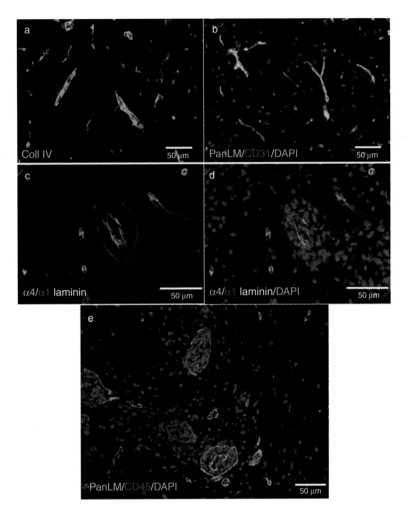

Figure 11.2 (a) Collagen IV and (b) panlaminin antibodies are used to identify brain blood vessels often in combination with EC markers such as CD31 since panlaminin will also identify parenchymal membrane (see e). (c and d) At sites of local inflammation, the vascular BM and parenchymal BM are distinguishable due to leukocyte infiltration (DAPI label, panel d; CD45 label, panel e) and can be visualized by α4 and α1 laminin antibody, respectively. Figures c–e were kindly provided by Dr. Eva Korpos and Prof. Lydia Sorokin, University of Munster, Germany.

delineation of BM: for example, in visualizing leukocyte transmigration across BBB (Figure 11.2d,e) (Graesser et al., 2002; Sixt et al., 2005).

Visualization of Blood Vessels in 3D

Visualization of blood vessels in thick sections for thin-focal plane 3D scanning as required with unbiased stereology requires infusion of the systemic circulation with EC-specific marker such as CD31, carbohydrate-binding lectins, or with cell membrane-binding lypohilic dyes and space-occupying compounds such as dextran, resin, or India ink. These approaches with direct intraluminal labeling avoid the issues of poor antibody penetration through thick sections. Factors in the selection of visualization method include cost of reagents, ease of procedure, and availability of equipment suitable for visualization of fine vessels such as the capillary network or vessels surrounding a specific cellular milieu.

Space-occupying compounds, for example, resin and India ink, have been replaced by advances in microscopy optics, improvement in filters, stability of fluorescent dyes, and greater effectiveness in identifying cell lineages, such as with double or triple cell labeling; hence, space-occupying dyes and resins are not covered here. Fluorescent dyes permit thick tissue sectioning (30–100 µm) and subsequent acquisition of images for stereology studies using computerized stereology systems that combined computer hardware, high resolution microscopy, and software. The following section will briefly address the current methodological approaches to visualizing 3D vascular networks.

Lectins

Lectins are specific nonenzymatic and nonimmune carbohydrate-binding glycoproteins that covalently bind to a carbohydrate moiety expressed on ECs. For example, *Bandeirea simplicifolia* binds to galactose present on mammalian ECs (Alroy et al., 1987), whereas *Lycopersicon esculentum* binds to trimers and tetramers of N-acetylglucosamine oligomers, glycoprotein glycophorin, and Tamm–Horsfall glycoprotein (Nachbar et al., 1980). Injection of approximately 100 µL of relatively inexpensive, azide-free biotinylated or fluorescently conjugated lectin, such as *Lycopersicon esculentum* (tomato lectin, used mostly in mouse) and *Bandeirea simplicifolia* (commonly used in rats) via the tail vein or heart chamber into anesthetized mice 5–10 minutes prior to euthanasia and subsequent perfusion with 4% paraformaldehyde, enables identification of all patent blood vessels within tissues or organs (Bergers et al., 2003).

Removal of lectin infused brain tissue and subsequent sectioning into 50- to 100-µm frozen sections permit confocal study and z-stack acquisition that enables 3D reconstruction of the vascular network within the tissue. Lectin infusion has been successfully demonstrated in brain stroke models whereby the cerebral vascular perfusion was assessed *in vivo* by fluorescein isothiocyanate (FITC)-conjugated lectin angiography (Thiyagarajan et al., 2008) and blood vessel malformations in mouse brain AVMs (Murphy et al., 2008). The use of lectins to immunolabel blood vessels in thin brain tissue sections is hindered by their extensive labeling of microglial cells (Streit and Kreutzberg, 1987) and leukocytes (Matsumoto et al., 2007).

DiI and Tetramethylrhodamine (TMR)

Lypophilic carbocyanine dye DiI has been successfully used to visualize 100-µm-thick brain sections with the aid of confocal microscopy (Li et al., 2008). DiI is a purple compound which, when infused systemically, can be seen macroscopically in larger vessels perfused with DiI. When viewed under a rhodamine filter, DiI stains intensely red. The lipophilic nature of DiI and its lateral diffusion permit its interaction with the cell lipid bilayer and enables labeling of angiogenic sprouts and pseudopodia of angiogenic ECs. Similarly, two-photon microscopy of TMR, a red-orange fluorophore used for protein labeling, perfused mouse cortical vasculature showed that TMR-perfused capillaries (~4–8 nm in diameter) and small arterioles and venules (10–60 mm in diameter) occupy between 3–4% and 4–6% of brain volume, respectively (Zlokovic, 2008).

Dextran

Dextrans are hydrophilic polysaccharides that can be conjugated to fluorophores such as FITC, Alexa Fluor ®, or Cy dyes. Due to their poly-(D-1,6-glucose) linkages, dextrans are biologically inert and, when injected into an animal, act as space-occupying compounds within vessels (Smith et al., 1994; Li et al., 2008). Fluorochrome-conjugated dextrans can be purchased in several molecular weight ranges which facilitates their use in assessing vascular permeability (Bellhorn et al., 1977), *in vivo* assessment of tumor vascularization (Kurozumi et al., 2007), and visualization of the relationship between preexisting brain blood vessels and the developing brain metastasis (Kienast et al., 2010).

Conclusion

Accurate quantification of vascular parameters using unbiased stereology requires clear and accurate delineation of blood vessels from the surrounding tissue. The availability of vascular-specific markers allows investigators to label and quantify vessels within defined reference spaces. Targeting of ECs may be combined with vSMC and BM markers to identify vascular structures, particularly in tissues where their identification is obscured by immunolabeling or tissue processing artifacts, fixation, sectioning plane, and so on.

Vascular stereology enables quantification of alteration of the vascular networks within human tissues or research models by providing the information on vascular volume, surface area, length, and number of vascular structures, as well as number of vessel segments, segment length, vessel diameter, vessel cross-sectional area, diffusion distance, vessel wall thickness, and vessel network branching. Such data provide information on the effect of CNS pathological process on the brain vasculature, as well as the role of specific vascular components in the genesis of diseases. Data of this type carry the promise of enhanced understanding of disease progression and the identification of new therapeutic strategies for disease management.

Acknowledgment

The author thanks Associate Professor Geraldine Mitchell for critical reading of the manuscript and her helpful comments.

References

Alitalo, K., Tammela, T., Petrova, T. V. 2005. Lymphangiogenesis in development and human disease. *Nature* **438** (15): 946–952.

Allen, I. V., McQuaid, S., McMahon, J., Crangle, K., McConnell, R. 1996. The expression of the endothelial cell antigen CD34 in demyelinating disease. *Neuropathol Appl Neurobiol* **22** (2): 101–107.

Alroy, J., Goyal, V., Skutelsky, E. 1987. Lectin histochemistry of mammalian endothelium. *Histochemistry* **86** (6): 603–607.

Bailey, T. L., Rivara, C. B., Rocher, A. B., Hof, P. R. 2004. The nature and effects of cortical microvascular pathology in aging and Alzheimer's disease. *Neurol Res* **26** (5): 573–578.

Baluk, P., McDonald, D. M. 2008. Markers for microscopic imaging of lymphangiogenesis and angiogenesis. *Ann N Y Acad Sci* **1131**: 1–12.

Bardin, N., Anfosso, F., Masse, J. M., Cramer, E., Sabatier, F., Le Bivic, A. et al. 2001. Identification of CD146 as a component of the endothelial junction involved in the control of cell-cell cohesion. *Blood* **98** (13): 3677–3684.

Baumhueter, S., Dybdal, N., Kyle, C., Lasky, L. A. 1994. Global vascular expression of murine CD34, a sialomucin-like endothelial ligand for L-selectin. *Blood* **84** (8): 2554–2565.

Bellhorn, M. B., Bellhorn, R. W., Poll, D. S. 1977. Permeability of fluorescein-labelled dextrans in fundus fluorescein angiography of rats and birds. *Exp Eye Res* **24** (6): 595–605.

Bergers, G., Song, S., Meyer-Morse, N., Bergsland, E., Hanahan, D. 2003. Benefits of targeting both pericytes and endothelial cells in the tumor vasculature with kinase inhibitors. *J Clin Invest* **111** (9): 1287–1295.

Chaubal, A., Paetau, A., Zoltick, P., Miettinen, M. 1994. CD34 immunoreactivity in nervous system tumors. *Acta Neuropathol* **88** (5): 454–458.

Chekenya, M., Hjelstuen, M., Enger, P. O., Thorsen, F., Jacob, A. L., Probst, B. et al. 2002. NG2 proteoglycan promotes angiogenesis-dependent tumor growth in CNS by sequestering angiostatin. *FASEB J* **16** (6): 586–588.

Copland, I., Sharma, K., Lejeune, L., Eliopoulos, N., Stewart, D., Liu, P. et al. 2008. CD34 expression on murine marrow-derived mesenchymal stromal cells: impact on neovascularization. *Exp Hematol* **36** (1): 93–103.

Crisan, M., Yap, S., Casteilla, L., Chen, C. W., Corselli, M., Park, T. S. et al. 2008. A perivascular origin for mesenchymal stem cells in multiple human organs. *Cell Stem Cell* **3** (3): 301–313.

Cruz-Orive, L. M., Weibel, E. R. 1990. Recent stereological methods for cell biology: a brief survey. *Am J Physiol* **258** (4 Pt 1): L148–L156.

Dallas, N. A., Samuel, S., Xia, L., Fan, F., Gray, M. J., Lim, S. J. et al. 2008. Endoglin (CD105): a marker of tumor vasculature and potential target for therapy. *Clin Cancer Res* **14** (7): 1931–1937.

Dejana, E., Giampietro, C. 2012. Vascular endothelial-cadherin and vascular stability. *Curr Opin Hematol* **19** (3): 218–223.

Dellavalle, A., Sampaolesi, M., Tonlorenzi, R., Tagliafico, E., Sacchetti, B., Perani, L. et al. 2007. Pericytes of human skeletal muscle are myogenic precursors distinct from satellite cells. *Nat Cell Biol* **9** (3): 255–267.

DeLisser, H. M., Christofidou-Solomidou, M., Strieter, R. M., Burdick, M. D., Robinson, C. S., Wexler, R. S. et al. 1997. Involvement of endothelial PECAM-1/CD31 in angiogenesis. *Am J Pathol* **151** (3): 671–677.

Dockery, P., Fraher, J. 2007. The quantification of vascular beds: a stereological approach. *Exp Mol Pathol* **82**: 110–120.

Duda, D. G., Cohen, K. S., di Tomaso, E., Au, P., Klein, R. J., Scadden, D. T. et al. 2006. Differential CD146 expression on circulating versus tissue endothelial cells in rectal cancer patients: implications for circulating endothelial and progenitor cells as biomarkers for antiangiogenic therapy. *J Clin Oncol* **24** (9): 1449–1453.

Engelhardt, B., Sorokin, L. 2009. The blood-brain and the blood-cerebrospinal fluid barriers: function and dysfunction. *Semin Immunopathol* **31** (4): 497–511.

Ervin, J. F., Pannell, C., Szymanski, M., Welsh-Bohmer, K., Schmechel, D. E., Hulette, C. M. 2004. Vascular smooth muscle actin is reduced in Alzheimer disease brain: a quantitative analysis. *J Neuropathol Exp Neurol* **63** (7): 735–741.

Farrell, C. L., Yang, J., Pardridge, W. M. 1992. GLUT-1 glucose transporter is present within apical and basolateral membranes of brain epithelial interfaces and in microvascular endothelia with and without tight junctions. *J Histochem Cytochem* **40** (2): 193–199.

Fina, L., Molgaard, H. V., Robertson, D., Bradley, N. J., Monaghan, P., Delia, D. et al. 1990. Expression of the CD34 gene in vascular endothelial cells. *Blood* **75** (12): 2417–2426.

Fujimoto, T., Singer, S. J. 1987. Immunocytochemical studies of desmin and vimentin in pericapillary cells of chicken. *J Histochem Cytochem* **35** (10): 1105–1115.

Garlanda, C., Dejana, E. 1997. Heterogeneity of endothelial cells. Specific markers. *Arterioscler Thromb Vasc Biol* **17** (7): 1193–1202.

Gavard, J., Gutkind, J. S. 2008. VE-cadherin and claudin-5: it takes two to tango. *Nat Cell Biol* **10** (8): 883–885.

Gerhart, D. Z., LeVasseur, R. J., Broderius, M. A., Drewes, L. R. 1989. Glucose transporter localization in brain using light and electron immunocytochemistry. *J Neurosci Res* **22** (4): 464–472.

Goretzki, L., Burg, M. A., Grako, K. A., Stallcup, W. B. 1999. High-affinity binding of basic fibroblast growth factor and platelet-derived growth factor-AA to the core protein of the NG2 proteoglycan. *J Biol Chem* **274** (24): 16831–16837.

Goretzki, L., Lombardo, C. R., Stallcup, W. B. 2000. Binding of the NG2 proteoglycan to kringle domains modulates the functional properties of angiostatin and plasmin(ogen). *J Biol Chem* **275** (37): 28625–28633.

Graesser, D., Solowiej, A., Bruckner, M., Osterweil, E., Juedes, A., Davis, S. et al. 2002. Altered vascular permeability and early onset of experimental autoimmune encephalomyelitis in PECAM-1-deficient mice. *J Clin Invest* **109** (3): 383–392.

Hall, A. P. 2006. Review of the pericyte during angiogenesis and its role in cancer and diabetic retinopathy. *Toxicol Pathol* **34** (6): 763–775.

Howard, C. V., Reed, M. G. 2005. *Unbiased Stereology*, 3nd ed. Oxon: BIOS Scientific Publishers, Taylor and Francis Group.

Hubbard, B. D., Lazarides, E. 1979. Copurification of actin and desmin from chicken smooth muscle and their copolymerization in vitro to intermediate filaments. *J Cell Biol* **80** (1): 166–182.

Hughes, S., Chan-Ling, T. 2004. Characterization of smooth muscle cell and pericyte differentiation in the rat retina in vivo. *Invest Ophthalmol Vis Sci* **45** (8): 2795–2806.

Hughes, S. W. 2005. Archimedes revisited: a faster, better, cheaper method of accurately measuring the volume of small objects. *Physics Educ* **40** (5): 468–474.

Hyde, D. M., Tyler, N. K., Plopper, C. G. 2007. Morphometry of the respiratory tract: avoiding the sampling, size, orientation, and reference traps. *Toxicol Pathol* **35** (1): 41–48.

Ilan, N., Madri, J. A. 2003. PECAM-1: old friend, new partners. *Curr Opin Cell Biol* **15** (5): 515–524.

Jackson, D. E. 2003. The unfolding tale of PECAM-1. *FEBS Lett* **540** (1–3): 7–14.

Johnson, J. P., Rothbacher, U., Sers, C. 1993. The progression associated antigen MUC18: a unique member of the immunoglobulin supergene family. *Melanoma Res* **3** (5): 337–340.

Johnson, J. P., Bar-Eli, M., Jansen, B., Markhof, E. 1997. Melanoma progression-associated glycoprotein MUC18/MCAM mediates homotypic cell adhesion through interaction with a heterophilic ligand. *Int J Cancer* **73** (5): 769–774.

Kienast, Y., von Baumgarten, L., Fuhrmann, M., Klinkert, W. E., Goldbrunner, R., Herms, J. et al. 2010. Real-time imaging reveals the single steps of brain metastasis formation. *Nat Med* **16** (1): 116–122.

Kurozumi, K., Hardcastle, J., Thakur, R., Yang, M., Christoforidis, G., Fulci, G. et al. 2007. Effect of tumor microenvironment modulation on the efficacy of oncolytic virus therapy. *J Natl Cancer Inst* **99** (23): 1768–1781.

Kutzner, H. 1993. Expression of the human progenitor cell antigen CD34 (HPCA-1) distinguishes dermatofibrosarcoma protuberans from fibrous histiocytoma in formalin-fixed, paraffin-embedded tissue. *J Am Acad Dermatol* **28** (4): 613–617.

Lamagna, C., Bergers, G. 2006. The bone marrow constitutes a reservoir of pericyte progenitors. *J Leukoc Biol* **80** (4): 677–681.

Lazarides, E., Hubbard, B. D. 1976. Immunological characterization of the subunit of the 100 A filaments from muscle cells. *Proc Natl Acad Sci U S A* **73** (12): 4344–4348.

Lee, G. D., Aruna, J. H., Barrett, P. M., Lei, D.-L., Ingram, D. K., Mouton, P. R. 2005. Stereological analysis of microvasculature parameters in a double transgenic model of Alzheimer's disease. *Brain Res Bull* **65**: 317–322.

Levine, J. M. 1994. Increased expression of the NG2 chondroitin-sulfate proteoglycan after brain injury. *J Neurosci* **14** (8): 4716–4730.

Li, Y., Song, Y., Zhao, L., Gaidosh, G., Laties, A. M., Wen, R. 2008. Direct labeling and visualization of blood vessels with lipophilic carbocyanine dye DiI. *Nat Protoc* **3** (11): 1703–1708.

Li, Z., Mericskay, M., Agbulut, O., Butler-Browne, G., Carlsson, L., Thornell, L. E. et al. 1997. Desmin is essential for the tensile strength and integrity of myofibrils but not for myogenic commitment, differentiation, and fusion of skeletal muscle. *J Cell Biol* **139** (1): 129–144.

Lo, E. H., Dalkara, T., Moskowitz, M. A. 2003. Mechanisms, challenges and opportunities in stroke. *Nat Rev Neurosci* **4** (5): 399–415.

Lokmic, Z., Mitchell, G. M. 2011. Visualisation and stereological assessment of blood and lymphatic vessels. *Histol Histopathol* **26** (6): 781–796.

Lokmic, Z., Lammermann, T., Sixt, M., Cardell, S., Hallmann, R., Sorokin, L. 2008. The extracellular matrix of the spleen as a potential organizer of immune cell compartments. *Semin Immunol* **20** (1): 4–13.

Maher, F., Vannucci, S. J., Simpson, I. A. 1994. Glucose transporter proteins in brain. *FASEB J* **8** (13): 1003–1011.

Matsubara, S., Bourdeau, A., terBrugge, K. G., Wallace, C., Letarte, M. 2000. Analysis of endoglin expression in normal brain tissue and in cerebral arteriovenous malformations. *Stroke* **31** (11): 2653–2660.

Matsumoto, H., Kumon, Y., Watanabe, H., Ohnishi, T., Shudou, M., Ii, C. et al. 2007. Antibodies to CD11b, CD68, and lectin label neutrophils rather than microglia in traumatic and ischemic brain lesions. *J Neurosci Res* **85** (5): 994–1009.

McAllister, K. A., Grogg, K. M., Johnson, D. W., Gallione, C. J., Baldwin, M. A., Jackson, C. E. et al. 1994. Endoglin, a TGF-beta binding protein of endothelial cells, is the gene for hereditary haemorrhagic telangiectasia type 1. *Nat Genet* **8** (4): 345–351.

Miettinen, M., Lindenmayer, A. E., Chaubal, A. 1994. Endothelial cell markers CD31, CD34, and BNH9 antibody to H- and Y-antigens–evaluation of their specificity and sensitivity in the diagnosis of vascular tumors and comparison with von Willebrand factor. *Mod Pathol* **7** (1): 82–90.

Morgello, S., Uson, R. R., Schwartz, E. J., Haber, R. S. 1995. The human blood brain barrier glucose transporter (GLUT1) is a *glucose transporter of gray matter astrocytes*. *Glia* **14** (1): 43–54.

Mouton, P. R. 2011. *Unbiased Stereology: A Concise Guide*. Baltimore, MD: The John Hopkins University Press.

Murphy, P. A., Lam, M. T., Wu, X., Kim, T. N., Vartanian, S. M., Bollen, A. W. et al. 2008. Endothelial Notch4 signaling induces hallmarks of brain arteriovenous malformations in mice. *Proc Natl Acad Sci U S A* **105** (31): 10901–10906.

Nachbar, M. S., Oppenheim, J. D., Thomas, J. O. 1980. Lectins in the U.S. diet. Isolation and characterization of a lectin from the tomato (*Lycopersicon esculentum*). *J Biol Chem* **255** (5): 2056–2061.

Nagasawa, K., Chiba, H., Fujita, H., Kojima, T., Saito, T., Endo, T. et al. 2006. Possible involvement of gap junctions in the barrier function of tight junctions of brain and lung endothelial cells. *J Cell Physiol* **208** (1): 123–132.

Newman, P. J., Albelda, S. M. 1992. Cellular and molecular aspects of PECAM-1. *Nouv Rev Fr Hematol* **34** (Suppl): S9–S13.

Nishiyama, A., Yang, Z., Butt, A. 2005. Astrocytes and NG2-glia: what's in a name? *J Anat* **207** (6): 687–693.

Paradis, H., Liu, C. Y., Saika, S., Azhar, M., Doetschman, T., Good, W. V. et al. 2002. Tubedown-1 in remodeling of the developing vitreal vasculature in vivo and regulation of capillary outgrowth in vitro. *Dev Biol* **249** (1): 140–155.

Parsons-Wingerter, P., Lwai, B., Yang, M. C., Elliott, K. E., Milaninia, A., Redlitz, A. et al. 1998. A novel assay of angiogenesis in the quail chorioallantoic membrane: stimulation by bFGF and inhibition by angiostatin according to fractal dimension and grid intersection. *Microvasc Res* **55** (3): 201–214.

Pickl, W. F., Majdic, O., Fischer, G. F., Petzelbauer, P., Fae, I., Waclavicek, M. et al. 1997. MUC18/MCAM (CD146), an activation antigen of human T lymphocytes. *J Immunol* **158** (5): 2107–2115.

Privratsky, J. R., Newman, D. K., Newman, P. J. 2010. PECAM-1: conflicts of interest in inflammation. *Life Sci* **87** (3–4): 69–82.

Ruggeri, Z. M. 2003. von Willebrand factor. *Curr Opin Hematol* **10** (2): 142–149.

Shovlin, C. L., Hughes, J. M., Scott, J., Seidman, C. E., Seidman, J. G. 1997. Characterization of endoglin and identification of novel mutations in hereditary hemorrhagic telangiectasia. *Am J Hum Genet* **61** (1): 68–79.

Simmons, D. L., Satterthwaite, A. B., Tenen, D. G., Seed, B. 1992. Molecular cloning of a cDNA encoding CD34, a sialomucin of human hematopoietic stem cells. *J Immunol* **148** (1): 267–271.

Sixt, M., Engelhardt, B., Pausch, F., Hallmann, R., Wendler, O., Sorokin, L. M. 2001. Endothelial cell laminin isoforms, laminins 8 and 10, play decisive roles in T cell recruitment across the blood-brain barrier in experimental autoimmune encephalomyelitis. *J Cell Biol* **153** (5): 933–946.

Sixt, M., Kanazawa, N., Selg, M., Samson, T., Roos, G., Reinhardt, D. P. et al. 2005. The conduit system transports soluble antigens from the afferent lymph to resident dendritic cells in the T cell area of the lymph node. *Immunity* **22** (1): 19–29.

Skalli, O., Pelte, M. F., Peclet, M. C., Gabbiani, G., Gugliotta, P., Bussolati, G. et al. 1989. Alpha-smooth muscle actin, a differentiation marker of smooth muscle cells, is present in microfilamentous bundles of pericytes. *J Histochem Cytochem* **37** (3): 315–321.

Smith, L. E., Wesolowski, E., McLellan, A., Kostyk, S. K., D'Amato, R., Sullivan, R. et al. 1994. Oxygen-induced retinopathy in the mouse. *Invest Ophthalmol Vis Sci* **35** (1): 101–111.

Song, S., Ewald, A. J., Stallcup, W., Werb, Z., Bergers, G. 2005. PDGFRbeta+ perivascular progenitor cells in tumours regulate pericyte differentiation and vascular survival. *Nat Cell Biol* **7** (9): 870–879.

Sorrentino, A., Ferracin, M., Castelli, G., Biffoni, M., Tomaselli, G., Baiocchi, M. et al. 2008. Isolation and characterization of CD146+ multipotent mesenchymal stromal cells. *Exp Hematol* **36** (8): 1035–1046.

Stallcup, W. B. 2002. The NG2 proteoglycan: past insights and future prospects. *J Neurocytol* **31** (6–7): 423–435.

Stallcup, W. B., Beasley, L. 1987. Bipotential glial precursor cells of the optic nerve express the NG2 proteoglycan. *J Neurosci* **7** (9): 2737–2744.

Stallcup, W. B., Dahlin, K., Healy, P. 1990. Interaction of the NG2 chondroitin sulfate proteoglycan with type VI collagen. *J Cell Biol* **111** (6 Pt 2): 3177–3188.

Stopa, E. G., Butala, P., Salloway, S., Johanson, C. E., Gonzalez, L., Tavares, R. et al. 2008. Cerebral cortical arteriolar angiopathy, vascular beta-amyloid, smooth muscle actin, Braak stage, and APOE genotype. *Stroke* **39** (3): 814–821.

Streit, W. J., Kreutzberg, G. W. 1987. Lectin binding by resting and reactive microglia. *J Neurocytol* **16** (2): 249–260.

Sundberg, C., Kowanetz, M., Brown, L. F., Detmar, M., Dvorak, H. F. 2002. Stable expression of angiopoietin-1 and other markers by cultured pericytes: phenotypic similarities to a subpopulation of cells in maturing vessels during later stages of angiogenesis in vivo. *Lab Invest* **82** (4): 387–401.

Thiyagarajan, M., Fernandez, J. A., Lane, S. M., Griffin, J. H., Zlokovic, B. V. 2008. Activated protein C promotes neovascularization and neurogenesis in postischemic brain via protease-activated receptor 1. *J Neurosci* **28** (48): 12788–12797.

Tigges, U., Welser-Alves, J. V., Boroujerdi, A., Milner, R. 2012. A novel and simple method for culturing pericytes from mouse brain. *Microvasc Res* **84** (1): 74–80.

Tormin, A., Li, O., Brune, J. C., Walsh, S., Schutz, B., Ehinger, M. et al. 2011. CD146 expression on primary nonhematopoietic bone marrow stem cells is correlated with in situ localization. *Blood* **117** (19): 5067–5077.

Vestweber, D., Broermann, A., Schulte, D. 2010. Control of endothelial barrier function by regulating vascular endothelial-cadherin. *Curr Opin Hematol* **17** (3): 230–236.

Virgintino, D., Girolamo, F., Errede, M., Capobianco, C., Robertson, D., Stallcup, W. B. et al. 2007. An intimate interplay between precocious, migrating pericytes and endothelial cells governs human fetal brain angiogenesis. *Angiogenesis* **10** (1): 35–45.

Weibel, E. R. 1973. A simplified morphometric method for estimating diffusing capacity in normal and emphysematous human lungs. *Am Rev Respir Dis* **107** (4): 579–588.

Weibel, E. R. 1975. Quantitation in morphology: possibilities and limits. *Beitr Pathol* **155** (1): 1–17.

Winkler, E. A., Bell, R. D., Zlokovic, B. V. 2011. Central nervous system pericytes in health and disease. *Nat Neurosci* **14** (11): 1398–1405.

Yamamoto, K., de Waard, V., Fearns, C., Loskutoff, D. J. 1998. Tissue distribution and regulation of murine von Willebrand factor gene expression in vivo. *Blood* **92** (8): 2791–2801.

Young, P. E., Baumhueter, S., Lasky, L. A. 1995. The sialomucin CD34 is expressed on hematopoietic cells and blood vessels during murine development. *Blood* **85** (1): 96–105.

Zlokovic, B. V. 2008. The blood-brain barrier in health and chronic neurodegenerative disorders. *Neuron* **57** (2): 178–201.

12   Blood Flow Analysis in Epilepsy Using a Novel Stereological Approach

Rocio Leal-Campanario, Luis Alarcon-Martinez, Susana Martinez-Conde, Michael Calhoun, and Stephen Macknik

Barrow Neurological Institute, Phoenix, AZ, USA

Background

Reports of human beings afflicted with epilepsy, a chronic neurological disorder characterized by unprovoked seizures, date to early Mesopotamia (ca. 2000 BC). About 200 years later, the oldest codified legal document in history, the *Hammurabi Code*, protected the rights of slave owners against defective goods with a full refund for any slave that suffers a seizure during the first lunar cycle after purchase. Ancient Egyptian medical texts (ca. 1700 BC) contained reports of seizures, while Hippocrates (460–370 AC), the father of Greek medicine, provided the first formal medical description (Hippocrates, 1849; Stol, 1993; Eadie and Bladin, 2001). The modern era of epileptology began with John Hughlings Jackson's (1835–1911) investigations into the pathology and anatomy of the disease and connections with various psychiatric symptoms. Our understanding of epilepsy advanced in the twentieth century with the identification of various gene mutations and the development of effective drugs and neuroimaging methods (Magiorkinis et al., 2010). Currently, 2.2 million people in the United States have a diagnosis of epilepsy, with approximately 150,000 new cases a year mostly in children and senior citizens (England et al., 2012).

Cell Death in Epilepsy

The link between epilepsy and neuronal damage first came to light about two centuries ago with reports of progressive neural degeneration, especially in the hippocampus, as well as more insidious damage in the form of sclerosis, cognitive decline, and death (Bouchet, 1825). Since that time, we have learned that seizures trigger a cascade of biochemical, anatomical, and functional changes that, in some cases, leads to cell death and apoptosis (Cavanagh and Meyer, 1956; Meldrum, 2002), with evidence of brain damage in over two-thirds of patients with temporal lobe epilepsy (Cavanagh and Meyer, 1956; Mathern et al., 2002; Thom et al., 2002). According to our current understanding, even brief seizures can cause permanent brain damage (Bengzon et al., 1997; Pretel et al., 1997; Zhang et al., 1998; Briellmann et al., 2000; Fuerst et al., 2001; Kotloski et al., 2002).

Neurostereology: Unbiased Stereology of Neural Systems, First Edition. Edited by Peter R. Mouton.
© 2014 John Wiley & Sons, Inc. Published 2014 by John Wiley & Sons, Inc.

Blood Flow versus Excitotoxicity

Controversies in the field of epilepsy revolve around the relative contributions of hypoxia and excitotoxicity to cell death, and whether seizures and cell death occur as a cascade in series, as multiple processes in parallel, or some combination of serial and parallel processes (Cole et al., 2002). Cell death from epilepsy is viewed traditionally as a consequence of glutamate-induced excitotoxicity that results in calcium overload and activates proapoptotic molecular cascades (Stavrovskaya and Kristal, 2005). A complication of this view is that ischemia activates the same proapoptotic pathways as excitotoxicity. While ischemic events in epileptic brains could contribute to apoptotic ictal neuronal degeneration, current models discount this possibility because seizure foci are macroscopically engorged with blood (Penfield et al., 1954)—hyperemia—and draining veins in the human epileptic brain contain oxygenated blood. This suggests hyperoxia rather than hypoxia within the epileptogenic focus (Penfield et al., 1954; Haglund et al., 1992; Tae et al., 2005).

Determining the relative contribution of excitotoxicity and hypoxia to cell death in epilepsy is complicated by the fact that consequences of excitotoxicity can be tested *in vitro*, whereas the impact of abnormal ictal hippocampal capillary vasodynamics can only be determined *in vivo*. Hyperemia may contribute to the malignant effects of individual capillary vasospasms by heightening metabolic rate, thereby maximizing the oxygen deficit in neurons that simultaneously suffer from localized capillary ischemia (Jespersen and Østergaard, 2012). The underlying vascular mechanisms of ischemia and hypoxia observed in regions that subsequently become epileptic foci are unknown (Bahar et al., 2006; Zhao et al., 2009, 2011).

Microscopic *In Vivo* Imaging in Epilepsy

In vivo fiber-optic-based confocal microscopy allows for investigations of capillary flow in any region, at any depth, of the brain—an achievement not possible with any other current form of microscopic imaging (Denk et al., 1994; Kleinfeld et al., 1998; Helmchen et al., 2001; Chaigneau et al., 2003; Larson et al., 2003; Hirase et al., 2004a,b; Schaffer et al., 2006). Specifically, the contribution of reduced flow rate from vascular changes, for example, ictal pericytic-capillary vasospasms—sudden constrictions, could be studied with regard to hippocampal neural degeneration. With a fiber-optic probe, the use of a blue laser for *in vivo* imaging is possible because the tip of the probe (objective), like a microelectrode, is positioned physically within 15 µm of tissue at any depth in the brain. As with *in vivo* two-photon imaging, one injects neurons with a fluorescent dye, for example, fluorescein dextrans, Oregon Green BAPTA-1, or quantum dots. The technique also works with the injection of a fluorescent dye into the bloodstream where serum, but red blood cells, takes up the dye. Although pericytes imaged *in vitro* and *in vivo* have been shown to constrict in response to drug applications (Hirase et al., 2004a,b; Peppiatt et al., 2006; Yemisci et al., 2009; Fernández-Klett et al., 2010), no prior studies have imaged spontaneous cerebral capillary vasospasms *in vivo*.

We studied Kv1.1 knockout (KO) mice (Smart et al., 1998; Zuberi et al., 1999), the only genetic model of human epilepsy that exists (episodic ataxia type 1) (Zuberi et al., 1999), making these studies directly relevant to human temporal lobe epilepsy. These findings in awake and spontaneously epileptic animals and their wild-type (WT) littermates indicate that pericytes drive normal and abnormal ictal hippocampal vasoconstrictions *in vivo*. To ensure generalization of these results to other forms of epilepsy, we recorded from WT animals rendered epileptic using the classic kainic-acid experimental model.

The Role of Stereology

We used standard and novel stereological approaches to test whether apoptotic neurons in epileptic animals are tightly coupled to the hippocampal microvasculature. Because excitotoxicity per se has no known spatial association to the vasculature, this observation in apoptotic but not healthy neurons indicates that abnormal capillary vasospasmic ischemia-induced hypoxia contributes to ictal neurodegeneration. In further support of this hypothesis, our results show that oral administration of nitric oxide (NO)-based compounds that regulate blood flow ameliorates ictal cell death and oxidative stress, suggesting that abnormal blood flow accounts for up to 54% of seizure-driven neurodegeneration in epilepsy.

Materials and Methods

General Surgical Methods

Before implanting a craniotomy chamber and head holder, we anesthetized mice with Ketamine-Xylazine (100 mg/kg–10 mg/kg i.p.) with continuous monitoring and controlling body temperature using a heating blanket and a rectal thermometer (TC-1000, CWE Inc., PA). A robotic stereotaxic drive (StereoDrive, Neurostar GmBH, Germany) implanted a 300 μm beveled fiber-optic bundle (5000–7000 3-μm-wide fibers) into the hippocampus (Figure 12.1), and green fluorescein lysine-fixable dextran (2MD, Invitrogen, Carlsbad, CA) was tail-vein injected (1 mL/kg of fluorescein 5% w/w).

Confocal Fiber-Optic Imaging

When the mice regained consciousness, we positioned the fiber-optic-coupled laser-scanning confocal microscope objective into the hippocampus of awake spontaneously seizing mice to

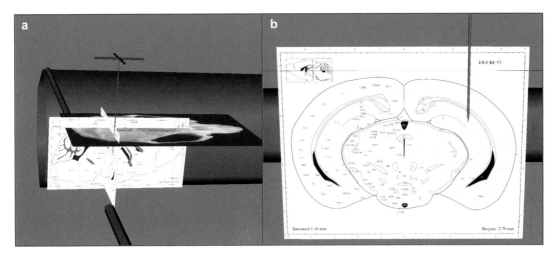

Figure 12.1   StereoDrive 3D software atlas view. (a) Sagittal view of the atlas and probe positioned for recordings. (b) Coronal view. Stereotactic coordinates of recording: anterior–posterior = 2.70 mm posterior to *Bregma*; lateral = 2.70 mm to the right side from the midline.

visualize blood flow dynamics during electroencephalography (EEG)-determined normal, ictal, or interictal periods of neural activity (Figure 12.2, Figure 12.3, and Figure 12.4).

During recordings, the mouse's head was immobilized with the surgical stereotaxic apparatus. Cellvizio (Leica, Bannockburn, IL, model FCM-1000) laser-scanning microscope targeted a 488 nm laser down the bundle (beveled at the tip to penetrate the tissue) at ≥12 Hz. Each fiber at the beveled surface captured the emitted fluorescence and the photons were descanned into an avalanche photodiode detector (Figure 12.4a) to record each movie.

Fiber-Coupled Confocal Image Analysis

To detect seizures, EEG recordings were continuously monitored (Figure 12.1). We used the Cellvizio's on-board image analysis software to create ROIs around each recorded vessel in order to analyze changes in fluorescence in each movie as a function of time (Figure 12.4). These data

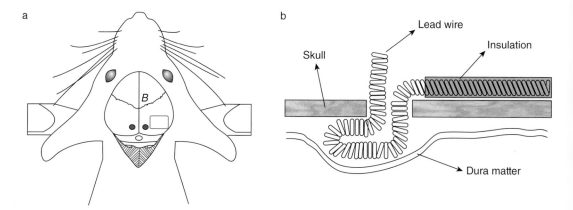

Figure 12.2 Surgical preparation. (a) Diagram of the mouse head positioned on the stereotaxic device, showing skull perforations performed to insert EEG recording electrodes (red and gray dots) as well as the craniotomy for the fiber-optic bundle used in the confocal microscopy (red rectangle). (b) Illustration of the coiled lead wire in contact with the dura for detection of EEG. B, Bregma point. We recorded a total of 67 seizures in our awake KO animals (none in WTs), with an average of 3.35 (+/−0.79) seizures per animal, occurring at a rate of 0.58 (+/−0.13) seizures per hour.

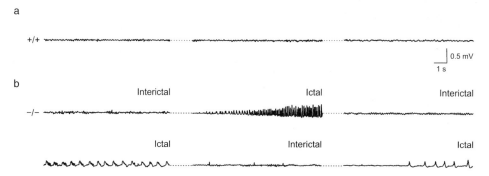

Figure 12.3 Typical spontaneous electroencephalographic (EEG) activity recorded with an implantable radiotelemetry transmitter in awake KO and WT mice. (a) Spontaneous EEG activity in WT mice. (b) Spontaneous ictal and interictal epileptiform activity in KO mice. Figure 12.2 shows the surgical preparation for the implantation of the recording system.

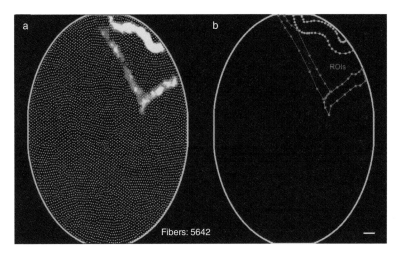

Figure 12.4 *In vivo* observation of hippocampus capillaries in awake mice. (a) Blood flow image with white dots overlaid to represent the position of each fiber on the bevel-cut surface of the fiber bundle. (b) ROIs created to determine fluorescence changes over time for each vessel. Scale bar = 20 μm.

allowed us to derive an independent measure ($\Delta F/F$) of fluorescence over time for each vessel (Figure 12.5a). From these fluorescence measures, we calculated the rate of vasospasms, the percentage of time that vessels vasospasmed, individual vasospasm duration, vasospasm magnitude, and onset and termination speeds (see Figure 12.5b–g).

Because only the KO mice have spontaneous seizures, the experimenter who collected the data was not blind and thus could identify KO or WT by the mouse's behavior or EEG. To control for experimenter bias, the image analyst stayed blind to the treatment group, and vasospasm internal dynamics were measured with an automatic and objective program custom programmed for this study in MATLAB (MathWorks, Natick, MA). The data were averaged across animals in each cohort for testing the significance of difference between cohorts using standard two-tailed unpaired Student's t-tests.

Seizure rate was assessed as a function of vasospasm onsets for each KO mouse ($n = 21$). We determined the pooled chance probability of seizure onset—the baseline seizure rate—by shuffling the seizure onset times with 10,000 random permutations, with the resultant correlation assigned to vasospasms as baseline (0% level) in the analysis. Actual seizure times were correlated to vasospasms to create a histogram of normalized seizure onset rates as a function of vasospasm onset time.

Immunohistochemical Procedures

After each recording session, mice were overdoses with Nembutal (100 mg/kg) and their brains were fixed in 4% paraformaldehyde. Every sixth hippocampus-containing cryosection cut at 50 μm was stained using rabbit anti-AIF (1:200) (Millipore, MA), rabbit antiactive Caspase-3 (1:250) (BD Pharmigen, NJ), mouse anti-Neu-N (1:200) (Millipore Corporation, MA), or rat antiendoglin (CD105) (1:250) (Developmental Studies Hybridoma Bank, IA) as primary antibodies. Secondary antibodies were sheep antirabbit IgG antibodies conjugated to Cy3 (1:500) (Sigma-Aldrich, St. Louis, MO) to stain apoptosis inducing factor (AIF+) and Caspase-3 + cells in red, goat antimouse IgG conjugated to Dylight-488 (Jackson ImmunoResearch, PA) (1:500) to stain Neu-N + cells in

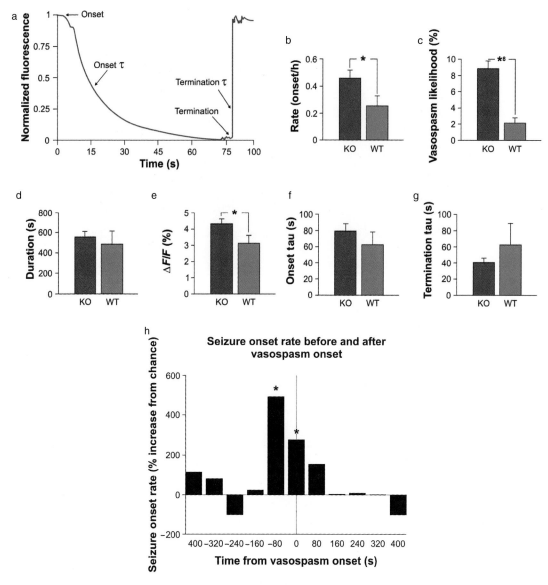

Figure 12.5 Vasodynamics in awake Kv1.1 KO versus WT littermates. KOs exhibited abnormal flow dynamics in several respects. (a) Capillary fluorescence ($\Delta F/F$) as a function of time during an ictal vasospasm, where F is fluorescence magnitude at $t = 0$ before each vasospasm. Notice that the onset proceeds more slowly than the termination. This is presumably due to local blood pressure working against the pericyte. The vessel opens more rapidly at the end of the vasospasm. (b–g) The vasospasm rate (number of vasospasm onsets measured per hour of recording), vasospasm likelihood per vessel (expressed as a percentage of the total recording time per vessel), and vasospasm magnitude were significantly higher in awake KO versus WT mice. See also Figure 12.14 for results from kainate-model epileptic mice. (h) Temporal difference between each seizure and vasospasm onset. In KO mice, seizure onset occurs with significantly higher frequency ($p < 0.05$) 80 seconds before vasospasm onset. A total of 1154 vessels were recorded in awake animals (703 vessels in KO mice and 451 in WT).

green, or biotin-tagged goat antirat IgG (1 : 200) (ABC Elite, Vector Laboratories, Burlingame, CA) completed by avidin–biotin/CY3 tyramide signal amplification (1 h) (CY3-TSA, Perkin Elmer Life Sciences, Inc., Boston, MA, Cat#: SAT704A001EA, 1:50) to stain the vessels in the animals that we did not injected the dye. Finally, sections were stained with fluorescent DNA-binding dye, 4′,6-diamidino-2-phenylindole dihydrochloride (DAPI, Sigma-Aldrich).

The general immunohistochemistry protocol included treatment of tissue sections for antigen retrieval for 15 minutes in phosphate-buffered saline (PBS)-containing TritonX-100 0.5% (Sigma-Aldrich); or, if necessary, in proteinase K (1 : 2 dilution, Dako, CA) in PBS 1× for 15 minutes. Sections were then washed in PBS 3 × 5 minutes and blocked in 80% PBS-containing Triton X-100 0.5%, 10% fetal bovine serum (PAA laboratories Inc., Canada), and 10% Gelatin of 2% (Sigma-Aldrich) for 1 hour at room temperature. Tissue was incubated in the primary antibody at appropriate dilution in blocking solution at 4°C overnight, washed in PBS, and incubated for 2 hour at room temperature (light shielded) in secondary antibody diluted with blocking solution. Sections were rewashed with PBS and incubated in DAPI for 2 minutes with a final wash in PBS for 10 minutes. Glass-mounted sections were cover slipped using Prolongold Antifade reagent (Invitrogen, CA).

Stereology Methods

We used the optical fractionator method (West et al., 1991; for a review of stereology methods, see Mouton, 2002) to quantify AIF+/− cells in 10 animals (5 KO and 5 WT) with the most consistent immunofluorescent staining. A random subsample of DAPI+ cells were analyzed to determine their proximity to blood vessels. This subsampling of up to a maximum of three cells per disector controlled for clustering, which occurred in some disector locations with as many as 17 DAPI+ neurons.

An algorithm was developed that masked the entire stack of green fluorescent vessels and then sequentially unmasked using concentric spheres in increasing steps of 2 μm radius, starting with a 2 μm radius sphere at the three-dimensional (3D) center of each subsampled DAPI+ nucleus (Figure 12.6). The smallest sphere that contained a green fluorescent blood vessel was determined to be the distance of the cell from the nearest vessel (maximum observed: 36 μm).

Each neuron–vessel distance was binned into one of four distributions depending on treatment group (KO or WT) and whether the neuron was AIF+ or AIF− (Figure 12.7, Figure 12.8, and Figure 12.9). We statistically tested mean differences (chi-square test for trend) on the raw data bins (Figure 12.7c–f, Figure 12.8a,b, and Figure 12.9); Gaussian curve fits and normalization (to the highest raw data point in each distribution) of the data in Figure 12.7a,b, Figure 12.8c,d, and Figure 12.9 were computed solely for graphical visualization purposes.

Whereas cytosolic AIF positivity indicates oxidative stress in neurons (Candé et al., 2004; Zhao et al., 2004) and serves as an excellent indicator of the spatial association between oxidative stress in cells and vessels, we further determined that a subset of AIF+ cells escalate from oxidative stress to death in two ways. Because *cytosolic* AIF labeling indicates oxidative stress, *nuclear-translocated* AIF labeling shows cells actively committed to apoptotic ischemic-cell death. Thus, for the transnuclear versus cytosolic AIF analysis, as well as the caspase and Neu-N analyses, we created images of the immunohistochemically stained sections with a Nikon Eclipse 80 microscope (Nikon Instruments, Melville, NY), equipped with a Nikon 100 W mercury light source for fluorescence illumination. A MAC5000 XYZ stage controller (Ludl Electronic Products, Hawthorne, NY) and a linear encoder (Heidenhain, Schaumburg, IL) affixed to the (Z movement was monitored to an accuracy of +/−0.1 μm) controlled stage movement. An average of 12 images at 2 μm Z spacing were taken from the top to bottom section surfaces for each channel separately,

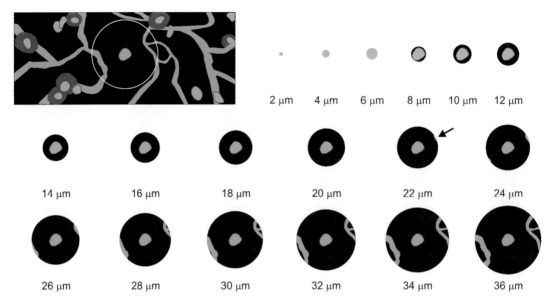

Figure 12.6 The logic of the novel 3D stereological method to determine cell–vessel distance. The blue spot in the cartoon depicts a DAPI+ pyramidal cell nucleus, as viewed from the top of a 3D reconstructed image stack. The white circle in the cartoon represents the radius of the largest sphere (36 μm) used in the analysis. The uppermost left 2-μm sphere is centered 3D at the center of the selected DAPI+ nucleus. The sphere becomes sequentially larger in 2-μm radius steps, and eventually unmasks the green fluorescein-stained vessel within the stack (at 22 μm in this example, see arrow). The distance of the nearest blood vessel to the central DAPI+ nucleus was determined as the radius of the smallest sphere that contained a vessel. We binned the cell counts by distance as a function of both cohort (KO vs. WT), and whether they were AIF+/–. These cell counts created the distance measurements in Figure 12.7, Figure 12.8, Figure 12.9, and Figure 12.13.

Figure 12.7 Stereological analysis of AIF+/– cell spatial correlation to vessels and the contribution of blood flow factors in ictal neurodegeneration. (a) KO AIF+/– normalized distributions of cell numbers as a function of distance from the nearest vessel. AIF+ cells are ~15% nearer to vessels as compared with AIF– cells (baseline) in KO mice (inset: *4 indicates statistical significance of $p < 0.000,01$ from a chi-square test). (b) WT AIF+/– distribution exhibits no significant difference. (c) Cell distributions of WT AIF+ cells treated with L-arginine, L-NAME, or untreated. L-NAME significantly displaced the distribution toward vessels (inset: *3 statistical significance of $p < 0.0001$), as compared with untreated mice (baseline). L-arginine was not significant. (d) Cell distributions of WT AIF– cells. L-NAME had no effect, whereas L-arginine dissociated cells from vessels (inset). (e) Cell distributions of KO AIF+ cells. L-NAME and L-arginine both dissociated cells from vessels (inset) and also reduced the number of AIF+ (oxidatively stressed) cells. (f) Cell distributions of KO AIF– cells. L-NAME and L-arginine both dissociated cells from vessels (inset) and also increased the number of AIF– (healthy) cells. (g) Contribution analysis of the sources of oxidative stress and cell death in KO animals. About 49% of cells were healthy (85% in untreated WT animals). Of the remaining 51% of dead and dying cells, 35% (15% of the total hippocampal cells) are cells that would normally be oxidatively stressed in untreated WT mice. The remaining 65% of the dead and oxidatively stressed cells (36% of the total) are related to seizures. Of these seizure-related AIF+ cells, 54% (18% of the total) are due to abnormal blood flow, whereas 46% (15% of the total) are due to other seizure-related effects, such as excitotoxicity.

at an *XY* spacing of 450 μm systematic-randomly spaced throughout the entire CA1-3 regions. Software facilitated both stage movement and stack capture. A MicroFire camera integrated with the PC/software via Firewire (Optronics, Goleta, CA) acquired high-resolution 8-bit grayscale images (1600 × 1200 pixels; 5.4 pixels/μm final magnification) in each fluorescence channel using a Nikon PlanApo 40×/0.95NA air objective. AIF images were acquired at a constant 500 ms exposure time, with adjusted exposure for DAPI (20–100 ms) and blood vessels (250–500 ms) to optimize the signal-to-noise ratio. All other instrument and configuration settings were held

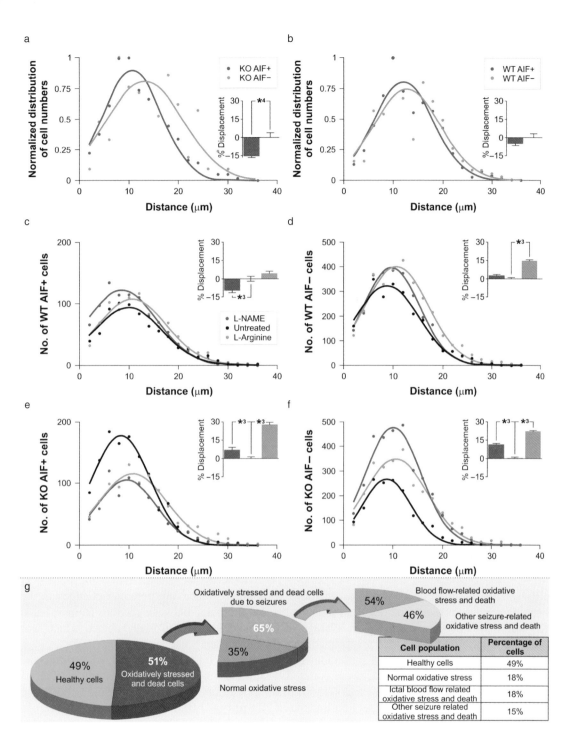

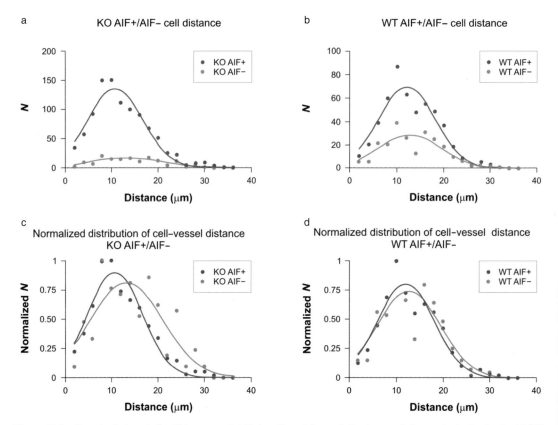

Figure 12.8 Stereological analysis of hippocampal AIF+/− cell spatial correlation to vessels in anesthetized animals. (a) KO AIF+/− distributions of cell numbers as a function of distance from the nearest vessel. (b) WT AIF+/− distributions as in panel (a). Note that the y-axis in a and b have differing scales. (c and d) AIF+/− normalized distributions of cell numbers as a function of distances from the nearest vessel for (c) KO and (d) WT mice, as in Figure 12.4a,b. The normalization in c and d adjusts the highest value on the y-axis from the entire distribution to be 1, and all other values become linearly scaled. N, number of cells.

constant for the duration of image acquisition. To counterbalance any potential changes in the imaging conditions over time (e.g., lamp intensity), we alternated between sections from WT and KO mice. This process produced an average of 60 stacks (+/−3 s.e.m.) per subject, which was subdivided into four (550 × 550 pixel) quadrants for further analysis.

For the stereology analysis of pyramidal neuron number, only large round nuclei within the pyramidal cell layers of CA1-313 were counted. Using the optical fractionator method, neurons that came into focus in a disector frame ($5600\,\mu m^2$) were counted within the middle $6\,\mu m$ of the section (average postprocessing section thickness: $22.8\,\mu m +/− 1.0$). For each subject, an average of 470 nuclei (+/−33 s.e.m.) were counted. The total number of DAPI+ neurons was calculated with sampling fractions of 1/6 for the sections (ssf), 1/36 for the area (asf), and 6/(mean thickness) in Z (tsf).

Classic Kainic-Acid Epilepsy Model

To ensure that the results could be generalized to other forms of epilepsy, we recorded from WT animals rendered epileptic in the classic kainic-acid experimental model. The non-N-methyl-D-

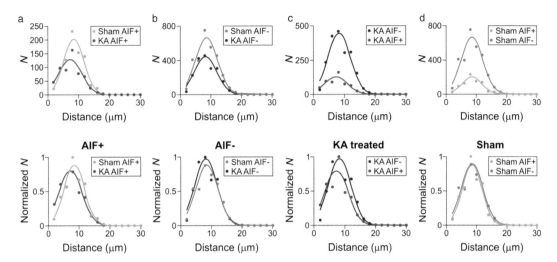

Figure 12.9 Stereological analysis of hippocampal AIF+/− cell spatial correlation to vessels in kainate injected (KA) animals versus sham. (a) Sham versus KA AIF+ cell distribution (*N*) as a function of distance from the nearest vessel (top). Normalized distribution (bottom). (b) Sham versus KA AIF− cell distribution (top). Normalized distribution (bottom). (c) Kainate AIF+/− cell distribution (top). Normalized distribution (bottom). (d) Sham AIF+/− cell distribution (top) and normalized distribution (bottom). The normalization in panels a–d, bottom, adjusts the highest value on the *y*-axis from the entire distribution to be 1, and all other values become linearly scaled. Note that the *y*-axes in the top row have differing scales.

aspartate (NMDA) receptor agonist kainic-acid (Sigma-Aldrich; K0250) or saline control solution was injected subcutaneously with 20–30 mg/kg of kainic acid or saline control solution. Mice were placed in the recording chamber with their head fixed to allow intrahippocampal recoding of the capillary beds and epidural EEG before kainic-acid injection.

To test the kainic-acid injection dose, we measured the seizure intensity after different injections for a group of mice. After the injection, the mice were placed in a clear plastic cage and monitored for locomotor activity and EEG. As described elsewhere (Schauwecker, 2000), seizure episodes started with automatisms, including staring, rigidity, and immobility, followed by jaw movements, blinking, head bobbing, and forelimb clonus. The next stage of seizure activity appeared in the form of rearing, forelimb/head clonus, tonic/clonic seizures, postural imbalance, uncontrolled running, and jumping that defined the latency to first maximal seizure. Seizure activity was scored using the Racine scale (Racine, 1972): Stage 1, immobility; Stage 2, forelimb and/or tail extension, rigid posture; Stage 3, repetitive movements, head bobbing; Stage 4, rearing and falling; Stage 5, continuous rearing and falling; Stage 6, severe tonic–clonic seizures. Finally, these animals were filled for studies of vasodynamics and stereological analyses (see Table 12.1).

The stereological study of the KA mice was done by selecting disectors spaced in a systematic-random manner through the entire hippocampus for 11 animals (6 sham and 5 KA animals) with consistent immunofluorescent staining (Table 12.1).

Oral Administration of Blood Flow Regulating Drugs

Nitric oxide (NO) is involved in regulating blood flow through vasodilatation and hypotension (Toda et al., 2009). Hence, we determined the mechanistic basis by which abnormal blood flow leads to cell death by treating for 21 days a new group of postnatal 21d-Kv1.1 KO mice and their

Table 12.1 Hippocampal regions CA1-3: Comparison between sham and kainate animals

	Subject cohort	Total number AIF+ cells	CE[a]	AIF+ cells	Total number AIF− cells	CE[a]	AIF− cells	Total number cells	CE[a]	Number of sections	Thickness (μm)
1	Sham	36,800	0.053	138	361,067	0.020	1354	397,867	0.017	9	32.10
2	Sham	37,164	0.064	146	248,436	0.024	976	285,600	0.021	11	30.10
3	Sham	47,163	0.051	147	481,250	0.020	1500	528,413	0.017	8	36.00
4	Sham	202,650	0.058	772	296,888	0.022	1131	499,538	0.019	8	33.00
5	Sham	44,800	0.065	240	203,467	0.025	1090	248,267	0.021	10	33.20
6	Sham	19,4571	0.069	681	246,286	0.026	862	440,857	0.023	7	36.00
	Mean	**93,858**	**0.060**	**354**	**306,232**	**0.023**	**1152**	**400,090**	**0.020**	**8.800**	**33.40**
7	KA	11,0473	0.018	454	256,473	0.009	1054	366,947	0.010	10	37.20
8	KA	81,389	0.021	293	232,778	0.010	838	314,167	0.012	9	34.40
9	KA	71,467	0.026	268	172,533	0.013	647	244,000	0.015	7	32.00
10	KA	94,500	0.021	405	214,667	0.011	920	309,167	0.012	9	32.60
11	KA	50,167	0.022	215	217,700	0.011	933	267,867	0.012	9	32.80
	Mean	**81,599**	**0.021**	**327**	**218,830**	**0.011**	**878**	**300,429**	**0.012**	**8.800**	**33.80**

[a]Coefficient of error (West et al., 1991).

Notes: Stereology counts for the total number of AIF+ cells (second column) and the total number of AIF− cells (fifth column) for two cohorts (sham and KA mice; first column). The coefficient of error (CE; third, sixth, and ninth columns) represents the precision of a population size estimate.

WT littermates with L-NAME (0.5 mg/mL; Sigma), a NO synthase inhibiting drug (Rees et al., 1990). To determine whether vasodilatation ameliorates ictal neurodegeneration, we orally administered L-arginine (1.25 g/L; Sigma), an NO donor and blood flow enhancer (Wiesinger, 2001) to a third cohort of Kv1.1 mice and their WT littermates, with the same protocols applied for the L-NAME and untreated cohorts.

For the stereological analysis of drug-treated animals, we selected systematic-random disectors through the hippocampus extent from 32 animals (5 WT and 5 KO, 6 WT-L-arginine, 4 KO-L-arginine, 6 WT-L-NAME, and 6 KO-L-NAME mice) with a consistent immunofluorescent staining for confocal stereological analyses (Table 12.2). Images of the immunohistochemically stained disectors were captured with a confocal microscope (LSM 5 Live, Zeiss, Germany) equipped with a diode laser of 405, 488, and 561 nm sources for fluorescence illumination (Zeiss, Germany). A motor-driven *XY* scanning stage with mark and find (*xyz*) and tile scan (mosaic scan) functions with a smallest increment of 1 μm (Zeiss, Germany), and a DC motor with optoelectronic coding (Zeiss, Germany) affixed to the stage (Z movement was monitored to an accuracy of +/−50 nm) controlled state movement. Images (2747 × 2747 μm) at 0.84 μm Z spacing were taken from the top to the bottom hippocampal surfaces, and the entire hippocampus was digitalized. Zen 2011 software (Zeiss, Germany) facilitated both stage movement and stack capture. A linear array camera integrated (Zeiss, Germany) acquired high-resolution 8-bit color images (512 × 512 pixels) in each fluorescence channel using a Zeiss PlanApo 20×/0.8NA air objective. We acquired AIF, DAPI, and blood vessel images by adjusting the laser intensity to optimize the signal-to-noise ratio. We kept all other instrument and configuration settings constant for the duration of image acquisition. We used the fractionator technique and the developed algorithm to quantify cell number and proximity to blood vessels, as detailed above.

With assistance from a computerized stereology system, Caspase-3, cytoplasmic AIF, and nuclear-translocated AIF expressing cells were counted using the optical disector method (West et al., 1991; for review, see Mouton, 2002). This image analysis system consists of a color camera

Table 12.2 Hippocampal regions CA1-3: Comparison between treated and nontreated animals

	Subject cohort	Total number AIF+ cells	CE[a]	AIF+ cells	Total number AIF− cells	CE[a]	AIF− cells	Total number cells	CE[a]	Number of sections	Thickness (µm)
1	WT	21,156	0.103	68	227,422	0.025	731	248,578	0.016	6	25.70
2	WT	14,444	0.091	50	255,667	0.023	885	270,111	0.014	6	32.80
3	WT	164,722	0.080	593	148,333	0.020	534	313,056	0.012	9	23.60
4	WT	75,733	0.083	284	259,733	0.021	974	335,467	0.013	6	24.30
5	WT	61,767	0.078	218	280,783	0.019	991	342,550	0.012	8	23.00
	Mean	**67,564**	**0.087**	**243**	**234,388**	**0.022**	**823**	**301,952**	**0.013**	**7.000**	**25.88**
6	KO	19,714	0.063	69	229,429	0.015	803	249,143	0.024	7	32.60
7	KO	12,7217	0.054	449	169,150	0.013	597	296,367	0.021	8	32.90
8	KO	113,158	0.053	367	183,458	0.013	595	296,617	0.020	8	27.90
9	KO	206,138	0.053	593	221,086	0.013	636	427,224	0.020	7	28.70
10	KO	228,890	0.053	677	171,414	0.013	507	400,305	0.020	7	22.70
	Mean	**139,024**	**0.055**	**431**	**194,907**	**0.013**	**628**	**333,931**	**0.021**	**7.400**	**28.96**
1	WT-L-arginine	101,852	0.019	293	260,714	0.014	750	362,567	0.010	7	34.90
2	WT-L-arginine	53,760	0.020	126	336,213	0.015	788	389,973	0.011	5	28.00
3	WT-L-arginine	54,000	0.018	180	267,600	0.014	892	321,600	0.010	9	32.90
4	WT-L-arginine	66,944	0.020	241	258,333	0.015	930	325,278	0.011	9	24.80
5	WT-L-arginine	73,775	0.025	227	187,525	0.019	577	261,300	0.013	8	36.10
6	WT-L-arginine	75,667	0.022	227	231,000	0.017	693	306,667	0.012	8	40.20
	Mean	**71,000**	**0.021**	**216**	**256,898**	**0.016**	**772**	**327,897**	**0.011**	**7.700**	**32.82**
7	KO-L-arginine	154,614	0.039	411	241,138	0.003	641	395,752	0.012	7	32.40
8	KO-L-arginine	42,858	0.041	139	248,825	0.004	807	291,683	0.012	8	34.00
9	KO-L-arginine	61,886	0.045	228	224,200	0.004	826	286,086	0.013	7	31.90
10	KO-L-arginine	112,744	0.052	278	246,983	0.004	609	359,728	0.015	6	28.00
	Mean	**93,026**	**0.044**	**264**	**240,287**	**0.004**	**721**	**333,312**	**0.013**	**7.000**	**31.58**
1	WT-L-NAME	39,950	0.033	141	189,550	0.019	669	229,500	0.016	8	28.60
2	WT-L-NAME	57,429	0.030	179	265,329	0.017	827	322,758	0.015	8	38.50
3	WT-L-NAME	93,944	0.031	285	172,067	0.018	522	266,011	0.015	9	30.10
4	WT-L-NAME	52,419	0.032	172	170,362	0.019	559	222,781	0.016	7	26.00
5	WT-L-NAME	84,600	0.029	282	217,200	0.016	724	301,800	0.014	8	30.20
6	WT-L-NAME	70,971	0.031	216	224,086	0.018	682	295,057	0.015	7	31.60

(Continued)

Table 12.2 (*Continued*)

Subject cohort	Total number AIF+ cells	CE[a]	AIF+ cells	Total number AIF− cells	CE[a]	AIF− cells	Total number cells	CE[a]	Number of sections	Thickness (μm)
Mean	**66,552**	**0.031**	**213**	**206,432**	**0.018**	**664**	**272,985**	**0.015**	**7.800**	**30.83**
7 KO-L-NAME	36,111	0.062	130	247,222	0.021	890	283,333	0.007	9	40.20
8 KO-L-NAME	27,188	0.067	87	260,313	0.023	833	287,500	0.008	8	28.70
9 KO-L-NAME	41,400	0.059	138	260,400	0.020	868	301,800	0.007	9	32.90
10 KO-L-NAME	44,089	0.063	124	267,733	0.022	753	311,822	0.007	6	28.40
11 KO-L-NAME	119,700	0.068	399	131,100	0.023	437	250,800	0.008	6	29.20
12 KO-L-NAME	46,500	0.071	155	245,100	0.024	817	291,600	0.008	8	34.20
Mean	**52,498**	**0.065**	**172**	**235,311**	**0.022**	**766**	**287,809**	**0.007**	**7.700**	**32.27**

[a]Coefficient of error (West et al., 1991).

Notes: Stereology results for numbers of AIF+ and AIF− cells from six cohorts (WT and KO mice treated with saline, L-arginine, and L-NAME. Coefficient of error (CE; third, sixth, and ninth columns) refers to the precision of a population size estimate.

(Imi Tech, model IMC-147FT, San Diego, CA), a personal computer (Dell, Austin, TX), a computer controlled motorized specimen stage for x-, y-, and z-axes (Applied Scientific Instrumentation, model MS-2000, Eugene, OR), and a microscope (Olympus, model BX53, MA) with a fluorescent light source (Polychrome V, TILL Photonics, Germany). For each section, the region of interest (reference space) was outlined as traced contours around the hippocampus CA1-3 region using low magnification objective (4×). After the software generated a random grid of virtual 3D counting frames (disectors) in the reference space, cells were counted in each group using a 60× objective with attention to unbiased counting rules for the optical disector (for review, see Mouton, 2002). Previous studies determined the counting frame area, disector height, and sampling grid area for efficient sampling. To measure the distance between caspase+ cells and vessels, we marked the cells in the center of each disector and created 3D reconstructions of the vessels and calculated the distance between each cell and the nearest vessel.

We verified the significance between the distance distributions with a two-tailed chi-square test for trend (Graphpad Prism 5.0, La Jolla, CA) (see Figure 12.7c–f).

Results

Kv1.1 KO Mice versus WT *In Vivo* Imaging

We used a fiber-optic-coupled laser-scanning confocal microscope to record 1154 vessels from Kv1.1 KO mice and their WT littermates (703 vessels in KO mice and 451 in WT littermates). A total of 9% of vessels exhibited pericyte-driven vasospasms in KOs as opposed to 2% in WTs (Figure 12.1, Figure 12.2, Figure 12.3, Figure 12.4, Figure 12.10, and Figure 12.11). The average rate of vasospasms was higher in KOs ($t(1004) = 2.11$; $p = 0.035$, labeled *), as was the likelihood

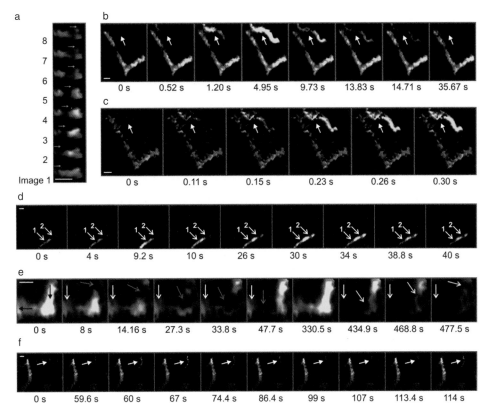

Figure 12.10 Fiber-coupled laser-scanning confocal imaging of hippocampal capillaries. (a) Eight sequential images of a length of capillary, recorded at 87.5 Hz. The arrows indicate a pair of red blood cells (black) flowing as a cluster to the right at 219 μm/s. (b) An occluded capillary releases from vasospasm rapidly and then slowly reconstricts over a 10-second period. Recorded at 11.7 Hz. (c) A later vasospasm releases in the same vessel, now recorded at 26.8 Hz. (d) An occlusion of a capillary due to a pericyte contraction in a KO mouse. The arrows point to pericytes (1 and 2). Pericyte 2 at first causes the vasospasm, and then releases at ~26 seconds. (e) High-speed (87.5 Hz) analysis of ictal vasospasms leading to red blood cell blockages in a capillary network. First frame (left) shows serum flow through the vessel network (black arrows). Eight seconds later, a vessel constriction appears (white arrow) due to an external (unstained) pericyte. Red blood cells clog the anastomosis (red arrows) over the following 40 seconds. The vessel then reopens and flows freely for ~5 minutes, followed by a second constriction event and a red blood cell blockage throughout the local network (yellow arrows). (f) Vasospasm of a WT mouse capillary (white arrow points to a pericyte shadow in the capillary), which begins the recording in vasospasm, releasing at time of 60 seconds, then vasospasming again at time of ~86 seconds, to release again at time of ~114 seconds. Scale = 20 μm (all panels).

of vasospasms per vessel expressed as a percentage of the total recording time per vessel ($t(1100) = 6.05$; $p < 1 \times 10^{-8}$, labeled *8) and the average vasospasm magnitude ($t(81) = 2.00$; $p = 0.049$, labeled *). There was no difference between cohorts for the average vasospasm duration ($t(55) = 0.52$; $p = 0.61$), or the average vasospasm onset ($t(52) = 0.93$; $p = 0.36$) and termination speeds ($t(36) = -0.084$; $p = 0.40$). See Figure 12.5.

Kv1.1 KO Mice versus WT Stereology

We found AIF+ cells more numerous in KO mice than in WT mice (Figure 12.12a,b). AIF+ cells were, on average, 15.17% (+/–0.07% s.e.m.) nearer to blood vessels than AIF– cells ($\chi^2(1,$

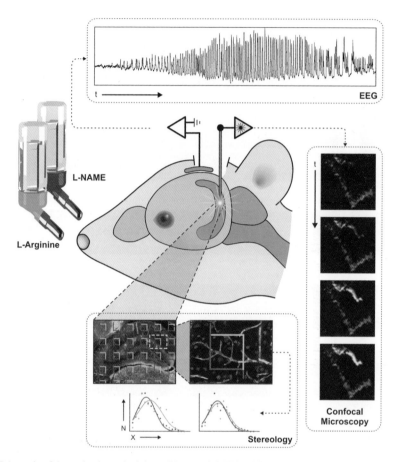

Figure 12.11 Schematic of the project's methodology. We recorded EEG while conducting confocal microscopy in hippocampal capillaries of awake epileptic mice and WT littermates. Some animals were given vasodilators (L-arginine) or vasoconstrictors (L-NAME) in the drinking water. Histological and stereological methods then determined that abnormal blood flow drives much of the cell death and oxidative stress caused by seizures.

$N = 1146) = 16.70, p < 0.0001$) in KO mice, whereas there was no difference ($\chi^2(1, N = 743) = 1.976$, $p = 0.1598$) in WT littermates (Figure 12.7a,b and Figure 12.8). AIF– cells were also not significantly farther from vessels in KO mice than in WT mice ($\chi^2(1, N = 388) = 1.287$, $p = 0.2566$), suggesting that nondegenerating cells in KO mice are normal. AIF+ cells near capillaries in KO mice were significantly closer to vessels than AIF+ cells in WT animals ($\chi^2(1, N = 1541) = 5.907$, $p = 0.0151$), supporting the idea that cells undergoing apoptosis in KO mice are more likely to die due to vascular effects.

To ensure that the oxidative stress measured with AIF occurred in neuronal cells, we stained interleaved sections of the same tissue with primary antibodies to the neuron-specific biomarker, Neu-N (Figure 12.12s,t). We found that an average of 87% (+/−23%) of the AIF+ cells are Neu-N+ neurons (Figure 12.13b). The AIF+/Neu-N+ count was not significantly different from the AIF+/DAPI+ cell count; therefore, we cannot rule out the possibility that all AIF+ cells were neurons.

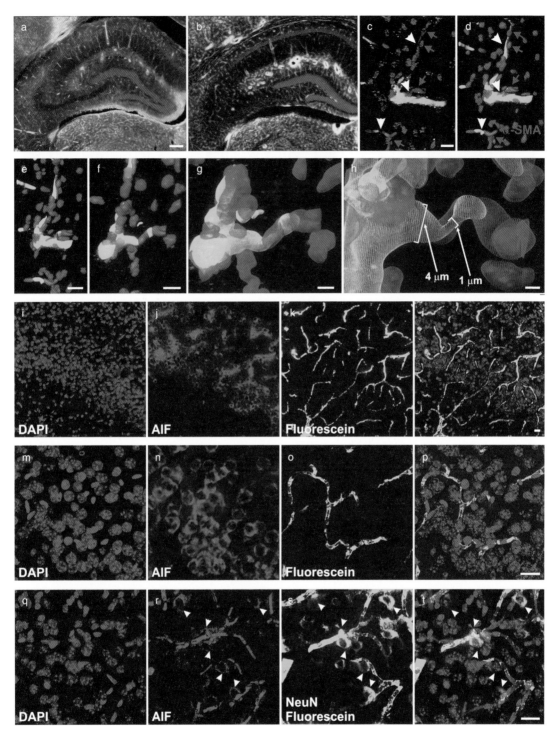

Figure 12.12 Contribution of abnormal capillary vasodynamics to neural degeneration in KO and WT mice. (a–t) Immuno-histochemistry of DAPI (blue) and fluorescein (green) in a KO hippocampus. KO (a) and WT (b) hippocampus with AIF labeled (red): scale = 150 μm. (c) KO hippocampus with alpha smooth muscle actin (α-SMA) (red) labeled to show pericytes (arrow-heads): scale = 10 μm. (d–h) 3D volumetric modeling of stack in panel c progressively reveals pericyte surrounding vessel and at vasospasmic constriction. (i) KO hippocampus filtering for blue fluorescence reveals DAPI-stained nuclei. (j) AIF-labeled red fluorescence reveals that AIF positivity clusters in nonrandom pattern. (k) Green fluorescence reveals capillaries that track clusters of AIF in panel j. (l) Composite of panels i–j. (m–p) KO hippocampus as in panels i–l. (q–t) KO hippocampus as in panels i–l, now with Neu-N positivity (vessels and Neu-N are both stained green in panels s and t) colocalized with AIF. Note that many AIF+ cells double label with Neu-N+ and are near vessels, meaning that cells dying near vessels are primarily neurons. See also Figure 12.13.

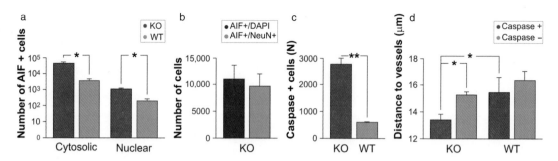

Figure 12.13 Stereological analysis of dying cells. (a) Number of AIF+ cells exhibiting cytosolic or nuclear labeling in KO versus WT. AIF positivity was higher in KO animals than in WT animals for both nuclear AIF staining (indicating imminent or complete cellular death) or cytosolic AIF staining (indicating oxidative stress that may lead to death). (b) We found that an average of 87% (+/–23%) of the AIF+ cells are Neu-N+ neurons. (c) Caspase positivity (indicating imminent or complete cellular death) is more prevalent in KO than in WT mice. (d) Caspase+ cells in KO mice lie nearer to vessels than Caspase– cells. Caspase+ cells in KO mice are nearer to vessels than Caspase+ cells in WT mice.

We also counted AIF cytosolic versus nuclear labeling (Figure 12.13a), as compared with AIF– cells (in both KO and WT cohorts), and found a significant number of neurons with both cytosolic and nuclear AIF labeling (two-way ANOVA $F(1, 14) = 9.70$; $p = 0.0076$). These AIF+ cell counts also revealed that WTs have fewer dying cells than KO mice ($F(1, 14) = 7.70$; $p = 0.0149$), and that there was a significant interaction between AIF labeling and cohort ($F(1, 14) = 7.07$; $p = 0.0187$), in which KO mice showed a significant difference between cytosolic and nuclear AIF staining (two-tailed $t(3) = 4.330$; $p < 0.01$ [Bonferroni corrected]), but WT animals did not. This indicates significantly more oxidative stress in KO animals than in WT animals.

Confirmation that the AIF+ population of neurons was dying was done by probing interleaved sections of the tissue with primary antibodies against active Caspase-3, one component in an AIF-independent proapoptotic molecular cascade important to both ischemic-cell death and excitotoxicity (Lipton, 1999; Friedlander, 2003). Our stereological analyses found that caspase+ cells were more prevalent in KO mice than in WT mice (two-tailed $t(4) = 5.979$; $p = 0.0039$), as well as spatially associated, that is, significantly closer, to vessels in KO mice (two-tailed Mann–Whitney U = 52,805; $p = 0.0040$), but not in WT mice (Figure 12.13c,d).

Classical Kainic-Acid Epilepsy Model: Imaging and Stereological Results

The classical awake kainic-acid mouse model of epilepsy rendered the same results as the KO mice (Figure 12.14), supporting the view that the observed effects are not specific to the Kv1.1 mutation, but rather generalize to other forms of epilepsy.

Hence, we recorded 147 vessels in KA and 120 in sham animals; 15.65% of the vessels in KA mice vasospasmed whereas only 3.33% vasospasmed in sham mice. The rate of vasospasm onsets ($t(265) = 2.42$; $p = 0.009$) and the percentage of recording time each vessel vasospasmed ($t(265) = 3.11$; $p < 0.0010$) were significantly higher in the treated than in the sham cohort (Figure 12.14). There was no difference between groups for average vasospasm duration ($t(34) = 0.24$; $p = 0.65$), average vasospasm magnitude ($t(34) = 0.97$; $p = 0.056$), and average vasospasm onset ($t(19) = 0.58$; $p = 0.20$) and termination speeds ($t(17) = -0.10$; $p = 0.85$). Further, seizures resulted in tighter association of AIF+ cells with vessels in the epileptic WT mice treated with kainic acid (Figure 12.9 and Table 12.1).

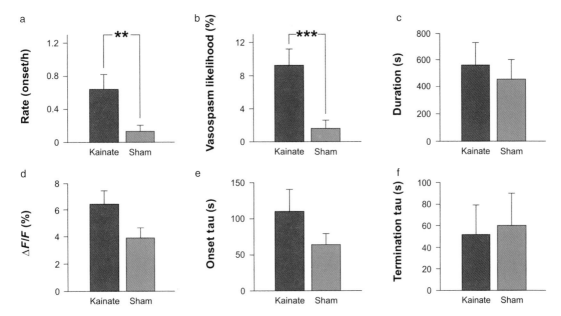

Figure 12.14   Kainate versus sham vasodynamics in awake mice. (a) Average vasospasm rate. (b) Percentage of recording time that vessels vasospasmed. (c) Average vasospasm duration. (d) Average vasospasm magnitude. (e) Average vasospasm onset speed. (f) Average vasospasm termination speed.

The Effects of Blood Flow Regulating Drugs

When healthy WT animals were treated with L-NAME, their AIF+ cells (Figure 12.7c, red) become more tightly associated with the vasculature as compared with their untreated counterparts (Figure 12.7c, black) ($\chi^2(1, N = 1492) = 13.72, p < 0.0002$). Moreover, we found a significant reduction in oxidative stress and vascular spatial dissociation in L-NAME-treated AIF+ neurons in KO animals, as compared with AIF+ neurons in untreated KO animals (Figure 12.7e, red) ($\chi^2(1, N = 1492) = 13.72, p < 0.0002$). This finding was further verified by a significant increase in survival—and vascular spatial dissociation of AIF− neurons—in L-NAME-treated KO animals compared with the untreated KO cohort (Figure 12.7f, red) ($\chi^2(1, N = 4863) = 56.82, p < 0.0001$).

Results of the third cohort of Kv1.1 mice and their WT littermates treated with L-arginine showed that the vasodilator significantly decreased the oxidative stress and increased the number of healthy cells in KO mice, leading to a reduction in oxidative stress and vascular spatial dissociation of L-arginine-treated AIF+ neurons in KO animals as compared with AIF+ neurons in untreated KO animals (Figure 12.7e, blue) ($\chi^2(1, N = 2154) = 86.01, p < 0.0001$), with a significant increase in survival and vascular spatial dissociation of AIF− neurons in the KO L-arginine-treated versus untreated cohorts (Figure 12.7f, blue) ($\chi^2 (1, N = 4293) = 134.2, p < 0.0001$).

A contribution analysis of the drug treatment results suggests that abnormal blood flow accounts for as much as 54% of the neurodegeneration caused by epilepsy (Figure 12.7g). We conclude that 51% of the cells in the hippocampus of KO mice are dead or dying, and that, of those dead and dying cells, 65% are due to epileptic seizures and the other 35% (18% of all hippocampal neurons) exhibit the same oxidative stress that is found in healthy WT mice (this value is the percentage of cells in healthy WT mice that exhibit AIF positivity). The difference between the number of dead and dying cells in the sham versus L-arginine-treated KO animals reveals that as much as 54% of ictal neurodegeneration is due to abnormal blood flow in the untreated animal (18% of all hippocampal cells), whereas 46% of the neurodegeneration (15% of all hippocampal cells) arises from other sources of death and oxidative stress, such as excitotoxicity.

Discussion

If excitotoxicity is the sole contributor to apoptosis, then cells undergoing apoptosis—measured with immunohistochemistry for AIF+—will not be associated with the vasculature because excitotoxicity would not associate with the blood supply. We tested this hypothesis by sectioning the hippocampus after each recording and preparing the tissue for histological analysis. Sections were stained with the fluorescent DNA-binding dye, DAPI (Naimski et al., 1980), to highlight cell nuclei in blue, and with AIF (Zhao et al., 2004; Culmsee et al., 2005) primary antibodies tagged with red fluorescent Cy3 secondary antibodies, to identify cells that have engaged apoptotic pathways (Figure 12.12a,b,i–t). Neurons depend on proximal capillaries for their oxygen supply, and 3D volumetric digital modeling created from 1-µm optical sections of the tissue with antibody labeling of pericytes (now against α-smooth muscle-actin (Yemisci et al., 2009) labeled red with Cy3) reveals that constrictions of capillary vessels occur at the sites of pericytes (Figure 12.12c–h).

Vessels were already stained green with fluorescein dextran during the fiber-coupled confocal recordings (Figures 12.12a,b,i–p). We used stereological methods to randomly sample and count neurons and developed a novel technique to measure the 3D distance between each individual hippocampal AIF+ or AIF– cell and its nearest blood vessel (Table 12.3 and Figure 12.6).

This model posits that cells near ischemic capillaries become hypoxic and add to the cell death brought about by excitotoxicity-driven apoptosis. This model can furthermore explain Wilder Penfield's observation of a hyperemic focus with hyperoxic draining veins, despite the presence of simultaneous hypoxia. We propose that local pockets of hypoxia ensue as a result of the vasospasms we find, leading to increased vascular irrigation in the focus (Gourley and Heistad, 1984). The hyperemic influx, however, is shunted through nonischemic vessels (because the vasospasm

Table 12.3 Hippocampal regions CA1-3 for stereological analyses

	Subject cohort	Total number	CE[a] (number)	DAPI+ cells	Number of sections	Thickness (µm)
1	KO	471,303	0.043	748	9	17.41
2	KO	423,425	0.082	471	10	24.84
3	KO	362,218	0.061	416	8	24.06
4	KO	473,834	0.082	457	9	28.65
5	KO	308,598	0.069	351	8	24.29
6	WT	330,920	0.119	452	8	20.23
7	WT	321,445	0.196	409	9	21.72
8	WT	370,354	0.063	459	7	22.29
9	WT	367,328	0.058	482	9	21.06
10	WT	394,038	0.066	456	8	23.88
	Mean	**382,346**	**0.084**	**470**	**8.500**	**22.84**

[a]Coefficient of error (West et al., 1991).

Notes: Stereology counts for total number of DAPI+ cells in two cohorts (KO and WT mice; second column from the left). The coefficient of error (CE; third column) represents the precision of a population size estimate.

keeps the oxygen from reaching the cells that need it), leading to increased metabolic rate in the focus. The surplus of oxygenated blood is then discarded via local draining veins, explaining the reports of macroscopic reddening of the draining veins, which were previously misinterpreted to mean that there was no ischemia in the ictal focus: our evidence shows that clearly there is. Capillaries, which are smaller in diameter than red blood cells, may become blocked—stopping the flow of serum entirely—due to the pericyte constrictions because the blood cells themselves clog the flow of serum at the point of constriction. A previous study has shown that activated pericytes can completely block capillary blood flow (Fernández-Klett et al., 2010). Capillaries may further become occluded when pericytes die, and once blocked, capillary reflow may be impaired or lead to further damage (Yemisci et al., 2009).

The novel model detailed in this report opens the possibility for new therapeutic interventions aimed at reducing ictal cell death in patients with epilepsy. These interventions to address abnormal blood flow dynamics could be especially important to patients with medically or surgically intractable forms of epilepsy, that is, absence epilepsy or generalized epilepsy, especially those vulnerable to ictal neural degeneration and hippocampal sclerosis.

References

Bahar, S., Suh, M., Zhao, M., Schwartz, T. H. 2006. Intrinsic optical signal imaging of neocortical seizures: the "epileptic dip". *Neuroreport* **17**: 499–503.

Bengzon, J., Kokaia, Z., Elmér, E., Nanobashvili, A., Kokaia, M., Lindvall, O. 1997. Apoptosis and proliferation of dentate gyrus neurons after single and intermittent limbic seizures. *Proc Acad Sci U S A* **94** (19): 10432–10437.

Bouchet, C. 1825. Epilepsie et l'alienation mentale. *Arch Gen Med* **9**: 510–542.

Briellmann, R. S., Berkovic, S. F., Jackson, G. D. 2000. Men may be more vulnerable to seizure-associated brain damage. *Neurology* **55** (10): 1479–1485.

Candé, C., Vahsen, N., Metivier, D., Tourriere, H., Chebli, K., Garrido, C., Tazi, J., Kroemer, G. 2004. Regulation of cytoplasmic stress granules by apoptosis-inducing factor. *J Cell Sci* **117**: 4461–4468.

Cavanagh, J. B., Meyer, A. 1956. Aetiological aspects of Ammon's horn sclerosis associated with temporal lobe epilepsy. *Br Med J* **2** (5006): 1403–1407.

Chaigneau, E., Oheim, M., Audinat, E., Charpak, S. 2003. Two-photon imaging of capillary blood flow during odor stimulation in olfactory bulb glomeruli. *Proc Natl Acad Sci U S A* **100** (22): 13081–13086.

Cole, A. J., Koh, S., Zheng, Y. 2002. Are seizures harmful: what can we learn from animal models? *Prog Brain Res* **135**: 13–23.

Culmsee, C., Zhu, C. H., Landshamer, S., Becattini, B., Wagner, E., Pellechia, M., Blomgren, K., Plesnila, N. 2005. Apoptosis-inducing factor triggered by poly(ADP-ribose) polymerase and Bid mediates neuronal cell death after oxygen-glucose deprivation and focal cerebral ischemia. *J Neurosci* **25**: 10262–10272.

Denk, W., Delaney, K. R., Gelperin, A., Kleinfeld, D., Strowbridge, B. W., Tank, D. W., Yuste, R. 1994. Anatomical and functional imaging of neurons using 2-photon laser scanning microscopy. *J Neurosci Methods* **54** (2): 151–162.

Eadie, M. J., Bladin, B. F. 2001. *A Disease Once Called Sacred. A History of the Medical Understanding of Epilepsy*, pp. 17–20. Eastleigh: John Libbey & Co.

England, M. J., Liverman, C. T., Schultz, A. M., Strawbridge, L. M., eds. 2012. *Epilepsy Across the Spectrum*. Washington DC: Institute of Medicine of the National Academy Press.

Fernández-Klett, F., Offenhauser, N., Dirnagl, U., Priller, J., Lindauer, U. 2010. Pericytes in capillaries are contractile in vivo, but arterioles mediate functional hyperemia in the mouse brain. *Proc Natl Acad Sci U S A* **107**: 22290–22295.

Friedlander, R. M. 2003. Apoptosis and caspases in neurodegenerative diseases. *N Engl J Med* **348**: 1365–1375.

Fuerst, D., Shah, J., Kupsky, W. J., Johnson, R., Shah, A., Hayman-Abello, B., Ergh, T., Poore, Q., Canady, A., Watson, C. 2001. Volumetric MRI, pathological, and neuropsychological progression in hippocampal sclerosis. *Neurology* **57** (2): 184–188.

Gourley, J. K., Heistad, D. D. 1984. Characteristics of reactive hyperemia in the cerebral circulation. *Am J Physiol* **246**: H52–H58.

Haglund, M. M., Ojemann, G. A., Hochman, D. W. 1992. Optical imaging of epileptiform and functional activity in human cerebral cortex. *Nature* **358**: 668–671.

Helmchen, F., Fee, M. S., Tank, D. W., Denk, W. 2001. A miniature head-mounted two-photon microscope: high-resolution brain imaging in freely moving animals. *Neuron* **31**: 903–912.

Hippocrates, L. E. 1849. *Hippocrate: De la Maladie Sacrée. Serie: Oeuvres completes d'Hippocrate*, 6. J-B. Baillère, Paris.

Hirase, H., Creso, J., Buzsáki, G. 2004a. Capillary level imaging of local cerebral blood flow in bicuculline-induced epileptic foci. *Neuroscience* **128** (1): 209–216.

Hirase, H., Creso, J., Singleton, M., Barthó, P., Buzsáki, G. 2004b. Two-photon imaging of brain pericytes in vivo using dextran-conjugated dyes. *Glia* **46**: 95–100.

Jespersen, S. N., Østergaard, L. 2012. The roles of cerebral blood flow, capillary transit time heterogeneity, and oxygen tension in brain oxygenation and metabolism. *J Cereb Blood Flow Metab* **32**: 264–277.

Kleinfeld, D., Mitra, P. P., Helmchen, F., Denk, W. 1998. Fluctuations and stimulus induced changes in blood flow observed in individual capillaries in layers 2 through 4 of rat neocortex. *Proc Natl Acad Sci U S A* **95**: 15741–15746.

Kotloski, R., Lynch, M., Lauersdorf, S., Sutula, T. 2002. Repeated brief seizures induce progressive hippocampal neuron loss and memory deficits. *Prog Brain Res* **135**: 95–110.

Larson, D. R., Zipfel, W. R., Williams, R. M., Clark, S. W., Bruchez, M. P., Wise, F. W., Webb, W. W. 2003. Water-soluble quantum dots for multiphoton fluorescence imaging in vivo. *Science* **300** (5624): 1434–1436.

Lipton, P. 1999. Ischemic cell death in brain neurons. *Physiol Rev* **79**: 1431–1568.

Magiorkinis, E., Sidiropoulou, K., Diamantis, A. 2010. Hallmarks in the history of epilepsy: epilepsy in antiquity. *Epilepsy Behav* **17** (1): 103–108.

Mathern, G. W., Adelson, P. D., Cahan, L. D., Leite, J. P. 2002. Hippocampal neuron damage in human epilepsy: Meyer's hypothesis revisited. *Prog Brain Res* **135**: 237–251.

Meldrum, B. S. 2002. Concept of activity-induced cell death in epilepsy: historical and contemporary perspectives. *Prog Brain Res* **135**: 3–11.

Mouton, P. R. 2002. *Principles and Practices of Unbiased Stereology: An Introduction for Bioscientists*. Baltimore, MD: The John Hopkins University Press.

Naimski, P., Bierzyński, A., Fikus, M. 1980. Quantitative fluorescent analysis of different conformational forms of DNA bound to the dye, 4′,6-diamidine-2-phenylindole, and separated by gel electrophoresis. *Anal Biochem* **106**: 471–475.

Penfield, W., Jasper, H. H., McNaughton, F. 1954. *Epilepsy and the Functional Anatomy of the Human Brain*. London: Churchill.

Peppiatt, C. M., Howarth, C., Mobbs, P., Attwell, D. 2006. Bidirectional control of CNS capillary diameter by pericytes. *Nature* **443**: 700–704.

Pretel, S., Applegate, C. D., Piekuy, D. 1997. Apoptotic and necrotic cell death following kindling induced seizures. *Acta Histochem* **99** (1): 71–79.

Racine, R. J. (1972). Modification of seizure activity by electrical stimulation. II. Motor seizure. *Electroencephalogr Clin Neurophysiol* **32** (3): 281–294.

Rees, D. D., Palmer, R. M., Schulz, R., Hodson, H. F., Moncada, S. 1990. Characterization of three inhibitors of endothelial nitric oxide synthase in vitro and in vivo. *Br J Pharmacol* **101**: 746–752.

Schaffer, C. B., Friedman, B., Nishimura, N., Schroeder, L. F., Tsai, P. S., Ebner, F. F., Lyden, P. D., Kleinfeld, D. 2006. Two-photon imaging of cortical surface microvessels reveals a robust redistribution in blood flow after vascular occlusion. *PLoS Biol* **4** (2): e22.

Schauwecker, P. E. 2000. Seizure-induced neuronal death is associated with induction of c-Jun N-terminal kinase and is dependent on genetic background. *Brain Res* **884**: 116–128.

Smart, S. L., Lopantsev, V., Zhang, C. L., Robbins, C. A., Wang, H., Chiu, S. Y., Schwartzkroin, P. A., Messing, A., Tempel, B. L. 1998. Deletion of the K(V)1.1 potassium channel causes epilepsy in mice. *Neuron* **20** (4): 809–819.

Stavrovskaya, I. G., Kristal, B. S. 2005. The powerhouse takes control of the cell: is the mitochondrial permeability transition a viable therapeutic target against neuronal dysfunction and death? *Free Radic Biol Med* **38**: 687–697.

Stol, M. 1993. *Epilepsy in Babylonia*. Amsterdam: Brill Publishers.

Tae, W. S., Joo, E. Y., Kim, J. H., Han, S. J., Suh, Y. L., Kim, B. T., Hong, S. C., Hong, S. B. 2005. Cerebral perfusion changes in mesial temporal lobe epilepsy: SPM analysis of ictal and interictal SPECT. *Neuroimage* **24**: 101–110.

Thom, M., Sisodya, S. M., Beckett, A., Martinian, L., Lin, W.-R., Harkness, W., Mitchell, T. N., Craig, J., Duncan, J., Scaravilli, F. 2002. Cytoarchitectural abnormalities in hippocampal sclerosis. *J Neuropathol Exp Neurol* **61** (6): 510–519.

Toda, N., Ayajiki, K., Okamura, T. 2009. Cerebral blood flow regulation by nitric oxide: recent advances. *Pharmacol Rev* **61**: 62–97.

West, M. J., Slomianka, L., Gundersen, H. J. 1991. Unbiased stereological estimation of the total number of neurons in the subdivisions of the rat hippocampus using the optical fractionator. *Anat Rec* **231**: 482–497.

Wiesinger, H. 2001. Arginine metabolism and the synthesis of nitric oxide in the nervous system. *Prog Neurobiol* **64**: 365–391.

Yemisci, M., Gursoy-Ozdemir, Y., Vural, A., Can, A., Topalkara, K., Dalkara, T. 2009. Pericyte contraction induced by oxidative-nitrative stress impairs capillary reflow despite successful opening of an occluded cerebral artery. *Nat Med* **15**: 1031–1037.

Zhang, L. X., Smith, M. A., Li, X. L., Weiss, S. R., Post, R. M. 1998. Apoptosis of hippocampal neurons after amygdala kindled seizures. *Brain Res Mol Brain Res* **55** (2): 198–208.

Zhao, H., Yenari, M. A., Cheng, D., Barreto-Chang, O. L., Sapolsky, R. M., Steinberg, G. K. 2004. Bcl-2 transfection via herpes simplex virus blocks apoptosis-inducing factor translocation after focal ischemia in the rat. *J Cereb Blood Flow Metab* **24**: 681–692.

Zhao, M., Ma, H., Suh, M., Schwartz, T. H. 2009. Spatiotemporal dynamics of perfusion and oximetry during ictal discharges in the rat neocortex. *J Neurosci* **29**: 2814–2823.

Zhao, M., Nguyen, J., Ma, H., Nishimura, N., Schaffer, C. B., Schwartz, T. H. 2011. Preictal and ictal neurovascular and metabolic coupling surrounding a seizure focus. *J Neurosci* **31**: 13292–13300.

Zuberi, S. M., Eunson, L. H., Spauschus, A., De Silva, R., Tolmie, J., Wood, N. W., McWilliam, R. C., Stephenson, J. P. B., Kullmann, D. M., Hanna, M. G. 1999. A novel mutation in the human voltage-gated potassium channel gene (Kv1.1) associates with episodic ataxia type 1 and sometimes with partial epilepsy. *Brain* **122** (Pt 5): 817–825.

13   AD-Type Neuron Loss in Transgenic Mouse Models

Kebreten F. Manaye[1] and Peter R. Mouton[2]

[1] *Department of Physiology and Biophysics, College of Medicine, Howard University, Washington, DC, USA*
[2] *Department of Pathology and Cell Biology, Byrd Alzheimer's Disease Institute, University of South Florida, Tampa, FL, USA*

Background

According to the most recent data from the World Health Organization (WHO), Alzheimer's disease (AD) remains the most prevalent cause of dementia in developed countries. AD is an age-related neurodegenerative disorder characterized by the insidious onset of dementia typically in the fifth or sixth decade of life followed by inexorable progression to severe dementia and premature death. The diagnosis of probable AD is confirmed at postmortem examination based on the presence of gross and microscopic brain changes such as marked cortical and whole brain atrophy (Mouton et al., 1998; McDonald et al., 2009), high densities of β-amyloid (Aβ)-containing plaques and neurofibrillary tangles (NFT) in cortical tissue (Alzheimer, 1907; Price et al., 1991; Mirra et al., 1993; Price, 1997; Norton et al., 1998), widespread neurogliosis (Xiang et al., 2006), and severe neuron loss in brain regions associated with cognitive function (Chan-Palay and Asan, 1989; West, 1993; West et al., 1994, 2000; Busch et al., 1997; Grudzien et al., 2007; Giannako-poulos et al., 2009). Evidence of focal neuroinflammation and strong correlations between cortical degeneration and severity of cognitive decline suggest anti-inflammatory approaches may provide an important avenue for future research (Norton et al., 1998; McGeer and McGeer, 2001; Xiang et al., 2006). Because the full pattern of AD-associated neuropathology does not occur during normal (nondemented) aging (Mouton et al., 1994; West et al., 1994; Ohm et al., 1997), AD appears to arise from a distinct disease process, rather than accelerated aging (West et al., 1994).

A major challenge in the field of AD research is to identify the mechanisms underlying the distinctive pattern of neuropathology, with the ultimate goal to slow or block this process in the growing worldwide population of elderly people. Among the consistent neuropathology found in brains from AD cases compared with age-matched, nondemented controls is significant loss of pyramidal cells in the CA1 subregion of hippocampus and noradrenergic tyrosine-immunopositive (TH+) neurons in the locus coeruleus (LC), two brain regions that play key roles in modulating cognitive functions (Squire, 1992; Ridley et al., 1995; Yu and Dayan, 2005; Doya, 2008; Weinshenker, 2008; Sara, 2009). In contrast to the age-related stability of cortical brain volumes (Mouton et al., 1998; McDonald et al., 2009) and total number of neurons in LC (Mouton et al., 1994; Ohm et al., 1997) and CA1 (West, 1993), the classical diagnostic markers of AD—amyloid plaques and NFTs—occur to a greater or lesser extent during normal (nondemented) brain aging

---

Neurosterology: Unbiased Stereology of Neural Systems, First Edition. Edited by Peter R. Mouton.

(Alzheimer, 1907; Price et al., 1991; Mirra et al., 1993; Price, 1997; Norton et al., 1998). Thus, a distinct pattern of neuron loss in CA1 and LC, together with particular distributions of amyloid plaque deposits and NFT in cortical tissue, may be essential for the onset of cognitive impairment in AD.

About 10–15% of patients with AD express mutations associated with early-onset, familial forms of the disease (Alzheimer, 1907; Berridge and Waterhouse, 2003; Lee et al.,2005; Manaye et al., 2007; Liu et al., 2008; Mastrangelo and Bowers, 2008; McDonald et al., 2009; Manaye et al., 2010). The identification and cloning of these familial mutations associated with AD together with the availability of transgenic technology for the cross-species transfer of cloned genetic mutations led to the development of heuristically useful mouse models with one or more of the neuropathological features of AD. These mouse models express mutant human Aβ peptides in cortical brain areas and form amyloid plaques that are histologically identical to those in AD (Games et al., 1995; Hsiao et al., 1995, 1996; Calhoun et al., 1998; Duyckaerts et al., 2008).

A common feature in the majority of transgenic murine models of AD is the overexpression of amyloid precursor protein (APP) that undergoes downstream cleavage to mutant Aβ peptides, leading to the deposition of AD-type amyloid plaques in neocortical tissue. The overexpression of a single APP mutations leads to deposition of mutant Aβ peptides, neurogliosis, and amyloid plaque formation starting in middle age, with progressive deposition through old age and death (Games et al., 1995; Hsiao et al., 1995; Schenk et al., 1997; Calhoun et al., 1998; Oakley et al., 2006). However, quantitative morphometric studies of the brains from these mice report little or no neuron AD-type loss in hippocampus (Irizarry et al., 1997; Johnson-Wood et al., 1997; Calhoun et al., 1998; Kurt et al., 2001). Co-overexpression of mutant APP peptides and a mutation for presenilin 1 (PS1) leads to greater amyloid deposition at earlier ages than single expression of APP alone (Borchelt et al., 1996, 1997; Duff et al., 1996; Holcomb et al., 1998; Younkin et al., 1998; McGowan et al., 1999; Gordon et al., 2002). In the double transgenic line developed by Borchelt and Lee at Johns Hopkins in Baltimore, coexpression of APPA246E and PS1ΔE9 mutations produces relatively heavy, highly fibrillar Aβ deposits starting about 5–7 months of age (Ohm et al., 1997; Norton et al., 1998; Oddo et al., 2003a,b; Oakley et al., 2006; O'Neil et al., 2007; Overk et al., 2009; Oh et al., 2010), several months earlier than mice expressing single APP mutations either alone or in combination with non-ΔE9 PS1 mutations. By middle age (12–15 months), dtg APPswe/PS1ΔE9 show significant age-related losses of TH+ neurons in the LC (O'Neil et al., 2007), and by 18 months of age, significant losses of pyramidal neurons in the CA1 subregion of hippocampus (Manaye et al., 2010). Furthermore, there is a strong correlation between total Aβ-containing plaque volume (amyloid load) and pyramidal neuron loss in the CA1 region of hippocampus of the dtg APPswe/PS1ΔE9 mice (Patel et al., 2005). Other studies in the dtg APPswe/PS1ΔE9 mice report disruptions in vascular structure, altered synapse number and size in the striatum radiatum region of the hippocampus, and lack of AD-type cortical atrophy (Lee et al., 2005; Manaye et al., 2007; West et al., 2008). Thus, the dtg APPswe/PS1ΔE9 line recapitulates some but not all of the critical neuropathologies associated with AD.

The dtg APPswe/PS1ΔE9 line has proven useful for assessing possible nutritional and pharmaceutical interventions to mitigate the progression of AD-type neuropathology. We assessed whether caloric restriction (CR) blocks the deposition of Aβ in cortical tissue. After 18 weeks of balanced diets with 40% fewer calories than *ad libitum*-fed controls, middle-aged (13- to 14-month-old) dtg APPswe/PS1ΔE9 mice were killed and brains were processed for stereological quantification of total volume of Aβ in the hippocampal formation and the overlying neocortex. Computerized stereology confirmed a significant one-third reduction in total Aβ volume in hippocampus and neocortex in the caloric restricted group compared with controls (Mouton et al., 2009). These results extend the neuroprotective effects of CR to middle-aged mice with heavy amyloid load, building on previous reports that CR inhibits relatively amyloid deposition in young tg APPswe and dtg APPswe/PS1ΔE9 mice (Patel et al., 2005). Neuroprotection studies report that long-term treatment with 17-alpha estradiol, a relatively noncarcinogenic, nonfeminizing analog of 17-β estradiol, blocks the loss of CA1 neurons in female dtg APPswe/PS1ΔE9 mice compared with vehicle-treated controls (Manaye et al., 2010). Studies with single APPswe and dtg APPswe/ PS1ΔE9 mice have also been useful to assess pharmaceutical approaches to target the underlying cause of AD neuropathology. Noradrenergic innervation from TH+ neurons in the LC is thought to modulate cognitive tone in the mammalian brain (Berridge and Waterhouse, 2003; Weinshenker, 2008; Sara, 2009). Studies in mice that express a single APPswe mutation have report that removal of noradrenergic innervation through chemical lesioning with the selective neurotoxin N-(2-chloroethyl)-N-ethyl-2 bromobenzylamine (DSP-4) causes significant increases in the total load of amyloid plaques in cortical tissue (Heneka et al., 2006). At 9 months of age, of mice, cortical regions in brains of norepinephrine-depleted mice showed a fivefold increase in Aβ-containing amyloid plaques, along with increased levels of APP C-terminal cleavage fragments and elevated levels of neuroglial activation compared with that in untreated mice that showed low accumulation of amyloid plaques (Heneka et al., 2006; Kalinin et al., 2007; Jardanhazi-Kurutz et al., 2010). These findings suggest that early loss of noradrenergic innervation promotes amyloid deposition and modulates the activation state of inflammatory cells, which may precede the formation of neuropathology in AD.

Comparisons between the distinct patterns of neuropathologies in transgenic mouse models may provide further insight into the possible causes for the cognitive decline in AD. Our group and others have also investigated AD-type neuropathology in mouse with three mutations related to AD, the so-called 3xTg line developed at the University of California, Irvine (Mastrangelo and Bowers, 2008). Microinjection of APPswe and tauP301L mutations into single cells derived from monozygous PS1M146V knock-in mice results in the 3xTg line that includes numerous neuropathologies associated with AD, including Aβ plaque formation, intracellular Aβ deposition, and phosphorylated tau (phospho-tau), a precursor to the formation of NFTs (Oddo et al., 2003a,b; Oh et al., 2010). The distribution of phospho-tau pathology, which closely recapitulates the distribution of tangles found in AD, follows Aβ deposition in these 3xTg mice (Oddo et al., 2003b; Overk et al., 2009). Taken together, these studies support the view that deposition of insoluble Aβ peptides likely plays a key, early role in the neuropathology that leads to cognitive decline in AD.

The present study used computerized stereology studies to assess whether 3xTg mice show AD-type loss of neurons in pontine LC and CA1 region of the hippocampus. These results are contrasted and compared with our earlier findings of neuron loss in LC and CA1 in dtg APPswe/ PS1ΔE9 mice. Finally, we analyze these findings with respect to the distinct patterns of extracellular and intracellular Aβ deposits in 3xTg mice and dtg APPswe/PS1ΔE9 mice. In contrast to the loss of TH+ LC neurons and pyramidal cells in the CA1 region of hippocampus in the dtg APPswe/ PS1ΔE9 mice, we report that the brains of 3xTg mice undergo loss of TH+ in LC neurons only. The remarkably higher ratio of extracellular-to-intracellular Aβ deposits in hippocampus, combined with the stability in number of CA1 neurons in 3xTg mice, suggests that experimental strategies to increase the ratio of intracellular-to-extracellular Aβ peptides could block or delay CA1 neuron loss in dtg APPswe/PS1ΔE9 and, by analogy, the brains of patients with AD.

Materials and Methods

Mice

3xTg mice were obtained by Dr. Scott Turner from the colony at the Georgetown University Medical Center in Washington, D.C. To assess age-related changes in AD-type neuropathology,

$n = 16$ female 3xTg mice were divided into three age groups: young (8 months, $n = 6$), middle aged (12 months, $n = 5$), and late middle age (15 months, $n = 5$). Brains were fixed *in situ* by intra-arterial perfusion and processed for immunocytochemistry and computerized stereology by Dr. Manaye's laboratory at Howard University College of Medicine in Washington, DC. All protocols and procedures were in strict compliance with animal care and handling guidelines from the National Institutes of Heath and the Animal Care and Use Committees at the Georgetown University Medical Center and the Howard University College of Medicine in Washington, D.C.

For comparison purposes, we report results from previous studies (O'Neil et al., 2007) in female dtg APPswe/PS1ΔE9 and nontransgenic littermate control (non-tg) mice bred from founders donated by Dr. David Borchelt and Dr. Michael Lee at the Johns Hopkins University School of Medicine (Borchelt et al., 1996, 1997). These mice were raised from birth in the vivarium at the Laboratory of Experimental Gerontology at the Gerontology Research Center (GRC, NIA/ NIH, Baltimore, MD). These dtg APPswe/PS1ΔE9 mice and non-tg controls were group housed ($n = 2$–5) in plastic cages with corncob bedding with *ad libitum* access to food (NIH formula 07) and filtered water. Conditions within the vivarium were maintained at a 12:12 h light:dark cycle and temperature of $22 \pm 2°C$. Animal husbandry and maintenance were carried out in accordance with the National Institutes of Health Guide for the Care and Use of Laboratory Animals.

Tissue Preparation

Tissue processing for quantification of the 3xTg mice followed the same protocol as used previously for computerized stereology of hippocampus and LC in mouse brains (Manaye et al., 2007; O'Neil et al., 2007). On the day of sacrifice, mice were anesthetized and killed by intracardial perfusion with 0.9% saline followed by 4% paraformaldehyde. Brains were removed, postfixed in 4% paraformaldehyde, and cryoprotected in a 30% sucrose solution before being stored at −80°C until sectioning. Each brain was serially sectioned in the coronal plane from the frontal pole through the brainstem at a microtome setting of 40 μm. A set of systematic-random sections throughout the LC and hippocampus, respectively, were collected in 12-well plates and washed in 0.1 M phosphate buffered saline (PBS), incubated in 1% hydrogen peroxide for 30 min at room temperature (RT), washed again in 0.1 M PBS, and placed in 0.3% Triton X-100 for 10 min at RT. Sections were transferred into 5% normal goat serum in 0.1 M PBS for 30 min at RT to block nonspecific binding, then incubated overnight in rabbit antityrosine hydroxylase antibody (polyclonal, Chemicon International, Temecula, CA) diluted to 1:1000 with 2% normal goat serum and 0.3% Triton X-100 in 0.1 M PBS at 4°C. After incubation, sections were washed in 0.1 M PBS and incubated in biotinylated secondary goat antirabbit antibody (1:400, Vector Laboratories, Burlingame, CA) with 1% normal goat serum in 0.1 M PBS for 90 min at RT. Sections were washed in 0.1 M PBS and reincubated for another 90 min in ABC solution (Vector Laboratories, Burlingame, CA) at RT, rinsed in 0.1 M PBS, and colorized using DAB (Vectastain kit, Vector Laboratories, Burlingame, CA) for 6–10 min. All sections for TH immunocytochemistry were lightly counterstained in a 0.1% solution of cresyl violet, rinsed, dehydrated through an ascending graded series of alcohol, cleared in xylene, and coverslipped. For estimation of total number of pyramidal neurons in CA1, a set of 8–12 sections through the hippocampus were sampled in a systematic-random manner and histochemically stained with 0.1% cresyl violet, dehydrated through an ascending alcohol series, cleared in xylene, and coverslipped. Adjacent sets of sections through hippocampus were processed using immunocytochemistry to visualize intracellular amyloid deposits (mouse anti-6E10 monoclonal antibody, Covance, Princeton, NJ) and phospho-tau (mouse anti-PHF-tau, clone AT8, Thermo Scientific Pierce, Rockford, IL) diluted to 1:1000 and 1:100, respectively. To quantify load (total volume) of extracellular amyloid plaques, a set of systematic-random sections through the hippocampus was counterstained with Congo red histochemistry (Squire, 1992). The average postprocessing section thickness ranged from 15 to 19 μm, with an average of 17 μm.

Computerized stereology studies were carried out using well-established protocols and methods (for review, see Mouton, 2011). Serial sections were subsampled in a systematic-random manner to generate 8–10 sections through CA1 and LC, as identified using a standard mouse brain atlas (Franklin and Paxinos, 2008). Because TH immunoreactivity was not confined to specific or readily definable LC subnuclei, we quantified the entire LC region, including the nucleus subcoeruleus (SubC)-containing TH+ neurons to avoid arbitrary delineation. All stereological parameters were quantified with assistance from a computerized stereology system by a trained user blind to treatment. Briefly, reference spaces on each sampled section were outlined under low power magnification (4×), and volume of Aβ and total numbers of pyramidal neurons in CA1 of the hippocampus and TH+ neurons in LC quantified using a high-resolution oil immersion objective (60×, 1.4 numerical aperture). Mean total neuron numbers were estimated using the optical fractionator method (West et al., 1991). The sampling fractions consisted of the following: section-sampling fraction (ssf, the number of sections sampled divided by the total number of sections); the area-sampling fraction (asf, the area of the sampling frame divided by the area of the x–y sampling step); and, the thickness-sampling fraction (tsf, the height of the disector divided by the section thickness). Neurons were distinguished from other cell types on the basis of neuronal phenotype, that is, nucleolus, a well-formed nuclear membrane and, in the case of noradrenergic neurons in the LC, TH immunoreactivity. To avoid artifacts, for example, lost caps, at the sectioning surface, a guard volume where no cells were counted was observed 2–3 μm above and below the disector. The total volume of Aβ-containing amyloid plaques (amyloid load), which appeared as pinkish red deposits on Congo red-stained sections throughout the hippocampus, was quantified using area fraction and the Cavalieri-point counting method (Mouton et al., 2009; Mouton, 2011). Briefly, total amyloid load was calculated as the amyloid area (Aamyloid) divided by total area of tissue sampled (Asampled):

$$\text{Area fraction} = \sum \text{Aamyloid} \Big/ \sum \text{Asampled} = \left[\sum \text{Pamyloid} \cdot a(p)\right] \Big/ \left[\sum \text{Psampled} \cdot a(p)\right],$$
(13.1)

where $a(p)$ = distance between points in x direction · distance between points in y direction on the point grid, $\sum$ Pamyloid = sum of points hitting amyloid, and $\sum$ Psampled = sum of points in point grid.

According to the Delesse principle, area fraction on random sections is equivalent to the volume fraction, that is, $A_A = V_v$. Amyloid load, as expressed by total amyloid volume (Total Vamyloid), was calculated as the product of the volume fraction (Vamyloid/Vsampled) and the volume of the reference space (Vref) obtained using the Cavalieri-point counting method:

$$\text{Total Vamyloid } (\mu m^3) = (\text{Vamyloid/Vsampled}) \cdot \text{Vref}$$
(13.2)

Since shrinkage of each reference space is equivalent in both Vref and the denominator of Vamyloid/Vsampled, this shrinkage cancels in their product, leading to an unbiased estimate of Total Vamyloid.

Sampling for all stereology parameters was continued to a mean coefficient of error (CE) of 0.05–0.10, according to Gundersen et al. (1999).

Statistical Analysis

ANOVA was used to test for age-related differences in mean total number of pyramidal neurons in CA1 and TH+ neurons in LC of female 3xTg mice at different ages, and female dtg APPswe/PS1ΔE9 mice and age- and gender-matched non-tg controls at different ages. The Pearson Product Moment was used to assess correlations between neuron loss and amyloid plaque load. Statistical differences required $p < 0.05$ for significance.

Results

Congo red histochemistry and immunocytochemistry on sections from hippocampus and neocortical regions revealed age-related increases in extracellular and intracellular deposits of Aβ peptides, amyloid plaques, and phospho tau in brains of adult (6–8 months, $n = 6$) through late middle age (13–15 months, $n = 5$) 3xTg mice. In these mice, Congo red staining showed extracellular amyloid deposits primarily restricted to the subiculum region of the hippocampal formation and layer V of neocortex, with evidence of intracellular Aβ-immunopositive deposits (6E10 and 4G8) in the pyramidal neuron layer of CA1, a region without extracellular plaques stained by Congo red (Figure 13.1, Figure 13.2, and Figure 13.3). In contrast, the dtg APPswe/PS1ΔE9 mice had a distinctly different pattern of age-related accumulation of extracellular Aβ peptide deposits and amyloid plaques within neocortical and hippocampal regions (Figure 13.1).

Figure 13.2 shows images of tissue sections through hippocampus-stained immunostained with Abeta-40, PHF-tau and both immunoprobes combined in 3xTg mice at 8, 12, and 15 months of age.

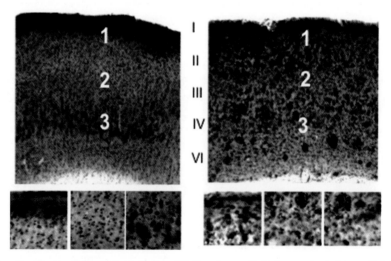

Figure 13.1   Deposits of extracellular Aβ in neocortex of 3xTg mice are limited to neocortical layer V (left), while plaque deposition in dtg APPswe/PS1ΔE9 mice extends throughout all neocortical layers (right). The insets below each image provide high magnification views that correspond to the numbered locations.

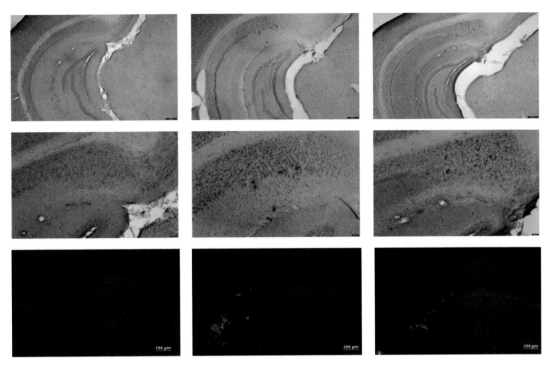

Figure 13.2 Stained sections through hippocampus of 3xTg mice. (A) Images of sections through hippocampus stained with Aβ-40 (left column, 4×), PHF-tau (middle column), and combined staining (right column) of 3xTg mice at 8 months (top row), 12 months (middle row), and 15 months of age (bottom row).

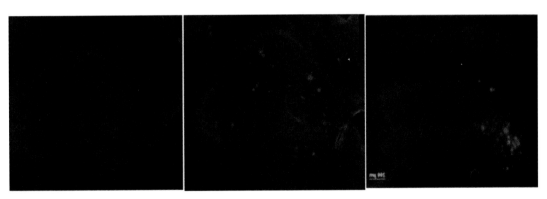

Figure 13.3 Differential pattern of hippocampal intracellular Aβ deposition between mouse strains. 6E10 staining reveals that intracellular Aβ plaques are absent in nontransgenic mice (left), distributed throughout the hippocampus in dtg APP/PS1 mice (middle), and present only in the subiculum of 3xTg mice (right). Magnification bar = 200 mm.

Intracellular Aβ Deposits in Hippocampus

Immunostaining for 6E10 in the 3xTg mice confirmed intracellular Aβ-immunopositive deposits in the pyramidal neuron layer, a region without extracellular plaques stained by Congo red.

As shown in Figure 13.3, intracellular Aβ deposits were present in cortical neurons of 3xTg mice, while 6E10 and 4G8 immunoreactivity in cortical brain regions of dtg APPswe/PS1ΔE9 mice showed no evidence of intracellular Aβ. Thus, there was a predominance of intracellular-to-extracellular Aβ peptides in cortical brain regions of female 3xTg compared with that in age-matched female dtg APPswe/PS1ΔE9 mice.

Loss of TH+ Neurons in LC

Female mice from the 3xTg and dtg APPswe/PS1ΔE9 lines showed significant age-related losses of TH+ neurons in LC. As shown in Figure 13.4 and Figure 13.5, between 8 and 12 months of age 3xTg mice undergo severe loss of TH+ neurons in LC, with a slight increase in severity at 15 months of age.

Using the same immunostaining and stereology approach as in the present study (optical fractionator), our group and others have previously reported significant age-related loss of TH-positive neurons in dtg APPswe/PS1ΔE9 mice compared with nontransgenic controls (O'Neil et al., 2007; Liu et al., 2008). Figure 13.5 summarizes this loss of TH+ neurons in LC across

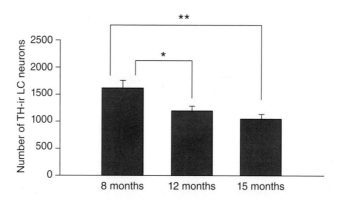

Figure 13.4   Age-related loss of TH+ neurons in LC for 12- and 15-month compared to 8-month-old 3xTg mice; *$p < 0.01$; **$p < 0.05$.

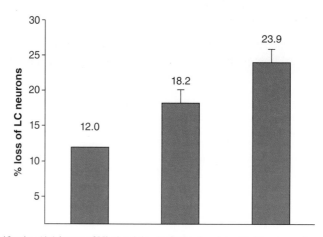

Figure 13.5   Low magnification (4×) image of Nissl staining in CA1 subregion of 3xTg mice and results of stereology analysis of pyramidal neurons at 8 months ($n = 6$), 12 months ($n = 5$), and 15 months ($n = 5$).

four different cohorts of female dtg APPswe/PS1ΔE9 and age- and gender-matched non-tg controls.

Age-Related Loss of Noradrenergic LC Neurons

At each age, there was significant loss of TH+ neurons in LC of dtg APPswe/PS1ΔE9 mice compared with age- and gender-matched controls (Figure 13.4).

In 3xTg mice and dtg APPswe/PS1ΔE9 mice age, the severity of TH+ neuron loss increased up to about 37% and 24%, respectively, in the oldest groups compared with that in 8-month-old adults. The more severe loss of TH+ neurons in LC of the 3xTg mice can be attributed to more rapid degeneration between 8 and 12 months of age. During this interval, there was a 26% loss of TH+ neurons in the 3xTg mice compared with about 4% for the dtg APPswe/PS1ΔE9 mice. Thus, age-related loss of TH+ neurons in LC was somewhat more severe in 3xTg mice than in dtg APPswe/PS1ΔE9 mice between adult and middle ages.

Loss of Pyramidal Neuron in CA1 Subregion of Hippocampus

There was only a nonsignificant 0.3% change in total number of CA1 pyramidal neurons for the 8- to 15-month-old groups of female 3xTg mice.

Furthermore, the loss of CA1 pyramidal neurons in female dtg APPswe/PS1ΔE9 mice was strongly correlated to the increasing amyloid load in hippocampal molecular layers ($n = 6$; $R2 = 0.914$, $p < 0.01$). There were no differences in the total numbers of pyramidal cells in the CA2/3 hippocampal subregions for either 3xTg or dtg APPswe/PS1ΔE9 mice, and no correlations between CA2/3 pyramidal neuron number and Aβ load in molecular layers of the hippocampus (data not shown).

Qualitative examination of neurogliosis at age of 12 months showed robust astrocytosis and microgliosis through the hippocampus of female dtg APPswe/PS1ΔE9 mice, compared with only moderate levels of astrocytosis and microgliosis limited to the subiculum in brains of age- and gender-matched 3xTg mice.

Discussion

AD is characterized by a severe loss of neurons that regulate neural circuits critical for cognitive function. Understanding the factors that mediate this neuron loss may hold the key to prevent or delay the onset of the disease. Toward this goal, studies to characterize the phenotype of transgenic mouse models of AD have concentrated on biochemical, morphological, and behavioral correlates to AD, with the ultimate goal of modeling AD as closely as possible. In particular, neuron loss has emerged as an important endpoint for pharmaceutical, nutritional, and immunological strategies to delay or block the onset of AD (Dickson, 2004; German and Eisch, 2004).

One brain region that undergoes severe neuron loss in AD is the LC, which provides the tonic noradrenergic innervation to hippocampus and other cortical brain regions and plays an important role in the regulation of normal cognitive abilities such as attention, learning, and memory. During normal aging, these cognitive functions remain generally stable in concert with stability in the total number of TH-positive neurons in LC (Mouton et al., 1994; Ohm et al., 1997). In the brains of persons with AD, cognitive abilities diminish as a function of LC neurodegeneration (Chan-Palay and Asan, 1989; Weinshenker, 2008). In contrast, dopaminergic neurons in substantia nigra

(SN) and ventral tegmental area (VTA) appear to be relatively spared in AD, along with the extra-pyramidal motor abilities controlled by these neuronal populations.

Although the presence of amyloid plaques, NFTs, and neuroinflammation are characteristic findings in the autopsied brains of patients with AD, the severity of these markers fail to correlate with the severity of cognitive decline. In contrast, the neuronal circuits mediated by noradrenergic LC neurons and pyramidal neurons in CA are thought to play a central role in the progressive dementia of AD. Transgenic mouse models with AD-type neuron loss in these brain regions that modulate cognitive function provide the opportunity to better understand the neurobiological basis of dementia in AD, as well as develop novel strategies for the therapeutic management of afflicted patients.

A wide spectrum of behavioral abnormalities in AD, including apathy, agitation, anxiety, irritability, dysphoria and aberrant motor behavior, delusion, disinhibition, anxiety, and hallucinations, may be related to disruptions in the noradrenergic projections from LC to cortical brain regions and loss of CA1 neurons in hippocampus. The majority of studies conclude that the loss of noradrenergic neurons in the LC and pyramidal neurons in hippocampal CA1 shows strong correlations with severity of dementia in AD. Importantly, unbiased stereology studies have reported that loss of neurons in LC and CA1 does not occur during normal brain aging (Hsiao et al., 1996; Holcomb et al., 1998; Heneka et al., 2006).

The present study revealed several remarkable differences in the extent and pattern of AD-type changes in the female dtg APPswe/PS1ΔE9 developed by Borchelt et al., (1996, 1997) and female 3xTg mouse line developed by Oddo et al. (2003a). We report that female 3xTg mice undergo significant age-related loss of TH+ neurons that is somewhat more severe than that previously reported in female dtg APPswe/PS1ΔE9 mice. In both the dtg APPswe/PS1ΔE9 and 3xTg mice, the severity of this noradrenergic neuron loss was correlated to increasing accumulation of extracellular amyloid plaques.

The lack of age-related loss of CA1 neurons distinguishes the 3xTg line from both the dtg APPswe/PS1ΔE9 (Manaye et al., 2010) and others (Casas et al., 2004; Schmitz et al., 2004), which show significant loss of pyramidal neurons in CA1 at 13 and 17 months of age, respectively. During the ages of 8 and 12 months in the 3xTg mice, there was less than 1% (0.3%) difference in total number of pyramidal neurons in CA1 and a 26% loss of pyramidal neurons in CA1 sub-region of hippocampus of dtg APPswe/PS1ΔE9 mice during the same age period. There was no evidence of CA1 neuron loss in 3xTg mice up to 15 months of age; however, the possibility remains that precipitous loss of CA1 neurons may occur at later ages. Nevertheless, the present study suggests that neuroprotective mechanisms, which are not well understood at this time, may protect the 3xTg mice from CA1 neuron loss found in the dtg APPswe/PS1ΔE9 mice.

In parallel with these differences in CA1 neuron loss, the spatiotemporal pattern of amyloid plaques and intracellular-to-extracellular Aβ deposition in cortical tissue of 3xTg varied from that in dtg APPswe/PS1ΔE9 mice. Stereology analysis of 3xTg mice in the present study indicates age-related increases in intraneuronal Aβ-immunoreactive deposits in the subiculum and, to a lesser extent, in the neocortex and hippocampal CA1 region. In contrast, none of the dtg APPswe/PS1ΔE9 mice showed evidence of intraneuronal Aβ immunoreactivity in the subiculum, hippocampus or neocortex. Thus, the presence of intraneuronal Aβ immunoreactivity may be one key to the neuroprotection against CA1 neuron loss in 3xTg mice.

In addition to age-related accumulation of intraneuronal Aβ peptides in the subiculum in the 3xTg mice, there is progressive deposition of extracellular Aβ immunoreactivity in the subiculum and occasionally in hippocampus and entorhinal cortex starting around age of 8 months, that is, about 4 months later than the appearance of extracellular Aβ in the dtg APPswe/PS1ΔE9 mice (Savonenko et al., 2005). In the dtg APPswe/PS1ΔE9 mice, there was early deposition of Aβ-immunoreactive deposits in hippocampus, with spread to subiculum and neocortex regions, whereas Aβ-immunoreactive deposits in 3xTg mice were primarily limited to the subiculum. Compared with age-matched dtg APPswe/PS1ΔE9 mice, there were noticeably diminished levels of peak amyloid staining and Aβ deposition as evidenced by Congo red histochemistry and immunocytochemistry for 6E10 and 4G8 in hippocampus of 3xTg mice. The two lines of mice showed distinct spatial and temporal patterns of deposition of intracellular Aβ, extracellular Aβ, as well as different rates of amyloid plaque formation in the hippocampus and neocortex. This finding indicates that extracellular deposition of Aβ peptides may be a trigger for reactive neurogliosis and neuron death in CA1 region of dtg APPswe/PS1ΔE9 mice, which, thus, diminished inflammatory reactivity coincident with reduced extracellular deposition of mutant human Aβ peptides. In support of this idea, there were markedly reduced levels of astrocytic activation, as evidenced by reduced glial fibrillary acidic protein (GFAP) immunoreactivity in the molecular layers of the CA1 region, as compared with that in dtg APPswe/PS1ΔE9 mice.

Age-related increases in deposits of phospho-tau were present in hippocampal regions of 3xTg mice. However, a prior study with a line of 3xTg mice expressing a repressible human tau variant indicates that these phospho-tau deposits are not associated with cognitive decline. These 3xTg mice overexpress mutant tau by 7- to 13-fold, which leads to a tauopathy with NFTs and impaired cognitive function (Santacruz et al., 2005). Prior to the extracellular deposition of AD-like distributions of Aβ and NFTs, the 3xTg mice develop long-term potentiation in association with intracellular Aβ immunoreactivity. After suppression of transgenic tau, the concomitant cognitive decline recovered despite continued accumulation of NFTs. Thus, NFTs alone are not likely to account for the cognitive decline in this 3xTg model of tauopathy. Although no morphometric studies were carried out in that study, the observed cognitive impairment could result from loss of noradrenergic innervation to cortical brain regions.

An important finding in this study is that the high levels of intracellular Aβ peptides in 3xTg mice did not block loss of TH+ neurons in LC, but appeared to protect against loss of pyramidal neurons in the CA1 region, suggesting that the loss of noradrenergic innervation to cortical regions could be responsible for the cognitive impairments reported in both the 3xTg mice and the dtg APPswe/PS1ΔE9 mice. The results from this study, therefore, support the hypothesis that relatively high levels of intracellular Aβ peptides in the 3xTg mice may protect against pyramidal neuron loss in CA1, but not protect against neuron loss in LC. Finally, these findings suggest that pharmacological strategies using noradrenergic agonists may effectively promote cognitive tone that may slow the progression of cognitive decline in AD.

In summary, there are remarkable differences in the pattern of neuron loss and spatiotemporal distribution of Aβ peptides in brains of 3xTg and dtg APPswe/PS1ΔE9 mice. Our findings suggest that relatively high levels of intracellular Aβ peptides may be protective against the loss of pyramidal neurons in the CA1 subregion. Because loss of CA1 neurons only occurred in dtg APPswe/PS1ΔE9 mice with high levels of extracellular Aβ peptides, strategies to maintain high intracellular-to-extracellular ratios of Aβ peptides in hippocampus could ameliorate neuroinflammatory mechanisms in cortical neuropil, and therefore slow the degeneration of pyramidal neurons that regulate cognitive function. The consistent finding of TH+ neuron loss in LC in both dtg APPswe/PS1ΔE9 mice and 3xTg mice suggests that pharmacologic strategies that stimulate central noradrenergic activity may slow cognitive decline in patients afflicted with AD.

Acknowledgments

The authors wish to acknowledge support from NIH/NINDS, Grant number U54 NS42867, the Public Health Service (NIH extra mural grants MH076541-02A1 and NS039407-06A1), Dr. David

R. Borchelt and Dr. Michael K. Lee for development and donation of founders for this study, and the NIA Intramural Program in Baltimore, Maryland.

References

Alzheimer, A. 1907. Ueber eine eigenartige Erkrankung der Hirnrinde. *Allg Z Psychiatr* **64**: 146–148.

Berridge, C. W., Waterhouse, B. D. 2003. The locus coeruleus-noradrenergic system: modulation of behavioral state and state-dependent cognitive processes. *Brain Res Rev* **42** (1): 33–84.

Borchelt, D. R., Thinakaran, G., Eckman, C. B., Lee, M. K., Davenport, F., Ratovitsky, T., Prada, C. M., Kim, G., Seekins, S., Yager, D., Slunt, H. H., Wang, R., Seeger, M., Levey, A. I., Gandy, S. E., Copeland, N. G., Jenkins, N. A., Price, D. L., Younkin, S. G., Sisodia, S. S. 1996. Familial Alzheimer's disease-linked presenilin 1 variants elevate Abeta1-42/1-40 ratio in vitro and in vivo. *Neuron* **17**: 1005–1013.

Borchelt, D. R., Ratovitski, T., van Lare, J., Lee, M. K., Gonzales, V., Jenkins, N. A., Copeland, N. G., Price, D. L., Sisodia, S. S. 1997. Accelerated amyloid deposition in the brains of transgenic mice coexpressing mutant presenilin 1 and amyloid precursor proteins. *Neuron* **19**: 939–945.

Busch, C., Bohl, J., Ohm, T. G. 1997. Spatial, temporal and numeric analysis of Alzheimer changes in the nucleus coeruleus. *Neurobiol Aging* **18** (4): 401–406.

Calhoun, M. E., Wiederhold, K. H., Abramowski, D., Phinney, A. L., Probst, A., Sturchler-Pierrat, C., Staufenbiel, M., Sommer, B., Jucker, M. 1998. Neuron loss in APP transgenic mice. *Nature* **395**: 755–756.

Casas, C., Sergeant, N., Itier, J. M., Blanchard, V., Wirths, O., van der Kolk, N., Vingtdeux, V., van de Steeg, E., Ret, G., Canton, T., Drobecq, H., Clark, A., Bonici, B., Delacourte, A., Benavides, J., Schmitz, C., Tremp, G., Bayer, T. A., Benoit, P., Pradier, L. 2004. Massive CA1/2 neuronal loss with intraneuronal and N-terminal truncated Abeta42 accumulation in a novel Alzheimer transgenic model. *Am J Pathol* **165**: 1289–1300.

Chan-Palay, V., Asan, E. 1989. Quantitation of catecholamine neurons in the locus coeruleus in human brains of normal young and older adults and in depression. *J Comp Neurol* **287** (3): 357–372.

Dickson, D. W. 2004. Building a more perfect beast: APP transgenic mice with neuronal loss. *Am J Pathol* **164**: 1143–1146.

Doya, K. 2008. Modulators of decision making. *Nat Neurosci* **11** (4): 410–416.

Duff, K., Eckman, C., Zehr, C., Yu, X., Prada, C. M., Perez-tur, J., Hutton, M., Buee, L., Harigaya, Y., Yager, D., Morgan, D., Gordon, M. N., Holcomb, L., Refolo, L., Zenk, B., Hardy, J., Younkin, S. 1996. Increased amyloid-beta42(43) in brains of mice expressing mutant presenilin 1. *Nature* **383** (6602): 710–713.

Duyckaerts, C., Potier, M. C., Delatour, B. 2008. Alzheimer disease models and human neuropathology: similarities and differences. *Acta Neuropathol* **115** (1): 5–38.

Franklin, K. B. J., Paxinos, G. 2008. *The Mouse Brain in Stereotaxic Coordinates*, 3rd ed. Boston: Elsevier/Academic Press, Amsterdam.

Games, D., Adams, D., Alessandrini, R., Barbour, R., Berthelette, P., Blackwell, C., Carr, T., Clemens, J., Donaldson, T., Gillespie, F., Guido, T., Hagopian, S., Johnson-Wood, K., Khan, K., Lee, M., Leibowitz, P., Lieberburg, I., Little, S., Masliah, E., McConlogue, L., Montoya-Zavala, M., Mucke, L., Paganini, L., Penniman, E., Power, M., Schenk, D., Seubert, P., Snyder, B., Soriano, F., Tan, H., Vitale, J., Wadsworth, S., Wolozin, B., Zhao, J. 1995. Alzheimer-type neuropathology in transgenic mice overexpressing V717F B-amyloid precursor protein. *Nature* **373**: 523–527.

German, D. C., Eisch, A. J. 2004. Mouse models of Alzheimer's disease: insight into treatment. *Rev Neurosci* **15** (5): 353–369.

Giannakopoulos, P., Kovari, E., Gold, G., von Gunten, A., Hof, P. R., Bouras, C. 2009. Pathological substrates of cognitive decline in Alzheimer's disease. *Front Neurol Neurosci* **24**: 20–29.

Gordon, M. N., Holcomb, L. A., Jantzen, P. T., DiCarlo, G., Wilcock, D., Boyett, K. W., Connor, K., Melachrino, J., O'Callaghan, J. P., Morgan, D. 2002. Time course of the development of Alzheimer-like pathology in the doubly transgenic PS1+APP mouse. *Exp Neurol* **173**: 183–195.

Grudzien, A., Shaw, P., Weintraub, S., Bigio, E., Mash, D. C., Mesulam, M. M. 2007. Locus coeruleus neurofibrillary degeneration in aging, mild cognitive impairment and early Alzheimer's disease. *Neurobiol Aging* **28** (3): 327–335.

Gundersen, H. J., Jensen, E. B., Kieu, K., Nielsen, J. 1999. The efficiency of systematic sampling in stereology reconsidered. *J Microsc* **193**: 199–211.

Heneka, M. T., Mutiah, R., Jacobs, A. H., Dummitrescu-Ozimek, L., Bilkei-Gorzo, A., Debeir, T., Sastre, M., Galldiks, N., Zimmer, A., Hoehn, M., Heiss, W., Klockgether, T., Staufenbiel, M. 2006. Locus ceruleus degeneration promotes Alzheimer pathogenesis in APP23 transgenic mice. *J Neurosci* **26** (5): 1343–1354.

Holcomb, L., Gordon, M. N., McGowan, E., Yu, X., Benkovic, S., Jantzen, P., Wright, K., Saad, I., Mueller, R., Morgan, D., Sanders, S., Zehr, C., O'Campo, K., Hardy, J., Prada, C., Eckman, C., Younkin, S., Hsiao, K., Duff, K. 1998. Accelerated Alzheimer-type phenotype in transgenic mice carrying both mutant amyloid precursor protein and presenilin 1 transgenes. *Nat Med* **4**: 97–100.

Hsiao, K. K., Borchelt, D. R., Olson, K., Johannsdottir, R., Kitt, C., Yunis, W., Xu, S., Eckman, C., Younkin, S., Price, D., Iadecola, C., Clark, H. B., Carlson, G. 1995. Age-related CNS disorder and early death in transgenic FVB/N mice over-expressing Alzheimer amyloid precursor proteins. *Neuron* **15** (5): 1203–1218.

Hsiao, K. K, Chapman, P., Nilsen, S., Eckman, C., Harigaya, Y., Younkin, S., Yang, F., Cole, G. 1996. Correlative memory deficits, AB elevation, and amyloid plaques in transgenic mice. *Science* **274**: 99–102.

Irizarry, M. C., McNamara, M., Fedorchak, K., Hsiao, K., Hyman, B. T. 1997. APPSw transgenic mice develop age-related A beta deposits and neuropil abnormalities, but no neuronal loss in CA1. *J Neuropathol Exp Neurol* **56**: 965–973.

Jardanhazi-Kurutz, D., Kummer, M. P., Terwel, D., Vogel, K., Dyrks, T., Thiele, A., Heneka, M. T. 2010. Induced LC degeneration in APP/PS1 transgenic mice accelerates early cerebral amyloidosis and cognitive deficits. *Neurochem Int* **57** (4): 375–382.

Johnson-Wood, K., Lee, M., Motter, R., Hu, K., Gordon, G., Barbour, R., Khan, K., Gordon, M., Tan, H., Games, D., Lieberburg, I., Schenk, D., Seubert, P., McConlogue, L. 1997. Amyloid precursor protein processing and AB42 deposition in a transgenic mouse model of Alzheimer's disease. *Proc Natl Acad Sci U S A* **94**: 1550–1555.

Kalinin, S., Gavrilyuk, V., Polak, P. E., Vasser, R., Zhao, J., Heneka, M. T., Feinstein, D. L. 2007. Noradrenaline deficiency in brain increases beta-amyloid plaque burden in an animal model of Alzheimer's disease. *Neurobiol Aging* **28** (8): 1206–1214.

Kurt, M. A., Davies, D. C., Kidd, M., Duff, K., Rolph, S. C., Jennings, K. H., Howlett, D. R. 2001. Neurodegenerative changes associated with beta-amyloid deposition in the brains of mice carrying mutant amyloid precursor protein and mutant presenilin-1 transgenes. *Exp Neurol* **171**: 59–71.

Lee, G. D., Aruna, J. H., Barrett, P. M., Lei, D. L., Ingram, D. K., Mouton, P. R. 2005. Stereological analysis of microvascular parameters in a double transgenic model of Alzheimer's disease. *Brain Res Bull* **65** (4): 317–322.

Liu, Y., Yoo, M. J., Savonenko, A., Stirling, W., Price, D. L., Borchelt, D. R., Mamounas, L., Lyons, W. E., Blue, M. E., Lee, M. K. 2008. Amyloid pathology is associated with progressive monoaminergic neurodegeneration in a transgenic mouse model of Alzheimer's disease. *J Neurosci* **28**: 13805–13814.

Manaye, K. F., Wang, P. C., O'Neil, J. N., Huang, S. Y., Xu, T., Lei, D. L., Tizabi, Y., Ottinger, M. A., Ingram, D. K., Mouton, P. R. 2007. Neuropathological quantification of dtg APP/PS1: neuroimaging, stereology, and biochemistry. *Age* **29**: 87–96.

Manaye, K. F., Kalifa, S., Drew, A. C., Edossa, A., Lei, D. L., Ingram, D. K., Mouton, P. R. 2010. 17-Alpha estradiol mitigates loss of pyramidal neurons in hippocampus of dtg APP/PS1 mice. *J Alzheimers Dis* **23** (4): 629–639.

Mastrangelo, M. A., Bowers, W. J. 2008. Detailed immunohistochemical characterization of temporal and spatial progression of Alzheimer's disease-related pathologies in male triple-transgenic mice. *BMC Neurosci* **9**: 81.

McDonald, C. R., McEvoy, L. K., Gharapetian, L., Fennema-Notestine, C., Hagler, D. J., Jr., Holland, D., Koyama, A., Brewer, J. B., Dale, A. M. 2009. Regional rates of neocortical atrophy from normal aging to early Alzheimer disease. *Neurology* **73**: 457–465.

McGeer, E. G., McGeer, P. L. 2001. Chronic inflammation in Alzheimer's disease offers therapeutic opportunities. *Expert Rev Neurother* **1**: 53–60.

McGowan, E., Sanders, S., Iwatsubo, T., Takeuchi, A., Saido, T., Zehr, C., Yu, X., Uljon, S., Wang, R., Mann, D., Dickson, D., Duff, K. 1999. Amyloid phenotype characterization of transgenic mice overexpressing both mutant amyloid precursor protein and mutant presenilin 1 transgenes. *Neurobiol Dis* **6** (4): 231–244.

Mirra, S. S., Hart, M. H., Terry, R. D. 1993. Making the diagnosis of Alzheimer's disease. A primer for practicing pathologists. *Arch Pathol Lab Med* **117**: 132–144.

Mouton, P. R. 2011. *Unbiased Stereology: A Concise Guide.* Baltimore & London: The Johns Hopkins University Press.

Mouton, P. R., Pakkenberg, B., Gundersen, H. J., Price, D. L. 1994. Absolute number and size of pigmented locus coerulus neurons in young and aged individuals. *J Chem Neuroanat* **7** (3): 185–190.

Mouton, P. R., Martin, L. J., Calhoun, M. E., Dal Forno, G., Price, D. L. 1998. Cognitive decline strongly correlates with cortical atrophy in Alzheimer's dementia. *Neurobiol Aging* **19**: 371–377.

Mouton, P. R., Chachich, M. E., Quigley, C., Spangler, E., Ingram, D. K. 2009. Caloric restriction attenuates cortical amyloidosis in a double transgenic mouse model of Alzheimer's disease. *Neurosci Lett* **464**: 184–187.

Norton, J., Goate, A. M., Price, J. L., Gearing, M., Mirra, S. S., Saunders, A. M. 1998. Clinicopathologic studies in cognitively healthy aging and Alzheimer's disease: relation of histologic markers to dementia severity, age, sex, and apolipoprotein E genotype. *Arch Neurol* **55** (3): 326–335.

Oakley, H., Cole, S. L., Logan, S., Maus, E., Shao, P., Craft, J., Guillozet-Bongaarts, A., Ohno, M., Disterhoft, J., Van Eldik, L., Berry, R., Vassar, R. 2006. Intraneuronal beta-amyloid aggregates, neurodegeneration, and neuron loss in transgenic mice with five familial Alzheimer's disease mutations: potential factors in amyloid plaque formation. *J Neurosci* **26**: 10129–10140.

Oddo, S., Caccamo, A., Shepherd, J. D., Murphy, M. P., Golde, T. E., Kayed, R., Metherate, R., Mattson, M. P., Akbari, Y., LaFerla, F. M. 2003a. Triple-transgenic model of Alzheimer's disease with plaques and tangles: intracellular Abeta and synaptic dysfunction. *Neuron* **39** (3): 409–421.

Oddo, S., Caccamo, A., Kitazawa, M., Tseng, B. P., LaFerla, F. M. 2003b. Amyloid deposition precedes tangle formation in a triple transgenic model of Alzheimer's disease. *Neurobiol Aging* **24**: 1063–1070.

Oh, K. J., Perez, S. E., Lagalwar, S., Vana, L., Binder, L., Mufson, E. J. 2010. Staging of Alzheimer's pathology in triple transgenic mice: a light and electron microscopic analysis. *Int J Alzheimers Dis* **2010**: 1.

Ohm, T. G., Busch, C., Bohl, J. 1997. Unbiased estimation of neuronal numbers in the human nucleus coeruleus during aging. *Neurobiol Aging* **18** (4): 393–399.

O'Neil, J. N., Mouton, P. R., Tizabi, Y., Ottinger, M. A., Lei, D. L., Ingram, D. K., Manaye, K. F. 2007. Catecholaminergic neuronal loss in locus coeruleus of aged female dtg APP/PS1 mice. *J Chem Neuroanat* **34**: 102–107.

Overk, C. R., Kelley, C. M., Mufson, E. J. 2009. Brainstem Alzheimer's-like pathology in the triple transgenic mouse model of Alzheimer's disease. *Neurobiol Dis* **35** (3): 415–442.

Patel, N. V., Gordon, M. N., Connor, K. E., Good, R. A., Engelman, R. W., Mason, J., Morgan, D. G., Morgan, T. E., Finch, C. E. 2005. Caloric restriction attenuates Aβ-deposition in Alzheimer transgenic models. *Neurobiol Aging* **26**: 995–1000.

Price, J. L. 1997. Diagnostic criteria for Alzheimer's disease. *Neurobiol Aging* **18**: S67–S70.

Price, J. L., Davis, P. B., Morris, J. C., White, D. L. 1991. The distribution of tangles, plaques and related immunohistochemical markers in healthy aging and Alzheimer's disease. *Neurobiol Aging* **12** (4): 295–312.

Ridley, R. M., Timothy, C. J., Maclean, C. J., Baker, H. F. 1995. Conditional learning and memory impairments following neurotoxic lesion of the CA1 field of the hippocampus. *Neuroscience* **67** (2): 263–275.

Santacruz, K., Lewis, J., Spires, T., Paulson, J., Kotilinek, L., Ingelsson, M., Guimaraes, A., DeTure, M., Ramsden, M., McGowan, E., Forster, C., Yue, M., Orne, J., Janus, C., Mariash, A., Kuskowski, M., Hyman, B., Hutton, M., Ashe, K. H. 2005. Tau suppression in a neurodegenerative mouse model improves memory function. *Science* **309**: 476–481.

Sara, S. J. 2009. The locus coeruleus and noradrenergic modulation of cognition. *Nat Rev Neurosci* **10** (3): 211–223.

Savonenko, A., Xu, G. M., Melnikova, T., Morton, J. L., Gonzales, V., Wong, M. P., Price, D. L., Tang, F., Markowska, A. L., Borchelt, D. R. 2005. Episodic-like memory deficits in the APPswe/PS1dE9 mouse model of Alzheimer's disease: relationships to beta-amyloid deposition and neurotransmitter abnormalities. *Neurobiol Dis* **18** (3): 602–617.

Schenk, D., Masliah, E., Lee, M., Johnson-Wood, K., Seubert, P., Games, D. 1997. The PDAPP transgenic mouse as an animal model for AB-induced amyloidosis and neuropathology. *Alzheimers Dis Rev* **2**: 20–27.

Schmitz, C., Rutten, B. P., Pielen, A., Schafer, S., Wirths, O., Tremp, G., Czech, C., Blanchard, V., Multhaup, G., Rezaie, P., Korr, H., Steinbusch, H. W., Pradier, L., Bayer, T. A. 2004. Hippocampal neuron loss exceeds amyloid plaque load in a transgenic mouse model of Alzheimer's disease. *Am J Pathol* **164**: 1495–1502.

Squire, L. R. 1992. Memory and the hippocampus: a synthesis from findings with rats, monkeys, and humans. *Psychol Rev* **99** (2): 195–231.

Weinshenker, D. 2008. Functional consequences of locus coeruleus degeneration in Alzheimer's disease. *Curr Alzheimer Res* **5** (3): 342–345.

West, M. J. 1993. Regionally specific loss of neurons in the aging human hippocampus. *Neurobiol Aging* **14** (4): 287–293.

West, M. J., Slomianka, L., Gundersen, H. J. 1991. Unbiased stereological estimation of the total number of neurons in the subdivisions of the rat hippocampus using the optical fractionator. *Anat Rec* **231** (4): 482–497.

West, M. J., Coleman, P. D., Flood, D. G., Troncoso, J. C. 1994. Differences in the pattern of hippocampal neuronal loss in normal ageing and Alzheimer's disease. *Lancet* **344**: 769–772.

West, M. J., Kawas, C. H., Martin, L. J., Troncoso, J. C. 2000. The CA1 region of the human hippocampus is a hot spot in Alzheimer's disease. *Ann N Y Acad Sci* **908**: 255–259.

West, M. J., Bach, G., Soderman, A., Jensen, J. L. 2008. Synaptic contact number and size in stratum radiatum CA1 of APP/PS1DeltaE9 transgenic mice. *Neurobiol Aging* **30**: 1756–1776.

Xiang, Z., Haroutunian, V., Ho, L., Purohit, D., Pasinetti, G. M. 2006. Microglia activation in the brain as inflammatory biomarker of Alzheimer's disease neuropathology and clinical dementia. *Dis Markers* **22**: 95–102.

Younkin, S., Hsiao, K., Duff, K. 1998. Accelerated Alzheimer-type phenotype in transgenic mice carrying both mutant amyloid precursor protein and presenilin 1 transgenes. *Nat Med* **4**: 97–100.

Yu, A. J., Dayan, P. 2005. Uncertainty, neuromodulation, and attention. *Neuron* **46** (4): 681–692.

14 Quantification in Populations of Nonuniformly Distributed Cells in the Human Cerebral Cortex

William L. Maxwell

Department of Anatomy, School of Biological Sciences, University of Glasgow, Glasgow, UK

Background

A fundamental concept in design-based stereology is systematic-random sampling (Stuart, 1962; Miles and Davy, 1976), a straightforward application of the equal opportunity rule to cell sampling (Cruz Orive and Weibel, 1981; Geuna, 2000). That is, for counts of total cell number, all cells, regardless of their size, shape, and spatial orientation, should have the same chance of being sampled and therefore counted. An alternative approach, the biased "model-based" strategy, does not apply the equal opportunity rule, but uses "correction" factors based on false or nonverifiable assumptions, for example, all cells are spheres. The unreliability of results using biased sampling methods varies according to the magnitude of the discrepancies between the real situation and the assumptions and models in the approach.

An essential requirement for generating reliable estimates of biological objects in the brain is the delineation of anatomically well-defined reference spaces (region of interest), for example, the thalamus, the hippocampus, or the basal ganglia. Less anatomically bounded reference volumes such as the cortical fields of Brodmann or Von Economo present a challenge, one that may require the assistance of experts in cytoarchitectonics or specialized staining methods. Further complications may occur if one or part of the reference space is unavailable for sampling.

The wake of the Redfern Report and the Bristol Heart Inquiry into the retention of tissue at Alder Hey Hospital and Walton Hospital controversy in the mid-1990s led to enactment of the Human Tissue Act 2004 in the United Kingdom, which made consent from relatives for postmortem examination mandatory. These changes placed tight limits on the material used for the analyses of changes in volume and/or neuron number described in this chapter. In some cases, the material was considered so valuable that serial sectioning through the whole block was not possible, thus the demands of systematic-random sampling could not be satisfied.

Materials and Methods

Brain material was obtained from the tissue archive in the Department of Neuropathology, Southern General Hospital, from cases after full neuropathological examination. All cases were assessed

---

Neurostereology: Unbiased Stereology of Neural Systems, First Edition. Edited by Peter R. Mouton.
© 2014 John Wiley & Sons, Inc. Published 2014 by John Wiley & Sons, Inc.

using the Glasgow Outcome Score (Adams et al., 2001; Jennett et al., 2001). The brains of 11 patients with no history of brain damage or disease were investigated using stereological techniques. Patients had a mean age of 47.09 ± 19.96 years. For glial responses to traumatic brain injury (TBI), data were included from 13 moderately disabled (MoD), 12 severely disabled (SD), and 11 vegetative state (VS) patients (Maxwell et al., 2010). Approval for this study was obtained from The Research Ethics Committee of the Southern General Hospital.

A technician unaware of the clinical patient details collected all numerical data. Blocks containing part of the dorsolateral prefrontal (DLPF) (BA 10), ventromedial prefrontal (VMPF) (BA 11), anterior cingulate (AC) (BA 24a), and motor cortex (MC) (BA 4) were available from all patients in this study.

Histopathological Analysis

Following postmortem examination, all material was handled with care to minimize the incidence of "dark" neurons (Cammermeyer, 1961; Jortner, 2006), and the brains were fixed in 10% formal saline for at least 3 weeks prior to dissection. Optimal preservation and processing of material are highly desirable in order to minimize structural change or tissue deformation. Dorph-Petersen et al. (2001) suggested that deformation of biological tissues may occur either in a uniform or differential manner in different tissue compartments of a histological block, isotropically with deformation in only one direction or the same in all directions, anisotropically or differentially in different directions within a block, and either uniformly or nonuniformly. Collectively, these modes of deformation may result in a global deformation of the specimen. Global deformation may be readily estimated or monitored by changes in the total volume of a block. It was therefore desirable to obtain blocks of standard size and to carefully monitor changes in dimensions of the block during tissue processing, as well as collect all blocks at a single time point and process through dehydration and embedding for the same time to minimize differential shrinkage or other artifacts. One centimeter thick blocks were cut in the coronal plane from the cerebral hemispheres. Dissected blocks were embedded with an automated tissue processor. All blocks for Brodmann areas BA 24a and BA 4 were embedded in paraffin; and all blocks for BA 10 and BA 11 were embedded in celloidin. Harrison et al. (1995) reported that neuronal size and shape negatively correlated with the pH of the brain when blocks were taken. Brain pH was not recorded for the material in the present study and a correction factor could not be applied. Another source of deformation of a specimen, which may be minimized by maintenance of rigorous laboratory practice, occurs when a section is cut from a block. Block advance varies with the speed at which the block passes over the edge of the knife, the relative hardness of the block, and variation in the quality of infiltration of the tissue by the embedding medium (Rolls et al., 2010).

In the analysis of cerebral cortex, the thickness of sections was rigorously monitored by random sampling using a constant sampling fraction across the whole set of sections. Both the intrasection and the intersection coefficients of variation (CV = SD/mean) were estimated.

One member of the analytical team, not involved in data collection, coded the cases before sections were cut; subsequently, all material was examined "blind" to clinical and pathological data by another team member. After all quantitative data had been collected, the code was broken to allow identification of material from a specific patient for statistical analysis.

Serial sections (n = a minimum of 27) were cut and stained with Cresyl violet/Luxol fast blue (Kluver and Barrera, 1953) for stereology, thus ensuring that the plane of each starting section clearly displayed the stratified, hex-laminar organization characteristic of cerebral cortex. The first vertical oriented section provided a vertical uniform random (VUR) plane. Unbiased sampling on serial sections was achieved using "physical disectors" (Howard and Reed, 2005; Mouton, 2011).

The mean heights or thicknesses of the cortex and of individual layers of the cortex were determined. A counting frame was applied between physical disectors using only cells within each size group containing a discrete nucleolus within their nucleus, and the numerical density (N_v) of cells calculated. Serial sections of known thickness generated a projected area on the free surface of the brain and the mean number of cells lying within the column of cortex beneath the projected area was estimated. The entire area of each section was digitally photographed at 20× and a schema noted for the relations of respective fields was photographed. The images covering each section were printed on A4 sheets of paper to a standard magnification (≈1700×), and the printed images for each section were assembled to form a photomontage. Within each set of images for a single section, a photograph of a 1000 μm scale (Agar Aids) was photographed, enabling calculation of the final magnification for the micrographs. A grid series of squares equivalent to 300 μm × 300 μm after magnification adjustment was drawn on a large sheet of thin Perspex and overlaid on the photomontage, with one edge of the first grid box within a counting column lying over the superficial boundary of the molecular layer of the cerebral cortex. This provided columns of grid squares overlying the whole montage and allowed measurement across the vertical depth of cerebral cortex. A counting volume of 300 μm wide × thickness of the cortical layer high × 100 μm in depth was used across the full thickness of each cortical sample to form an "unbiased counting brick" (Howard and Reed, 2005). The sampling was therefore *de facto* biased for sites with a discrete laminar cortical structure. However, the relative position of the counting brick within any cortical field was randomized to provide an unbiased sample volume. A bias inherent to this nonuniform sampling was reduced variance and increased precision (Geuna, 2000; Benes and Lange, 2001; Schmitz and Hof, 2005).

The thicknesses of the cerebral cortex in VMPF, DLPF, AC, and MC were estimated as a mean value of three measurements from each section across the cortex from the pial surface of layer 1 to the junction between the inferior boundary of layer 6 and the subcortical white matter.

The first hypothesis tested was that the depth of each cortical layer differed between the four cortical zones (BA10, BA11, BA24a, BA4) with the first two being examples of granular cortex, the latter two being examples of nongranular cortex. The key features used for identification and discrimination between different cortical areas and cortical layers are summarized in the boxes in Table 14.1.

The second hypothesis tested was that the number of pyramidal and nonpyramidal neurons and the proportions of different sized neurons differed between cortical layers within the four cortical regions. In the simplest terms, there are two types of neurons within the cerebral cortex: the larger pyramidal neurons with axons passing into the subcortical white matter and to other parts of the brain and spinal cord; and the smaller nonpyramidal or local circuit neurons (Lewis, 2004). A marked variation in the size and/or somal volume of pyramidal neurons has been reported both between cortical layers and different areas of human cortex (Benes et al., 1986; Ong and Garey, 1991; Rajkowska et al., 1998; Rivara et al., 2003; Maxwell et al., 2010). As previously reported (Maxwell et al., 2010), we discriminated between big pyramidal (nuclear diameter = nd > 20 μm), medium (nd = 10 μm), and small pyramidal (nd < 10 μm) neurons. Pyramidal neurons were also classified as big (nd > 10 μm), medium (nd = 10^{-6} μm), and small (nd < 6 μm) cells. This novel approach, which has not been utilized in published sampling strategies, despite a number of published critiques (Williams and Rakic, 1988; Coggeshall and Lekan, 1996; Geuna, 2000), was adopted to minimize the influence of spatial differences in three-dimensional (3D) distributions between subtypes of neurons, as reported later. Each neuron subgroup was counted using appropriately sized counting boxes to obtain representative samples. Only neurons with a nucleus and a discrete nucleolus were counted. The number of cells within each layer of the cortex was estimated using the optical disector technique (Sterio, 1984), to ensure that the results obtained were not distorted by variations in cell size, shape, or orientation (Williams and Rakic, 1988; West

Table 14.1   The structural criteria form used to distinguish the six layers of VMPF (BA11), DLPF (BA10), AC (BA24a), and MC (BA4)

VMPF cortex (BA11)	DLPF cortex (BA10)
Layer 2:	Layer 2:
Widely spaced, small nonpyramidal neurons	Closely packed, medium nonpyramidal cells
	Poorly defined boundary with layer 3
Layer 3:	Layer 3:
Large pyramidal cells with a cell soma diameter of more than 31.5 μm	Large pyramidal cells form minicolumns
Medium pyramidal cells form minicolumns	Less extensive pale neuropil
Extensive pale neuropil	
Small pyramidal cells in groups of 4–6	
Layer 5:	Layer 5:
Pyramidal cells do not form minicolumns	Medium pyramidal cells form minicolumns
	Nonpyramidal cells closely packed
Layer 6:	Layer 6:
Few pyramidal cells	Medium and small pyramidal cells widely spaced
Horizontally oriented nonpyramidal cells	Fewer horizontally oriented nonpyramidal cells
AC cortex (BA24a)	MC (BA4)
Layer 2:	Layer 2:
Relatively high number of medium and small pyramidal neurons	Large, medium, and small pyramidal cells
	Greatest depth of the four cortical areas
	Poorly defined boundary with layer 3
Layer 3:	Layer 3:
Few large pyramidal cells	Pyramidal and nonpyramidal cells with lowest packing density of the four cortical areas
Large numbers of medium and small pyramidal cells. Low numbers of nonpyramidal cells.	
Layer 5a:	Layer 5a:
Relatively thin, minicolumns of pyramidal cells	Large, medium, and small pyramidal cells
Layer 5b:	Layer 5b:
Large pyramidal cells, spindle cells	Vertically oriented spindle pyramidal cells
Layer 6:	Layer 6:
Only small pyramidal and nonpyramidal	Low density of cells; extensive pale neuropil

Source: Maxwell et al. (2010).

et al., 1991; Howard and Reed, 2005; Mouton, 2011). All counts were undertaken in a standard counting volume (disector) in each cortical field.

The third hypothesis tested the spatial relationships between groups of neurons within cortical minicolumns (Schlaug et al., 1995; Buxhoeveden et al., 2000; Maxwell et al., 2010) and different cortical layers. Nearest neighbor analysis (NNA) was used to examine the distances between points, in this case, the nucleolus of a cell as a reference point, and the nearest point/nucleolus to it in another similar cell, and then compare that value with those for a random series of points with a complete spatial randomness (CSR) pattern (Diggle, 1990, 2003). The CSR value may be generated using two assumptions, starting with all points are equally likely to be encountered in a random section or volume; and second, all points are located independently of each other. The technique investigates second-order properties of spatial distribution in an identified subregional neighborhood pattern and compares it with the expected pattern if all points were uniformly or randomly distributed. The expected nearest neighbor distance (NND) based on a completely random distribution is defined as

$$Rn = 2d\sqrt{n/a}, \tag{14.1}$$

where Rn = description of distribution, d = the mean distance between the nearest neighbors, a = area under study, and n = total number of points; and the nearest neighbor index (NNI) (the ratio of the observed NND to the mean random distance) is

$$NNI = NND/NND \text{ random}, \tag{14.2}$$

with the consideration that when NNI is less than 1.0, the population is clustered, and if NNI is greater than 1.0, the observed population is dispersed. Use of the term clustered indicates that the population of points, in this case, the nucleoli of neurons, are more closely spaced that would be expected in a normal or uniform population, while the term scattered indicates that points are more widely spaced than expected. In practice, if the value of NNI lies between 0.81 and 1.19, the points/cells have no pattern and are randomly distributed (Diggle, 2003). The standard error (SE) over a sample may be calculated using Equation 14.3.

$$SE_{d(\text{ran})} = \sqrt{\left[\frac{(4-\pi)A}{4\pi N^2}\right]}$$
$$= \frac{0.26136}{\sqrt{\dfrac{N^2}{A}}}. \tag{14.3}$$

Within a randomly selected section from close to the midpoint of the unbiased disector used in this analysis, a randomly placed reference line was placed perpendicular to the pia mater through the upper and lower boundaries of each cortical region. Cells crossed by the reference line and within which a discrete nucleolus was visible were nominated the registered neuron. The surrounding tissue was then scanned in all directions within a counting volume consisting of serial sections to include at least 150–200 similar cells containing a discrete nucleolus. Methodologically, the nucleolus was used as a point—*vide supra*—for the measurement of distance between neighboring cells. The x–y–z coordinates of the nucleolus and the corresponding mean NND for each cell type or subtype was calculated. Calculation of the NNI (Equation 14.2) allowed statistically rigorous determination of whether neurons were clustered, randomly distributed, or scattered within each cortical layer of the four cortical regions across patients.

Statistical Analyses

Differences in the thickness of the cerebral cortex between VMPF, DLPF, AC, and MC in mature, adult humans were determined by ANOVA, followed by the Tukey–Kramer post hoc test. Differences in number of cells and spacing of neurons were analyzed using the Kruskal–Wallis test, the nonparametric analog of one-way analysis of variance, because the neurons analyzed did not follow a Poisson distribution. The test determined if there are "significant" differences among the population medians rather than the population means, and if the value of p is small, the differences between subjects are not due to random sampling. For post hoc testing, either the unpaired t-test with Welch correction or Dunn's posttest was used because the sample sizes were not equal.

To determine the direction and magnitude of differences between experimental groups, an effect size (ES) analysis was undertaken to provide an interpretable and statistically significant value for the direction and magnitude of a difference between two groups. The result of the ES and its confidence interval also gives an unambiguous indication about whether an outcome is worse or better in one group (Becker, 2000; Coe, 2002; Faraone, 2008). The ES (standardized mean difference) was calculated as

$$ES = \frac{[\text{mean of group 1}] - [\text{mean of group 2}]}{\text{pooled standard deviation}}. \tag{14.4}$$

In the Results section, the value of Hedge's g for ES is provided in parentheses. Hedge's g values were calculated rather than Cohen's d values because sample sizes were small and there was a good correlation (Spearman test) between and across groups.

Results

Differences in Thickness of Cortex at Four Cortical Areas in Normal (Control) Adult Brains

Significant differences were obtained for the entire thickness or depth of the cerebral cortex between the four different cortical regions examined (ANOVA $p < 0.0001$) (Table 14.2A) in control/uninjured patients. The thickness of the cerebral cortex differed across different cortical fields. In normal (uninjured) brains, the mean thickness of the cortex was approximately 2500 µm in VMPF, DLPF, and AC cortices (Table 14.2A, 3), and about 3750 µm in MC (Table 14.2B).

Comparison of cortical thickness using the Tukey–Kramer multiple comparisons test showed that MC differed markedly from VMPF, DLPF, and AC ($q = 165.30$). Further analysis (unpaired t-test with Welch correction) indicated that there were significant differences in thickness between VMPF and DLFC ($t = 4.89$, Table 14.2A), between VMPF and AC ($t = 6.96$, Table 14.2A), between VMPF and MC ($t = 89.59$), and between DLPF and MC ($t = 96.47$, Table 14.2A). On the other hand, the thickness of cortex in DLPF did not differ from that in AC (Table 14.2A).

When the thicknesses of separate individual cortical layers were compared in normal patients, for layer 1 or the cortical molecular layer, there were significant differences between all four cortical regions, VMPF, DLPF, AC, and MC (Table 14.3). The depth of layer 1 within DLPF was greater than in any other cortical region: $t = 4.825$ for VMPF, $t = 6.506$ for AC, and $t = 2.283$ for MC. For MC, although the depth in DLPF did not differ from the depth of layer 1 in MC, the

Table 14.2A   Differences in total thickness of cortex in normal (control) brains (unpaired t-test with Welch correction)

Comparison	t	p-value
VMPF vs. DLPF	4.89	$p < 0.0001$
VMPF vs. AC	6.96	$p < 0.0001$
VMPF vs. MC	89.59	$p < 0.0001$
DLPF vs. AC	1.99	$p = 0.051$
DLPF vs. MC	96.47	$p < 0.0001$
AC vs. MC	99.99	$p < 0.0001$
Mean	95% confidence interval	

Table 14.2B Numbers of pyramidal neurons (Pn) and nonpyramidal neurons (nP) within a column of tissue of 300 μm wide, the depth of each cortical layer high, and 100 μm across within cortical layers 1–6 in VMPF, DLPF, AC, and MC

	VLPF		DLPF		AC		MC	
	Pn	nP	Pn	nP	Pn	nP	Pn	nP
Layer 1	0	4955	0	1900	0	6320	0	5300
Layer 2	25,200	8360	27,600	6600	27,400	5700	0	7900
Layer 3	31,869	8584	34,000	13,700	37,400	8400	38100	13,800
Layer 4	18,620	5160	19,400	7900				
Layer 5	19,875	8950	18,100	7950				
Layer 5a					18,300	13,450	38,300	16,600
Layer 5b					20,100	7550	43,300	13,000
Layer 6	15,449	11,520	11,000	12,200	12,100	19,300	15,900	18,500

Note: Data obtained from brains of 11 adults with no history of brain injury or disease.

entire cortical thickness in MC was about 1.5 times greater than the total depth in the other three cortical regions (Table 14.3).

Layer 2, the external granular layer, differed in thickness between VMPF and DLPF (Welch's $t = 2.81$) being greater in the latter, VMPF and AC ($t = 3.088$), and MC ($t = 12.665$). Layer 3, the external pyramidal layer, was between 1.3 times and 1.48 times thicker than the sum of the thicknesses of layers 1 and 2 within DLPF and AC. However, layer 3 in VMPF and MC was between 2.02 times and 2.31 times thicker than the sums of the thickness of layers 1 and 2 in the respective regions.

There was also a highly significant difference in the thickness of cortical layer 3 between VMPF and DLPF ($t = 13.527$), VMPF and AC ($t = 18.994$), and VMPF and MC ($t = 22.848$) (Table 14.3).

Layer 4, the internal granular layer, is present in granular cortex only, which is in prefrontal cortex VMPF and DLPF in the present context. There was no difference in the thickness of layer 4 between VMPF and DLPF ($p = 0.39$, Welch's $t = 0.88$).

Layer 5, the internal pyramidal layer, is anatomically a single layer in granular cortex, but in agranular cortex is subdivided into layers 5A and 5B. There was no difference in thickness of layer 5 between VMPF and DLPF ($t = 1.731$, $p = 1.006$). Within AC, layer 5A contains minicolumns of intermediate sized pyramidal neurons, while vertically oriented, spindle shaped pyramidal neurons occur in layer 5B. A range of sizes of pyramidal neurons occur within layer 5A of MC, while within layer 5B, large pyramidal neurons occur. There was a major difference in the thicknesses of layers 5A and 5B within AC ($t = 29.58$, $p < 0.0001$) with layer 5B being some 3.5 times thicker than layer 5A (Table 14.3) There was also a difference in the thicknesses of layers 5A and 5B within MC ($t = 6.978$, $p < 0.0001$), together with a difference in the depth of layer 5A in AC compared with that of layer 5A in MC ($t = 29.576$). There was not, however, any difference in the thickness of layer 5B between AC and MC ($t = 0.4664$, $p = 0.6462$).

Differences in the depth of layer 6, the polymorphic or multiform layer, were highly significant between VMPF and DLPF ($t = 4.174$, $p = 0.0006$), VMPF and AC ($t = 4.532$, $p = 0.0002$), and VMPF and MC ($t = 10.447$, $p < 0.0001$); DLPF and MC ($t = 7.473$, $p < 0.0001$); AC and VMPF ($t = 4.53$, $p = 0.0002$) and MC ($t = 7.104$, $p < 0.0001$). However, the depth of layer 6 does not differ between DLPF and AC ($p = 0.68$, Table 14.3).

In the simplest terms, two types of neuron occur within mammalian cerebral cortex, excitatory pyramidal cells, and inhibitory nonpyramidal cells (Gaspard and Vanderhaeghen, 2011). The proportions of these cells change with posttraumatic survival following TBI (Maxwell et al., 2010). In the current study, it was decided to investigate the hypothesis that the ratios of the number of pyramidal cells to the number of nonpyramidal cells also differed within cortical layers in different

Table 14.3 Thickness (mean ± standard deviation in micrometer) by layer of cerebral cortex from 11 brains at four different cortical areas (VMPF = Brodmann, BA11; DLPF = BA10; AC = BA24a; MC = BA4)

	VMPF	DLPF	AC	MC
Layer 1	285 ± 22.80	336.3 ± 26.90	261.67 ± 26.90	310 ± 27.14
Cf VMPF		$t = 4.83$ $p = 0.0001$	$t = 2.194$ $p = 0.0408$	$t = 2.339$ $p = 0.0304$
Cf DLPF	$t = 4.83$ $p = 0.0001$		$t = 6.506$ $p < 0.0001$	$t = 2.283$ $p = 0.0341$
Cf AC	$t = 2.194$ $p = 0.0408$	$t = 4.825$ $p = 0.0001$		$t = 4.195$ $p = 0.0005$
Cf MC	$t = 2.34$ $p = 0.029$	$t = 2.28$ $p = 0.034$	$t = 4.19$ $p = 0.0005$	
Layer 2	161.3 ± 12.90	175.43 ± 10.53	145.8 ± 10.52	230 ± 12.54
Cf VMPF		$t = 2.814$ $p = 0.0111$	$t = 3.088$ $p = 0.0061$	$t = 12.665$ $p < 0.0001$
Cf DLPF	$t = 2.814$ $p = 0.0111$		$t = 6.602$ $p < 0.0001$	$t = 11.053$ $p < 0.0001$
Cf AC	$t = 3.088$ $p = 0.0061$	$t = 6.602$ $p < 0.0001$		$t = 11.053$ $p < 0.0001$
Cf MC	$t = 12.66$ $p < 0.0001$	$t = 11.05$ $p < 0.0001$	$t = 17.06$ $p < 0.0001$	
Layer 3	902 ± 37.8	691.11 ± 35.28	606.67 ± 35.28	1250 ± 33.51
Cf VMPF		$t = 13.527$ $p < 0.0001$	$t = 18.944$ $p < 0.0001$	$t = 22.848$ $p < 0.0001$
Cf DLPF	$t = 13.527$ $p < 0.0001$		$t = 5.613$ $p < 0.0001$	$t = 38.095$ $p < 0.0001$
Cf AC	$t = 18.944$ $p < 0.0001$	$t = 5.613$ $p < 0.0001$		$t = 43.851$ $p < 0.0001$
Cf MC	$t = 22.84$ $p < 0.0001$	$t = 38.09$ $p < 0.0001$	$t = 43.85$ $p < 0.0001$	
Layer 4	252 ± 20.16	258.75 ± 15.50		
Cf VMPF	ns	ns		
Layer 5a			170 ± 15.53	500 ± 33.59
			$t = 29.576$ $p < 0.0001$	$t = 6.978$ $p < 0.0001$
Layer 5	313.6 ± 25.08	335.42 ± 33.45		
	ns	ns		
Layer 5b			593.33 ± 33.45	600 ± 33.63
			ns	Ns
Layer 6	612.2 ± 48.97	690 ± 37.73	696.67 ± 37.73	825 ± 46.54
Cf VMPF		$t = 4.174$ $p = 0.0006$	$t = 4.532$ $p = 0.0002$	$t = 10.447$ $p < 0.0001$
Cf DLPF	$t = 4.174$ $p = 0.0006$		ns $p = 0.68$	$t = 7.473$ $p < 0.0001$
Cf AC	$t = 4.532$ $p = 0.0002$	ns $p = 0.68$		$t = 7.104$ $p < 0.0001$
Cf MC	$t = 10.45$ $p < 0.0001$	$t = 7.47$ $p < 0.0001$	$t = 7.10$ $p < 0.0001$	

Note: Since standard deviations differed across groups, differences in the thicknesses of cortical layers between Brodmann areas were determined by the unpaired t-test with Welch correction.

cortical regions of normal patients. However, a criticism sometimes made of published quantitative analyses is that results are quoted as ratios rather that finite numbers within a defined reference space (Huttenlocher, 1990; West and Gundersen, 1990). The values for the numbers of pyramidal and nonpyramidal neurons within a column of 300 μm by 100 μm and the depth of each cortical layer are provided in Table 14.2B. Although only undertaken using criteria of the shape and size of neuron subgroups (Figure 14.2), quantitative analysis provides support for this hypothesis.

Layer 1 of cerebral cortex or the molecular layer of DLPF and AC contained only small nonpyramidal neurons (sPn) (Figure 14.1a,c). However, in VMPF and MC, small (sPn) and medium (mPn) sized cells occurred, and the majority (circa 60%) were small cells (Figure 14.1a,d).

Layer 2 or the external granular layer contained Pns, and nPm and nPs nonpyramidal neurons in VMPF, DLPF, and AC (Figure 14.1a–c), and the majority (75–80%) were small pyramidal neurons. The external granular layer of MC, however, contained only nonpyramidal neurons and the majority (≈ 60%) were small cells (Figure 14.1d).

Layer 3 or the external pyramidal cell of granular cortex contained Pnb (≈0.047 for VMPF, ≈0.05 for DLPF), Pnm (≈0.23 for VMPF,≈ 0.22 for DLPF), and Pns (≈0.54 for VMPF, ≈0.44 for DLPF) pyramidal cells (Figure 14.2, Figure 14.1a,b), forming either ≈80% of all neurons in VMPF or ≈70% in DLPF. Within agranular cortex, the proportions of pyramidal cells were Pnb (≈0.05 for AC, ≈0.08 for MC), Pnm (≈0.22 for AC, ≈0.33 for MC), and Pns (≈0.54 for AC, ≈0.32 for MC), forming either ≈81% of all neurons in AC or ≈73% of all neurons in MC (Figure 14.1c,d). In general, pyramidal neurons outnumbered nonpyramidal neurons more than twice (3.76 : 1 for VMPF, 2.4 : 1 for DLPF, 4.5 : 1 for AC, and 2.7 : 1 for MC).

Layer 4 occurred only in granular cortex and the largest proportion (≈60%) of neurons were Pns (Figure 14.1a,b).

Within layer 5 or the internal pyramidal layer, of granular cortex, Pnm (≈26% for VMPF, ≈21% for DLPF) and Pns (≈41% for VMPF, ≈49% for DLPF) pyramidal neurons formed a large proportion of the total number of neurons (67% in VMPF, 70% in DLPF), while Pnb neurons were absent. In agranular cortex, within layers 5A and 5B of AC and MC (Figure 14.1c,d), small pyramidal neurons formed ≈65% and ≈72% of the total number of neurons within AC and ≈70% and ≈77% within MC. The largest pyramidal cells of any region occurred within layer 5B of MC (Figure 14.1d), where ≈10% of neurons were large or Betz cells. Rivara et al. (2003) reported that about 12% of the total number of pyramidal neurons in human MC of normal patients are Betz cells occurring within layer 5B. It is noteworthy, however, that Rivara et al. (2003) reported a considerable variability between members of their sample population, in which the proportion of large pyramidal Betz cells varied between 5.1% and 17% of the total number of pyramidal cells within layer 5B of MC.

Comparison of the proportion of Pnm and Pns neurons within layer 5B of AC and MC also indicated a difference (Table 14.2B). Within layers 5A and 5B of AC, Pns neurons formed the largest proportion of all neurons, 52% in layer 5A and 63% in layer 5B. But within layer 5B of MC, Pnm cells formed the larger proportion of neurons at 38% compared with 29% for small pyramidal neurons (Figure 14.1d), while Pns cells formed the majority in layer 5A (45%).

In layer 6, of all four cortical regions, around 40% of neurons were Pns cells. In VMPF cortex, the proportion of Pnb cells (≈21%) differed from that in DLPF (≈10%, $p < 0.001$) and AC/MC (≈16.5%, $p < 0.05$). In agranular cortex, nonpyramidal cells were in the majority (≈61% of the total number of neurons in AC, ≈54% of the total neuron number in MC) (Figure 14.1c,d), where the greatest proportions were nPm cells in agranular cortex (Figure 14.1c,d). On the other hand, within granular cortex, nPm cells were in the minority (7%) and nPb (21%) and nPs (15%) formed similar proportions of the nonpyramidal cell population (Figure 14.1a,b).

In conclusion, this study provides novel, statistically valid evidence that the proportion of pyramidal to nonpyramidal cells differed between different cortical layers and between different

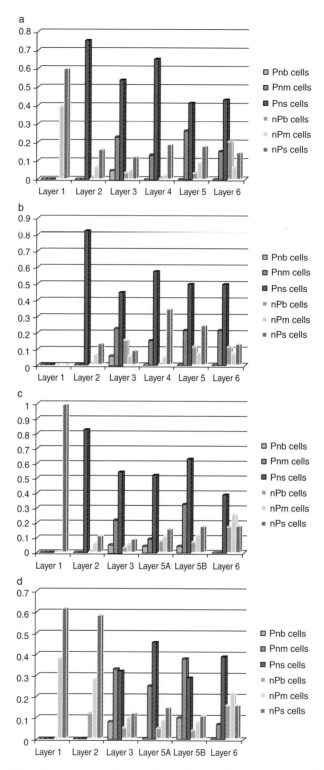

Figure 14.1 Bar graphs of the relative proportion of each subtype of neuron: big, medium, and small pyramidal neurons (Pnb, Pnm, and Pns) and big, medium, and small nonpyramidal neurons (nPb, nPm, and nPs) within each cortical layer of healthy cerebral cortex from (a) ventromedial prefrontal (VMPF), (b) dorsolateral prefrontal (DLPF), (c) anterior cingulate (AC), and (d) motor cortices (MCs).

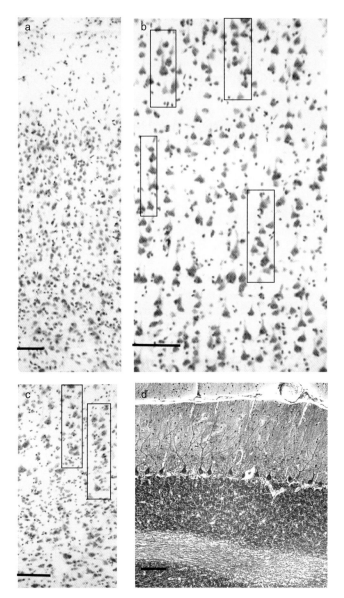

Figure 14.2 Photomicrographs of human cerebral cortex (a–c) and cerebellar cortex (d) to illustrate the characteristic nonuniform distribution of neurons. In all micrographs, the marker bar represents 100 μm. Panel a provides a low power overview of, from the top,cortical layer 1, layer 2, and part of layer 3 in ventromedial prefrontal cortex. Cell nuclei are relatively widely spaced in layer 1, are closely packed in layer 2, and tend to form vertically arranged groups in layer 3. Panel b shows a medium power field of part of cortical layer 3 from dorsolateral prefrontal cortex, and panel c shows part of layers 5 and 6 of ventromedial prefrontal cortex. Boxes outline columnar, vertically oriented aggregates of pyramidal neurons within which cells are more closely packed than in adjacent lucent regions between minicolumns. Panel d is medium power photomicrograph of a cortical region in cerebellum. The Purkinje cells, the large neurons with superiorly extending branched processes, form a single row of cells. The branching Purkinje cell processes extend into the molecular layer consisting of widely separated nuclei of cells. Deep to the layer of Purkinje cells occur a relatively thick, darkly stained layer containing numerous, very closely packed granule neurons and astrocytes.

types of cortex. Pyramidal neurons were between three and four times more numerous in layers 2 and 3 of VMPF, DLPF, and AC but not in MC (Table 14.2B). There was more than double the number of pyramidal neurons in layer 5 of granular cortex and layers 5A and 5B of agranular cortex (Table 14.2B). But within layer 6 of prefrontal cortex, pyramidal neurons outnumber nonpyramidal neurons to only a small degree. In agranular cortex, however, nonpyramidal neurons within layer 6 outnumber pyramidal neurons forming 54% of neurons in MC and 61% in AC.

Spatial Distribution of Neurons

A property of a population of neurons frequently quoted in many stereological reports of neuronal changes in a variety of clinically related analyses is that the density of neurons differs from that in normal or control patients. However, a frequent omission in a high proportion of such analyses has been the lack of precise details of the volume of a counting box or region examined in a study and whether the populations of cells were normally distributed. It may be that the latter has not been considered and routine, commercial programs have been used for estimation of numbers. Cell density has usually been provided in terms of number of neurons or cells per cubic millimeter of tissue. As a result, it has been unclear whether the data relate to the total volume of a region of cortex or other brain region such as the hippocampus, thalamus, corpus callosum, or just to the volume of the counting box used. Frequently, because a statement had not been provided as to how representative was the sample used of the full region of interest, a number of problems of interpretation may arise as reviewed in several publications (Huttenlocher, 1990; West and Gundersen, 1990; Geuna, 2000; Gardi et al., 2008).

We tested the hypothesis that the spacing or NND for different subgroups of neurons differed between cortical layers and cortical regions using SE analysis. Methodologically, the nucleolus was used as a point for the measurement of distance between neighboring cells.

Large pyramidal neurons (Pnb) in all four cortical regions were more widely spaced than would be expected for a Poisson distribution and are therefore scattered (Table 14.4). Medium sized

Table 14.4A   VMPF cortex

	Pnb	Pnm	Pns	nPb	nPm	nPs
Layer 1						0.289
Layer 2			1.61		0.303	0.135
Layer 3	2.4 horizontal 0.317 vertical	2.02	1.98	0.585	0.418	0.345
Layer 4		1.084	1.45		0.287	0.0953
Layer 5		3.371	1.470	0.815	0.572	0.461
Layer 6		1.5	2.368	1.01	0.761	0.506

Table 14.4B   DLPF cortex

	Pnb	Pnm	Pns	nPb	nPm	nPs
Layer 1						0.790
Layer 2			1.307		0.790	0.273
Layer 3	2.129	2.541	1.471	0.660	0.580	0.354
Layer 4		1.081	1.597		0.350	0.313
Layer 5		0.783	0.620	0.910	0.470	0.360
Layer 6			1.130	0.850	0.500	0.325

Table 14.4C AC cortex

	Pnb	Pnm	Pns	nPb	nPm	nPs
Layer 1						*1.405*
Layer 2			1.146		1.150	**0.587**
Layer 3	*1.437*	1.189	*1.413*	1.044	1.088	**0.540**
Layer 5a	*1.24*	1.127	*1.249*	1.010	1.085	**0.538**
Layer 5b	*1.62*	1.061	1.086	1.037	1.097	**0.547**
Layer 6		1.061	1.111	1.068	1.046	0.995

Table 14.4D MC

	Pnb	Pnm	Pns	nPb	nPm	nPs
Layer 1					1.040	**0.768**
Layer 2			**0.710**	1.043	1.011	0.923
Layer 3	*2.121*		*1.207*	*1.300*	1.042	0.986	**0.640**
Layer 5a		*3.893/9.44*	**0.533**	1.014	1.021	1.248
Layer 5b	*3.659 vert 9.76 hor*	*2.53*	*1.643*	*1.240*	1.002	1.017
Layer 6		1.12	**0.440**	1.000	1.009	**0.428**

pyramidal (Pnm) cells in layers 3–6 of prefrontal cortices, and layers 3, 5a, 5b, and 6 of AC and MCs were either scattered or randomly distributed within the neuropil (Table 14.4), except in layer 5 of DLPF, where medium sized pyramidal cells were clustered or more closely packed than expected for a Poisson distribution (Table 14.4). Small pyramidal neurons (Pns) were also scattered within all layers of the cerebral cortex except in layer 5 of DLPF and layers 2, 5a, and 6 of MC, where the cells were closely packed or clustered.

Large nonpyramidal cells were clustered in layer 3 of ventromedial and dorsolateral cortex, were randomly distributed in layers 5 and 6 of the same, and were randomly distributed in AC and MCs (Table 14.4). Medium sized nonpyramidal cells were clustered within all cortical layers of VMPF and DLPF (Table 14.4A,B) but were uniformly distributed within all layers of agranular cortex. Similarly, small nonpyramidal neurons (nPs) were clustered in all layers of granular prefrontal cortex with the exception of layer 4 of VMPF where cells were normally distributed. In agranular cortex, however, nPs cells were scattered in layer 1 of AC cortex, clustered in layers 2–5, and uniformly distributed within layer 6 (Table 14.4C). In MC, the spatial distribution of nPs cells differed in that cells were clustered in layers 1, 3, and 6, but uniformly distributed within layers 2, 5A, and 5B.

A major and important conclusion was that neurons within the four cortical regions investigated were not uniformly or randomly distributed within 3D space. Therefore, the use of stereological techniques which assume a uniform or random distribution of points and designed to provide an equal chance of each or any point being sampled can never give a meaningful estimate of number. Use of nonparametric techniques provided statistically validated data that the number of six subtypes of neurons differed between both cortical area and layers within those cortical areas. Use of 3D spacing techniques provided novel information that in normal patients of a mean age of 47.09 ± 16.95 years (range of 18–74 years), pyramidal neurons within all six cortical layers of granular and agranular cortices were scattered, while nonpyramidal neurons were clustered or had a lesser spacing between like cells than expected for a Poisson distribution. Furthermore, there was a more consistent lesser spacing between nonpyramidal neurons within granular cortex than in agranular cortex.

Spatial Distribution of Glial Cells

There are three types of glial or supporting cells within adult cerebral cortex, astrocytes, oligo-dendrocytes, and a variety of microglia. The literature concerning astrocytes and their function within intact and/or injured neuropil has expanded dramatically in the last decade, and it is now widely accepted that astrocytes have an intimate and wide-ranging physiological role in maintaining both an optimal physicochemical microenvironment for neurons within the CNS and in maintenance of the integrity of the blood–brain barrier (Benarroch, 2005; Otis and Sofroniew, 2008; Sofroniew and Vinters, 2010).

Astrocytes within paraffin and celloidin sections may be identified by their size and the observation that astrocytes possess a lucent or pale nucleus outlined by a discrete dark profile on the internal aspect of the nuclear envelop. However, the most widely used aid to recognition or identification of astrocytes in sections has utilized labeling with an antibody against glial fibrillary acidic protein (GFAP), an intermediate filament unique to astrocytes, which also allowed appreciation of the extent of processes arising from the cell body, use of immunocytochemistry for glutamate synthetase and S 100β (Li et al., 2012), or differential fixation and staining (Shehab et al., 1990). But Lyck et al. (2008) reported that GFAP labeling in long-term fixed human brain may be problematic. In the present study, astrocyte nuclear morphology was the criterion used during counting. Additionally, in the acute phase after brain injury, astrocytes frequently swell and are lucent, while "reactive astrocytes" become packed with GFAP over about a day after any injury and the cells may then be identified by means of immunocytochemical labeling as the cell assumes the state of reactive astrogliosis (Ridet et al., 1997; Chen and Swanson, 2003). The material available in the present study related only to chronic survivors of TBI and patients with no history of head injury. Under those conditions, use of GFAP immunohistochemistry to identify astrocytes may be problematic and inconsistent (Lyck et al., 2008). Nonetheless, characteristically, the glia limitans and the most superficial regions of cortical layer 1 contained small numbers of labeled astrocytes in postmortem material, and their number also increased with the age of a patient (Peters, 2007). The characteristic nuclear morphology of astrocytes referred to above was used during analysis of NNDs. The analysis suggested that astrocytes are distributed in a close to uniform pattern (Table 14.5) or scattered to a small degree within cortical layers 1, 3, 4, 5, or 5A and 5B in granular and nongranular cortices (Table 14.5). However, in layer 2 of VMPF, DLPF, AC, and MC, astrocytes were clustered (Table 14.5).

Microglial cells assume a range of reactive subtypes following injury and generate a wide range of cell surface activation molecules, for example, Toll-like receptors, major histocompatability complex (MHC) class 1, and innate cytokines (Town et al., 2005). In the absence of injury or infection, microglia normally exists in a quiescent or "resting" state being small and possessing branching or ramified processes when labeled using the CR4/43 antibody. Upon "activation," cell processes retract and the cell soma "rounds up," often referred to as being "ameboid," and increases in volume. Examples of rounded or ameboid cell bodies are illustrated (Figure 14.3) from subcortical white matter in a MoD patient that survived for 4 months after TBI. In this relatively low magnification micrograph, there is the impression that numbers of CR3/43 labeled cells are far more numerous in white matter than in the overlying gray matter of cortical layer 6. Estimation of the number of immunolabeled cells within a standard sized counting brick in cortical layer 5 and subcortical white matter was undertaken and a marked difference in number obtained (Table 14.7). Moreover, estimated counts of activated microglia within white matter from MoD ($n = 13$), severely disabled (SD) ($n = 12$), and vegetative state (VS) patients ($n = 11$) followed by Dunnett multiple comparisons test indicated that with increasing severity of brain injury, a greater number of activated microglia occurred within layer 5 gray matter in DLPF and VS MC (Table 14.7). However, the increase in number of CR3/43 positive microglia was much greater within subcortical white matter, where all changes were statistically significant ($p < 0.01$) across MoD,

Table 14.5   Values for NNDs and NNI for astrocytes within the six cortical layers of VMPF, DLPF, AC, and MC of healthy patients

VMPF cortex	Control astrocyte NND measurement	Calculated NND for cell number (control)	NNI
Layer 1	28	21.829	*1.28*
Layer 2	17.95	24.829	**0.72**
Layer 3	29.2	19.592	*1.49*
Layer 4	16.45	21.149	**0.77**
Layer 5	20.45	19.297	1.05
Layer 6	17.66	17.467	1.01
DLPF cortex	Control astrocyte NND measurement	Calculated NND for cell number (control)	NNI
Layer 1	21.85	21.917	0.99
Layer 2	20.35	24.273	0.84
Layer 3	33.193	19.903	*1.67*
Layer 4	24.65	20.547	1.19
Layer 5	26.68	19.229	*1.38*
Layer 6	29.90	17.568	*1.70*
AC cortex	Control astrocyte NND measurement	Calculated NND for cell number (control)	NNI
Layer 1	23.5	21.195	1.11
Layer 2	18.7	24.124	**0.77**
Layer 3	31.89	20.176	*1.58*
Layer 5a	22.63	20.822	1.08
Layer 5b	24.7	19.468	*1.27*
Layer 6	17.34	17.398	0.99
MC	Control astrocyte NND measurement	Calculated NND for cell number (control)	NNI
Layer 1	24.6	21.186	1.16
Layer 2	19.4	24.495	**0.79**
Layer 3	29.8	20.071	*1.48*
Layer 5a	23.7	19.685	*1.20*
Layer 5b	23.8	20.215	1.17
Layer 6	17.38	17.461	0.99

SD, and VS patients. The increasing value of q across MoD, SD, and VS patients (Table 14.7) demonstrated that with increasing severity of Glasgow Outcome Score (GOS), the number of activated or ameboid microglia increased within subcortical white matter.

Discussion

The results obtained provide statistically validated support for the hypotheses that the depth of each of the six layers of human cerebral cortex in a sample of 11 normal adults differed between four cortical regions, between ventromedial and dorsolateral prefrontal cortices, AC, and MC; that the proportion of pyramidal to nonpyramidal neurons differed between granular and agranular cortices; and that pyramidal neurons do not follow a Poisson distribution but were scattered or more widely spaced than might have been expected when compared with a normally distributed population of cells. Nonpyramidal neurons were, on the contrary, either normally dispersed or clustered more closely than would have been expected for a random, Poisson-type distribution.

A number of publications have reported changes in density of neurons within cerebral cortical layers both between primate species (Collins et al., 2010; Elston et al., 2011) and in a range of clinical conditions, for example, schizophrenia (Benes et al., 1986; Weinberger, 1988; Rajkowska et al., 1998; Selemon et al., 1998; Kolluri et al., 2005; Cullen et al., 2006; Smiley et al., 2011),

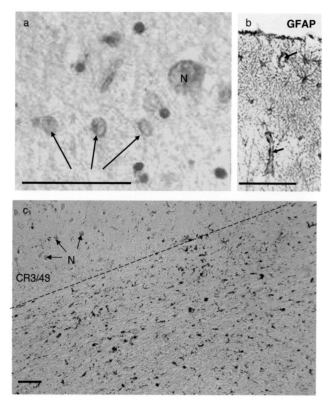

Figure 14.3 Micrographs of immunolabeled paraffin sections to illustrate the distribution of glial cells in a DLPF cortical area from a control patient (a and b) and an MoD patient 4 months (c) after TBI. The bar represents 50 μm. In panel a, three astrocyte nuclei (arrows) and a neuronal nucleus (N) are seen. The three astrocyte nuclei show the characteristic linear density at the periphery of the nucleus and a little heterochromatin within. In panel b, the section has been immunolabeled with anti-GFAP to illustrate the density of labeling in the superficial glia limitans and the stellate appearance of the radiating cell processes of astrocytes. A meshwork of fine astrocyte processes occurs within the most superficial part of the cortex, and this is characteristic of human material obtained at postmortem. Note also immunolabeling of the perivascular, glial foot processes of sections through two blood vessels (arrows). Photomicrograph (c) is a field from a slide from a 4-month survival MoD patient labeled with CR3/43 to demonstrate the occurrence of rounded up, activated microglia and cell processes. Note the discrete boundary indicated by the dotted line between the inferior part of cortical layer 6 containing a number of neuronal nuclei (arrows N) and the underlying white matter containing linearly arranged nerve fibers and immunolabeled activated microglia within the subcortical white matter.

AIDS (Ketzler et al., 1990; Gray et al., 1991), amyotrophic lateral sclerosis (Mochizuki et al., 2011), autism (Oblak et al., 2011), and TBI (Maxwell et al., 2010; Lifshitz and Lisembee, 2012). However, reports either did not distinguish between pyramidal and nonpyramidal neurons (Rajkowska et al., 1998; Toft et al., 2005; Tsai et al., 2009) or had selected only one of a few layers of the cortex (Cullen et al., 2006). A consistent feature of such studies was use of neuronal density without regard to possible differences in total reference volume, as highlighted by West and Gundersen (1990), "the second and much more problematic aspect of the data of earlier studies is that only the number of neurons per unit volume of tissue is reported, and nothing is known about the volume of the region or, consequently, about the total number of neurons." Stereological studies may only be meaningful in relation to biology if the characteristics assessed or estimated have been expressed in absolute numbers rather than ratios or densities (Huttenlocher, 1990; West and Gundersen, 1990; Wanke et al., 1994; Noori and Fornal, 2011). Reports of ratios alone, such as cell density without scaling to total cell number, fail to address whether observed changes relate to the particles of interest, the reference space volume or both, or even to correctly understand

Table 14.6 Values for NNDs and NNI for astrocytes within the six cortical layers of VMPF, DLPF, AC, and MC of healthy patients

VMPF cortex	Control astrocyte NND measurement	Calculated NND for cell number (control)	NNI
Layer 1	28	21.829	*1.28*
Layer 2	17.95	24.829	**0.72**
Layer 3	29.2	19.592	*1.49*
Layer 4	16.45	21.149	**0.77**
Layer 5	20.45	19.297	1.05
Layer 6	17.66	17.467	1.01

DLPF cortex	Control astrocyte NND measurement	Calculated NND for cell number (control)	NNI
Layer 1	21.85	21.917	0.99
Layer 2	20.35	24.273	0.84
Layer 3	33.193	19.903	*1.67*
Layer 4	24.65	20.547	1.19
Layer 5	26.68	19.229	*1.38*
Layer 6	29.90	17.568	*1.70*

AC cortex	Control astrocyte NND measurement	Calculated NND for cell number (control)	NNI
Layer 1	23.5	21.195	1.11
Layer 2	18.7	24.124	**0.77**
Layer 3	31.89	20.176	*1.58*
Layer 5a	22.63	20.822	1.08
Layer 5b	24.7	19.468	*1.27*
Layer 6	17.34	17.398	0.99

MC	Control astrocyte NND measurement	Calculated NND for cell number (control)	NNI
Layer 1	24.6	21.186	1.16
Layer 2	19.4	24.495	**0.79**
Layer 3	29.8	20.071	*1.48*
Layer 5a	23.7	19.685	*1.20*
Layer 5b	23.8	20.215	1.17
Layer 6	17.38	17.461	0.99

Table 14.7 Results for differences in estimated number of CR3/43 reactive activated microglia within a standard counting box in cortical layer 5 and subcortical white matter in 11 control, 13 MoD, 12 SD, and 11 VS patients

Cortical region	Control	MoD	SD	VP
VMPF L5	1.8 ± 1.1	$p > 0.05$, $q = 0.123$	$p > 0.05$, $q = 0.577$	$p > 0.05$, $q = 1.26$
Subcortical	4.6 ± 1.3	$p < 0.01$, $q = 4.071$	$p < 0.01$, $q = 5.51$	$p < 0.01$, $q = 8.68$
DLPF L5	7.5 ± 1.1	$p < 0.01$, $q = 4.74$	$p < 0.01$, $q = 6.80$	$p < 0.01$, $q = 14.27$
Subcortical	1.8 ± 1.1	$p < 0.01$, $q = 4.13$	$p < 0.01$, $q = 4.25$	$p < 0.01$, $q = 7.07$
AC L5	$1.8 + 1.1$	$p > 0.05$, $q = 0.206$	$p > 0.05$, $q = 0.743$	$p > 0.05$, $q = 1.86$
Subcortical	2.0 ± 1.1	$p < 0.01$, $q = 5.88$	$p < 0.01$, $q = 6.78$	$p < 0.01$, $q = 12.19$
MC L5	0.75 ± 1.1	$p > 0.05$, $q = 1.45$	$p > 0.05$, $q = 1.83$	$p < 0.01$, $q = 3.41$
Subcortical	3.7 ± 2.1	$p < 0.01$, $q = 5.16$	$p < 0.01$, $q = 6.79$	$p < 0.01$, $q = 9.42$

Note: Comparison carried out using the Dunnett multiple comparisons test against control values.

what the authors of a study meant by the somewhat loose term "density." For example, the British Standards Institute (BSI) (1991) and American Society for Testing and Materials (ASTM) (1994) list more than 14 and 40 definitions, respectively, of density based on mass per unit volume. Only when the reference volume is known can neuron density be part of a meaningful discussion of the functional capacity of a neural structure or network.

The reference trap is of particular significance for studies of patients and/or animals in disease states or models of human diseases. For example, the present study reports that thinning of cortical layers occurs during the chronic phase after TBI, extending previous nonquantitative magnetic resonance imaging (MRI) reports (Newcombe et al., 2011; Bigler and Maxwell, 2012). This finding is dependent on layer-by-layer analysis that would not be possible without mean cortical values for neuron size and spacing. The current study also indicates that a greater discrimination of detailed information about the range of sizes and spatial distribution of neurons across cortical layers may be clinically and pathologically important since neither pyramidal or nonpyramidal neurons within cerebral cortex exhibit a Poisson/unimodal Gaussian spatial distribution, and use of parametric, normal, or lognormal statistical techniques is probably inappropriate during interpretation of data.

The present study provides novel information in support of the hypothesis that astrocytes follow a Poisson distribution in cerebral cortex. In addition, we find changes in numbers of microglia in subcortical white matter after TBI, with no evidence to support increased numbers of reactive microglia in cortical gray matter during the chronic phase of TBI.

The present study extends our previous work (Maxwell et al., 2010) with the finding that the packing density of neurons differs both between different cortical regions and for different sizes of neurons, supporting the hypothesis that neurons within different cortical regions form different cortical networks. These findings illustrate the need for further work to fully define such networks and how they may change in response to positive or negative influences. This study also supports the view that astrocytes are normally distributed in cerebral cortex. A widely documented feature of injury or disease in the brain is a temporal increase in the number of reactive microglia. The present study extends that literature with the finding that in chronic stage TBI, numbers of reactive microglia remain elevated within subcortical white matter to a greater extent that within cerebral gray matter. Diffuse TBI has long been recognized as primarily injury to cerebral white matter, but there has been a recent appreciation that long-term degeneration of white matter may occur following changes in cortical neuronal number (Maxwell et al., 2010; Bigler and Maxwell, 2012). To date, no studies have quantified changes in numbers of myelinated nerve fibers in white matter. The novel data for long-term elevated numbers of reactive microglia in subcortical white matter present here provide indirect evidence for continued, chronic loss of white matter after TBI.

References

Adams, J. H., Graham, D. I., Jennett, B. 2001. The structural basis of moderate disability after traumatic brain injury. *J Neurol Neurosurg Psychiatry* **71** (6): 521–524.

ASTM. 1994. *Compilation of ASTM Standard Definitions*, 8th ed. Philadelphia: American Society for Testing and Materials.

Becker, L. A. 2000. *Effect Size (ES)*. Available at http://web.uccs.edu/lbecker/Psy590/es.htm (last accessed July 17, 2013).

Benarroch, E. E. 2005. Neuron-astrocyte interactions: partnership for normal function and disease in the central nervous system. *Mayo Clin Proc* **80** (10): 1326–1338.

Benes, F. M., Lange, N. 2001. Two-dimensional versus three-dimensional cell counting: a practical perspective. *Trends Neurosci* **24** (1): 11–17.

Benes, F. M., Davidson, J., Bird, E. D. 1986. Quantitative cytoarchitectural studies of the cerebral cortex of schizophrenics. *Arch Gen Psychiatry* **43** (1): 31–35.

Bigler, E. D., Maxwell, W. L. 2012. Neuroimaging correlates of functional outcome, Ch. 19, In *Brain Injury Medicine Principles and Practice*, 2nd ed, edited by N. Zasler, D. Katz, D. B. Arciniegas, M. Ross Bullock, and J. S. Kreutzer. New York: DemosMedical.

British Standards Institute. BS 2955, 1991. *Glossary of Terms Relating to Particle Technology*. London: British Standards Institute.

Buxhoeveden, D. P., Switala, A. E., Roy, E., Casanova, M. F. 2000. Quantitative analysis of cell columns in the cerebral cortex. *J Neurosci Methods* **97** (1): 7–17.

Cammermeyer, J. 1961. The importance of avoiding "dark" neurons in experimental neuropathology. *Acta Neuropathol (Berl)* **1** (3): 245–270.

Chen, Y., Swanson, R. A. 2003. Astrocytes and brain injury. Review article. *J Cereb Blood Flow Metab* **23** (2): 137–149.

Coe, R. 2002. Effect size calculator. How to use the spreadsheet 2002. ESCalcGuide pdf.

Coggeshall, R. E., Lekan, H. A. 1996. Methods for determining numbers of cells and synapses: a case for more uniform standards of review. *J Comp Neurol* **364** (1): 6–15.

Collins, C. E., Airey, D. C., Young, N. A., Leitch, D. B., Kaas, J. H. 2010. Neuron densities vary across and within cortical areas in primates. *Proc Natl Acad Sci U S A* **107** (36): 15927–15932.

Cruz Orive, L.-M., Weibel, E. R. 1981. Sampling designs for stereology. *J Microsc* **122** (3): 235–257.

Cullen, T. J., Walker, M. A., Eastwood, S. L., Esiri, M. M., Harrison, P. J., Crow, T. J. 2006. Anomalies of asymmetry of pyramidal cell density and structure in dorsolateral prefrontal cortex in schizophrenia. *Br J Psychiatry* **188** (1): 26–31.

Diggle, P. J. 1990. A point process modelling approach to raised incidence of a rare phenomenon in the vicinity of a specific point. *J R Statist Soc A* **153** (3): 349–362.

Diggle, P. J. 2003. *Statistical Analysis of Spatial Point Patterns*, 2nd ed. London: Arnold.

Dorph-Petersen, K.-A., Nyengaard, J. R., Gundersen, H. J. G. 2001. Tissue shrinkage and unbiased stereological estimation of particle number and size. *J Microsc* **204** (3): 232–246.

Elston, G. N., Benavides-Piccione, R., Elston, A., Manger, P. R., DeFelipe, J. 2011. Pyramidal cells in prefrontal cortex of primates: marked differences in neuronal structure among species. *Front Neuroanat* **5** (2): 1–17.

Faraone, S.V. 2008. Understanding effect size: how it's measured and what it means. *Medscape Psychiatry & Mental Health* © 2008 Medscape.

Gardi, J. E., Nyengaard, J. R., Gundersen, H. J. G. 2008. The proportionator: unbiased stereological estimation using biased automatic image analysis and non-uniform probability proportional to size sampling. *Comput Biol Med* **38** (3): 313–328.

Gaspard, N., Vanderhaeghen, P. 2011. Laminar fate specification in the cerebral cortex. *F1000 Biol Rep* **3** (6): 1–6.

Geuna, S. 2000. Appreciating the difference between design-based and model-based sampling strategies in quantitative morphology of the nervous system. *J Comp Neurol* **427** (3): 333–339. Erratum in 430(1):145.

Gray, F., Haug, H., Chimelli, L., Geny, C., Gaston, A., Scaravilli, F., Budka, H. 1991. Prominent cortical atrophy with neuronal loss as correlate of human immunodeficiency virus encephalopathy. *Acta Neuropathol (Berl)* **82** (3): 229–233.

Harrison, P. J., Heath, P. R., Eastwood, S. L., Burnet, P. W. J., McDonald, B., Pearson, R. C. A. 1995. The relative importance of premortem acidosis and postmortem interval for human brain gene expression studies: selective mRNA vulnerability and comparison with their encoded proteins. *Neurosci Lett* **200**: 151–154.

Howard, V., Reed, M. G. 2005. *Unbiased Stereology. Three-Dimensional Measurement in Microscopy*, 2nd ed. Oxon, UK: Garland Science/Bios Scientific Publishers.

Huttenlocher, P. R. 1990. Morphometric study of human cerebral cortex development. *Neuropsychologia* **28** (6): 517–527.

Jennett, B., Adams, J. H., Murray, L. S., Graham, D. I. 2001. Neuropathology in vegetative and severely disabled patients after head injury. *Neurology* **56** (2): 486–490.

Jortner, B. S. 2006. The return of the dark neuron. A histological artifact complicating contemporary neurotoxicalogic evaluation. *Neurotoxicology* **27** (4): 628–634.

Ketzler, S., Weis, S., Haug, H., Budka, H. 1990. Loss of neurons in the frontal cortex in AIDS brains. *Acta Neuropathol (Berl)* **80** (1): 92–94.

Kluver, H., Barrera, E. 1953. A method for the combined staining of cells and fibers in the nervous system. *J Neuropathol Exp Neurol* **12** (4): 311–406.

Kolluri, N., Sun, Z., Sampson, A. R., Lewis, D. A. 2005. Lamina-specific reductions in dendritic spine density in the prefrontal cortex of subjects with schizophrenia. *Am J Psychiatry* **162** (6): 1200–1202.

Lewis, D. A. 2004. Structure of the human prefrontal cortex. *Am J Psychiatry* **161** (8): 1366.

Li, D.-R., Zhang, F., Wang, Y., Tan, X.-H., Qiao, D.-F., Wang, H.-J., Michiue, T., Maeda, H. 2012. Quantitative analysis of GFAP- and S100 protein immunopositive astrocytes to investigate the severity of traumatic brain injury. *Leg Med* **14** (1): 84–92.

Lifshitz, J., Lisembee, A. M. 2012. Neurodegeneration in the somatosensory cortex after experimental diffuse brain injury. *Brain Struct Funct* **217** (1): 49–61.

Lyck, L., Dalmau, I., Chemnitz, J., Finsen, B., Schroder, H. D. 2008. Immunohistochemical markers for quantitative studies of neurons and glia in human neocortex. *J Histochem Cytochem* **56** (3): 201–221.

Maxwell, W. L., MacKinnon, M.-A., Stewart, J. E., Graham, D. I. 2010. Stereology of cerebral cortex after traumatic brain injury matched to the Glasgow Outcome Score. *Brain* **133** (1): 139–160.

Miles, R. E., Davy, P. J. 1976. Precise and general conditions for the validity of a comprehensive set of stereological fundamental formulae. *J Microsc* **107** (2): 211–226.

Mochizuki, Y., Mizutani, T., Shimizu, T., Kawata, A. 2011. Proportional neuronal loss between the primary motor and sensory cortex in amyotrophic lateral sclerosis. *Neurosci Lett* **503** (1): 73–75.

Mouton, P. R. 2011. *Unbiased Stereology: A Concise Guide*. Baltimore, MD: The Johns Hopkins University Press.

Newcombe, V., Chatfield, D., Outtrim, J., Vowler, S., Manktelow, A. et al. 2011. Mapping traumatic axonal injury using diffusion tensor imaging: correlations with functional outcome. *PLoS ONE* **6** (5): e19214.

Noori, H. R., Fornal, C. A. 2011. The appropriateness of unbiased optical fractionators to assess cell proliferation in the adult hippocampus. *Front Neurosci* **5**: Article 140.

Oblak, A. L., Rosene, D. L., Kemper, T. L., Bauman, M. L., Blatt, G. J. 2011. Altered posterior cingulate cortical cytoarchitecture, but normal density of neurons and interneurons in the posterior cingulate cortex and fusiform gyrus in autism. *Autism Res* **4** (1): 1–12.

Ong, W. Y., Garey, L. J. 1991. Ultrastructural characteristics of human adult and infant cerebral cortical neurons. *J Anat* **175** (1): 79–104.

Otis, T. O., Sofroniew, M. V. 2008. Glia get excited. *Nat Neurosci* **11** (2): 379–380.

Peters, A. 2007. The effects of normal aging on nerve fibers and neuroglia in the central nervous system, Chapter 5. In *Brain Aging: Models, Methods, and Mechanisms*, edited by D. R. Riddle. Boca Raton, FL: CRC Press. Available at http://www.ncbi.nlm.nih.gov/books/NBK3873/ (last accessed July 17, 2013).

Rajkowska, G., Selemon, L. D., Goldman-Rakic, P. S. 1998. Neuronal and glial somal size in the prefrontal cortex. *Arch Gen Psychiatry* **55** (3): 215–224.

Ridet, J. L., Malhotra, S. K., Privat, A., Gage, F. H. 1997. Reactive astrocytes: cellular and molecular cues to biological function. *Trends Neurosci* **20** (12): 570–577.

Rivara, C.-M., Sherwood, C. C., Bouras, C., Hof, P. R. 2003. Stereologic characterization and spatial distribution patterns of Betz cells in the human primary motor cortex. *Anat Rec* **270A** (1): 137–151.

Rolls, G. O., Farmer, N. J., Hall, J. B. 2010. Artifacts in histological and cytological preparation. *Scientia Leica Microsystems*. Available at http://www.leica-microsystems.com (last accessed July 17, 2013).

Schlaug, G., Schleicher, A., Zilles, K. 1995. Quantitative analysis of the columnar arrangement of neurons in the human cingulate cortex. *J Comp Neurol* **351** (3): 441–452.

Schmitz, C., Hof, P. R. 2005. Design-based stereology in neuroscience. *Neuroscience* **130** (4): 813–831.

Selemon, L. D., Rajkowska, G., Goldman-Rakic, P. S. 1998. Elevated neuronal density in prefrontal area 46 in brains from schizophrenic patients: application of a three-dimensional stereological counting method. *J Comp Neurol* **392** (3): 402–412.

Shehab, A. S., Cronly-Dillon, J. R., Nona, S. N., Stafford, C. A. 1990. Preferential histochemical staining of protoplasmic and fibrous astrocytes in rat CNS with GFAP antibodies using different fixatives. *Brain Res* **518** (1–2): 347–352.

Smiley, J. F., Rosoklija, G., Mancevski, B., Pergolizzi, D., Figarsky, K., Bleiwas, C., Duma, A., Mann, J. J., Javitt, D. C., Dwork, A. J. 2011. Hemispheric comparisons of neuron density in the planum temporal of schizophrenia and nonpsychiatric brains. *Psychiatry Res: Neuroimaging* **192** (1): 1–11.

Sofroniew, M. V., Vinters, H. V. 2010. Astrocytes: biology and pathology. *Acta Neuropathol (Berl)* **119** (1): 7–35.

Sterio, D. C. 1984. The unbiased estimation of number and sizes of arbitrary particles using the disector. *J Microsc* **134** (2): 127–136.

Stuart, A. 1962. *Basic Ideas of Scientific Sampling. Issue 4 of Griffin's Statistical Monographs & Courses*, 1st ed. London: Charles Griffin & Company.

Toft, M. H., Gredal, O., Pakkenberg, B. 2005. The size distribution of neurons in the motor cortex in amyotrophic lateral sclerosis. *J Anat* **2007** (4): 399–407.

Town, T., Nikolic, V., Tan, J. 2005. The microglial "activation" continuum: from innate to adaptive responses. *J Neuroinflammation* **2**: 24. Available at http://www.jneuroinflammation.com/content/2/1/24 (last accessed July 17, 2013).

Tsai, P. S., Kaufhold, J. P., Blinder, P., Friedman, B., Drew, P. J., Karten, H. J., Lyden, P. D., Kleinfeld, D. 2009. Correlations of neuronal and microvascular densities in murine cortex revealed by direct counting and colocalization of nuclei and vessels. *J Neurosci* **29** (46): 14533–14570.

Wanke, R., Weis, S., Kluge, D., Kahnt, E., Schenck, E., Brem, G., Hermanns, W. 1994. Morphometric evaluation of the pancreas of growth hormone transgenic mice. *Acta Stereologica* **13** (1): 3–8.

Weinberger, D. R. 1988. Schizophrenia and the frontal lobes. *Trends Neurosci* **11** (8): 367–370.

West, M. J., Gundersen, H. J. 1990. Unbiased stereological estimation of the number of neurons in the human hippocampus. *J Comp Neurol* **296** (1): 1–22.

West, M. J., Slomianka, L., Gundersen, H. J. G. 1991. Unbiased stereological estimation of the total number of neurons in the subdivisions of the rat hippocampus using the optical fractionator. *Anat Rec* **231** (4): 482–497.

Williams, R. W., Rakic, P. 1988. Three-dimensional counting: an accurate and direct method to estimate numbers of cells in sectioned material. *J Comp Neurol* **278**: 344–352. An updated version was also published in September 1999.

15   The Effects of High-Fat Diet on the Mouse Hypothalamus: A Stereological Study

Mohammad Reza Namavar,[1,2] Samira Raminfard,[2] Zahra Vojdani Jahromi,[2] and Hassan Azari[2]

[1] Histomorphometry and Stereology Research Center, Shiraz University of Medical Sciences, Shiraz, Iran
[2] Department of Anatomical Sciences, School of Medicine, Shiraz University of Medical Sciences, Shiraz, Iran

Background

Obesity, a chronic increase in stores of body fat, is defined as a body mass index (BMI) greater than $30 \, kg/m^2$ (Formiguera and Cantón, 2004; Townsend, 2008; Moraes et al., 2009). During the last 10 years, the prevalence of obesity has increased in the majority of developed countries (Rada et al., 2010). These data suggest that primary obesity is related to environmental, social, and behavioral changes, although genetic factors may also be involved (Townsend, 2008; Cammisotto and Bendayan, 2012).

Overconsumption of dietary fats resulting in an imbalance between caloric intake and energy expenditure ranks among the most important environmental causes of obesity (Rada et al., 2010). In rodents, high-fat diets (HFDs) in the range of 20–60% of caloric intake produce obesity similar to that seen in humans (Buettner et al., 2006; Townsend, 2008). Although the exact physiological mechanisms remain unclear, both experimental and human studies indicate that obesity is closely associated with chronic inflammation characterized by abnormal cytokine production, increased acute-phase reactants and other mediators, and activation of a network of inflammatory signaling pathways, with inflammatory markers correlated with the severity of obesity and insulin resistance (Pistell et al., 2010). Increased levels of serum lipids, such as cholesterol and saturated long-chain fatty acids, also activate inflammatory and innate immune responses (De Souza et al., 2005; Moraes et al., 2009; Pistell et al., 2010; Yi et al., 2011).

The majority of studies on the effects of HFDs on obesity have targeted mechanisms at the molecular levels in hypothalamic neurons that regulate body weight, appetite, and energy balance. Leptin resistance or deficiency in hypothalamic cells of rodents and humans results in obesity (Sahu, 2003; Unger, 2007; Townsend et al., 2008; Wang et al., 2010; Cammisotto and Bendayan, 2012), while lesions of the ventromedial hypothalamus and lateral hypothalamus cause hyperphagia/obesity and aphagia/starvation, respectively (Sahu, 2003). Because little is known about the effects of obesity on morphometric parameters in the hypothalamus, the present study accesses whether the consumption of HFD leads to structural changes in hypothalamic neuron numbers and the hypothalamic volume.

Neurostereology: Unbiased Stereology of Neural Systems, First Edition. Edited by Peter R. Mouton.
© 2014 John Wiley & Sons, Inc. Published 2014 by John Wiley & Sons, Inc.

Materials and Methods

This study was carried to assess the differential effects of either short-term (4 weeks, experiment I) or long-term (8 weeks, experiment II) exposure of mice to standard diet (control groups) or HFD (experimental groups). Male Balb-C mice (30 ± 3 g) were obtained from the Laboratory Animal House of Shiraz University of Medical Sciences (SUMS) at 6 weeks of age and housed in groups of two or three to acclimatize for 2 weeks prior to study under 12-h light/dark cycle with food and water *ad libitum*. The Ethical Committee of SUMS approved the procedures in this study.

Experimental Design

A total of 40 mice were used in two experiments. For the short-term study, 20 mice were randomized into control ($n = 10$) or HFD ($n = 10$) groups for 4 weeks. For the long-term study, an additional group of mice were randomized into control ($n = 10$) or HFD ($n = 10$) for 8 weeks. Body weights and BMI were determined in the beginning and the end of experiments.

Mice in the control groups remained on the same diet of regular rodent chow consisting of protein (15%), fat (9%), and carbohydrates (76%) throughout the study. The HFD (D12451 from Research Diets, New Brunswick, NJ) consisted of protein (20%), fat (45%), and carbohydrates (35%).

Histological Processing

After sampling of blood, mice were anesthetized and perfused transcardially with cold 0.09% saline followed by 10% buffered formalin. Brains were immediately removed and postfixed in the same fixative overnight at 4°C, transferred to 30% sucrose (Sigma-Aldrich, St. Louis, MO) in phosphate buffered saline for 48 h, and then frozen and stored at −20°C until sectioning. Brains were coronally sectioned on a cryostat (SLEE, Germany). Sections were cut in a serial manner through the entire hypothalamus at an instrument setting of 30 μm, immersed into a 12-well plate containing cryoprotectant solution and kept in a −20°C freezer until stereological analyses.

Stereological Procedures

Every sixth section (at interval of 180 μm) was mounted onto glass slides, stained with cresyl violet and coverslipped. The volume of the hypothalamus was estimated in an unbiased manner using the Cavalieri-point counting method (Howard and Reed, 1998; Abusaad et al., 1999; Mouton, 2011). Briefly, a grid of points was laid over the image of section on the monitor of a computer and the points falling on the hypothalamus were counted at a final magnification of 4.5×. The volume of the hypothalamus (V_{ref}) was calculated using the following formula: $V_{ref} = d \times t \times a(p) \times \Sigma P$, where $d = 0.18$ mm; $t = 0.030$ mm (cut section thickness); the area per point $[a(p)] = 0.10513$ mm^2; ΣP = number of points hitting the section of the hypothalamus. The precision of the estimates was expressed by the coefficient of error (CE). We calculated the CE of our measurement using the method of Gundersen et al. (1999) (Abusaad et al., 1999; Gundersen et al., 1999). An average of 9 (±1) sections was counted per brain. A total of ~132 (±7) points per brain provided a mean CE of 0.053 (CE = 5.3%) on the estimates of total volume.

The numerical density and number of neurons in the hypothalamus were estimated using the optical disector technique (Howard and Reed, 1998; Abusaad et al., 1999; Mouton, 2011). The stereology equipment consists of an Eclipse microscope (E200, Nikon, Japan) with a high-numerical-aperture (NA = 1.25) 60× oil-immersion objective, connected to a video camera transmitting the microscopic image to a monitor. An electronic microcator with digital readout (MT12, Heidnehain, Germany) was used to measure movements in the Z direction. A computer-generated counting frame was superimposed on the screen using a stereology software system (Stereolite, SUMS, Shiraz, Iran). Systematic-uniform-random sampling was used to ensure unbiased and efficient sampling through the hypothalamus.

The neuronal density was calculated as follows: $N_V = \Sigma Q/[\Sigma P \times a(f) \times h]$, where ΣQ is the number of neurons counted within the disectors; ΣP is number of disector; $a(f) = 0.001369 \, mm^2$, the summed areas of the sampling frames; and $h = 0.015 \, mm$, is the height of disector. Neuronal nuclei were counted in 9 (±1) sections, 77 (±5) optical disectors, and 475 (±40) neurons per hypothalamus in each mouse, providing a mean CE of 0.08 (8%) on the estimates of total number. Cells were identified as neurons if they had a nucleolus, dendritic processes, euchromatin material within the nucleus, and nuclei surrounded by cytoplasm (Benes et al., 2001; Korbo et al., 2003). Numerical density was converted to the total number of (Total N) neurons in the hypothalamus by calculating the product of numerical density (N_V) and the volume of the hypothalamus, that is, Total $N = N_V \cdot V_{ref}$ (Abusaad et al., 1999; Gundersen et al., 1999; Mouton, 2011).

Statistical Analysis

Statistical significance was determined by one-way ANOVA to compare the effects of short- versus long-term HFD treatment compared with control diet. Statistical analysis was performed using SPSS 15.0 (SPSS, Inc., Chicago, IL) and data expressed as mean ± standard error of mean (SEM). A probability of less than 0.05 ($p < 0.05$) for group mean comparisons was considered a significant difference.

Results

Mice in this study were maintained on HFD or control diets for either 4 (short term) or 8 weeks (long term). The results revealed significant increases in weight and BMI for both short-term and long-term treatment with HFD in comparison with their respective control groups ($p < 0.05$). Furthermore, there was a significant increase in weight and BMI in the mice treated with long-term HFD compared with short-term HFD ($p < 0.05$) (Table 15.1).

Table 15.1   Mean value ± SEM of the weight (g) and BMI (g/cm^2) of the mice fed with normal and high-fat diet (HFD) for short- and long-term periods

Variable groups	Weight before experiment	Weight after experiment	BMI before experiment	BMI after experiment
Short-term control	29 ± 0.96	28.5 ± 1.40	0.31 ± .01	0.31 ± .02
Short-term HFD	29 ± 1.08	35.7 ± 1.25[a]	0.29 ± .03	0.38 ± .01[a]
Long-term control	30.2 ± 1.20	31.4 ± 1.07	0.31 ± .01	0.32 ± .01
Long-term HFD	30.1 ± 0.73	40.42 ± 0.64[a,b,c]	0.28 ± .01	0.41 ± .01[a,b]

[a]Significant difference with short-term control group ($p < 0.05$).
[b]Significant difference with long-term control group ($p < 0.05$).
[c]Significant difference with short-term HFD group ($p < 0.05$).

Table 15.2 Mean value ± SEM of blood factors in the control and high-fat diet (HFD) groups in mice were fed with short- and long-term (mg/dL) periods

Variable groups	Triglyceride	Cholesterol	LDL
Short-term control	199.33 ± 21.07	177.67 ± 4.33	63.67 ± 14.90
Short-term HFD	152.75 ± 14.70	162.5 ± 2.60	80 ± 1.70
Long-term control	174.34 ± 10.72	150 ± 12.09	64.67 ± 5.36
Long-term HFD	173.50 ± 23.40	211.75 ± 15.80^{a,b}	93.25 ± 7.20^{a,c}

[a]Significant difference with long-term control group ($p < 0.05$).
[b]Significant difference with short-term HFD group ($p < 0.05$).
[c]Significant difference with short-term control group ($p < 0.05$).

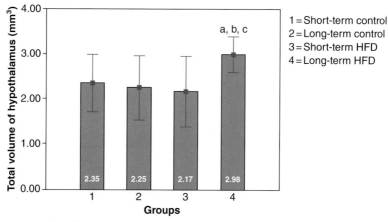

a Signifact difference with short-term control ($p<0.05$).
b Signifact difference with long-term control ($p<0.05$).
c Signifact difference with short-term HFD ($p<0.05$).

Figure 15.1 Mean value ± SEM of volume of the total hypothalamus in mice which were fed with normal and high-fat diet (HFD) for short- and long-term period (mm^3).

Based on blood samples obtained at the end of the study, mice in the long-term HFD group showed a significant elevation in serum cholesterol levels compared with long-term control ($p = 0.003$), as well as short-term HFD ($p < 0.006$). In addition, low density lipoprotein (LDL) levels for the long-term HFD group were significantly higher than the control groups ($p < 0.05$) (Table 15.2). Although triglyceride appeared to decrease in both short- and long-term HFD groups relative to their respective control, this decrease was not statistically significant (Table 15.2).

The total volume of hypothalamus for mice in the long-term HFD group was significantly greater than in control ($p < 0.028$) and in the short-term HFD groups ($p < 0.023$) (Figure 15.1). In the short-term HFD group, the volume of hypothalamus decreased on the right and left side and total hypothalamus, although this decrease was not statistically significant (Table 15.3, Figure 15.1). There were no significant differences between the volume of the right and the left sides of the hypothalamus for all control and experimental groups.

After 8 weeks of HFD, numerical density of neurons significantly decreased when compared with the short-term ($p < 0.005$) and the long-term ($p < 0.001$) controls (Table 15.3 and Figure 15.2). In the short-term HFD treatment group, there was a nonsignificant decrease in the numerical density of neuron on both sides of the hypothalamus (Table 15.3).

Table 15.3 Mean value ± SEM of numerical density and total number of neurons and volume of the right and left sides of hypothalamus in mice which were fed with normal and high-fat diet (HFD) for short- and long-term periods

Variable groups	Volume (mm³)		Numerical density × 10⁵ (neuron/mm³)		Neuron number × 10⁵	
	Right side	Left side	Right side	Left side	Right side	Left side
Short-term control	1.18 ± 0.12	1.16 ± 0.12	3.06 ± 0.08	3.23 ± 0.07	3.63 ± 0.39	3.76 ± 0.42
Short-term HFD	1.09 ± 0.13	1.06 ± 0.10	2.80 ± 0.05	2.83 ± 0.17	3.08 ± 0.44	3.03 ± 0.39
Long-term control	1.13 ± 0.12	1.10 ± 0.12	3.37 ± 0.02	3.45 ± 0.04	3.85 ± 0.42	3.84 ± 0.47
Long-term HFD	1.48 ± 0.07^{a,b}	1.49 ± 0.09^{a,b,c}	2.58 ± 0.15^{b,c,d}	2.54 ± 0.16^{c,d}	3.85 ± 0.33	3.80 ± 0.32

^{a}Significant difference with long-term control group ($p < 0.05$).
^{b}Significant difference with short-term HFD group ($p < 0.05$).
^{c}Significant difference with short-term control group ($p < 0.05$).
^{d}Significant difference with long-term control group ($p < 0.001$).

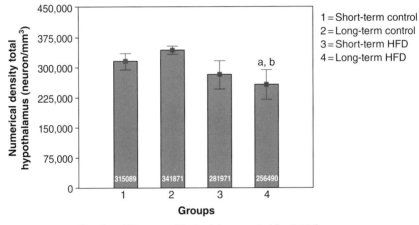

a Significat difference with short-term control ($p<0.005$).
b Significat difference with long-term control ($p<0.001$).

Figure 15.2 Mean value ± SEM of numerical density of neuron (neuron/mm³) in total hypothalamus of mice which were fed with normal and HFD for short- and long-term period.

There were no significant differences in total neuron number in the short- and long-term treatment groups compared with their respective controls (Table 15.3 and Figure 15.3).

Compare with control, consumption of HFD showed an apparent increase in the extracellular space (Figure 15.4, lower panel vs. upper panel), although no quantitative analysis of this parameter was carried out.

Discussion

Obesity has grown as one of the most important epidemiological problems in modern societies (De Souza et al., 2008; Cammisotto and Bendayan, 2012). Chronic consumption of a HFD is a contributing factor to the advent of obesity in humans and in animal models (Townsend, 2008). The hypothalamus plays a major part in the regulation of the food intake and destruction

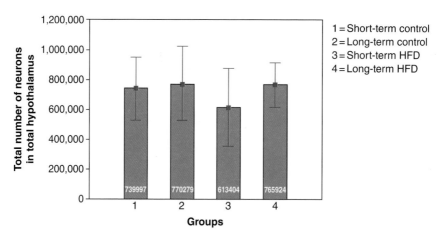

Figure 15.3 Mean value ± SEM of total number of neurons of the total hypothalamus in mice which were fed with control and HFD for short- and long-term periods.

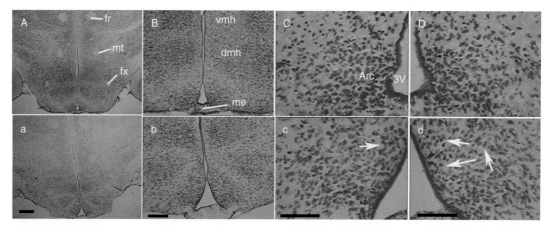

Figure 15.4 Cresyl violet staining of hypothalamus in normal (upper panel) and high-fat (lower panel) diet treated mice. An increase in extracellular space is evident in the hypothalamus of high-fat diet treated mouse (lower panel, arrows). 3v, third ventricle; Arc, arcuate hypothalamic nucleus; dmh, dorsomedial hypothalamic nucleus; fr, fasciculus retroflexus; fx, fornix; me, median eminence; mt, mammillothalamic tract; vmh, ventromedial hypothalamic nucleus. Scale bars: A = 400, B = 200, C and D = 100 μm. This figure represents the plate 49 in the mouse brain in stereotaxic coordinates (Paxinos and Franklin, 2001).

of distinct hypothalamic regions may induce hyperphagia or reduction in food intake (Park et al., 2004).

This is the first stereological study to compare the effects of HFD (45 kcal% fat) on neuron density and the total number in the hypothalamus of adult male mice. We report that HFD treatment for 8 weeks (long term) but not 4 weeks (short term) increases the total volume of the hypothalamus and reduces the numerical density of neurons in the hypothalamus. However, there was no change in the total number of neurons in hypothalamus for mice treated with HFD for either the short or long term as compared with their relative control groups.

As expected from previous studies (De Souza et al., 2008; Pirnik et al., 2008; Hsuchou et al., 2009; Pistell et al., 2010; Wang et al., 2010; Amin et al., 2011; Valladolid-Acebes et al., 2011), short- and long-term treatments with HFD significantly increased weight and BMI (Table 15.1). The finding of increased BMI after short-term HFD is exceptional since many studies have reported that a minimum of 12 days is required for divergence of normal diet and HFD mice, including treatment with diets very high in fat (Townsend, 2008). Blood assays in this study showed significant increases in LDL and cholesterol level (Table 15.2) in concert with previous studies (Granholm et al., 2008; Amin et al., 2011).

Although regional brain volumes give rather unspecific information about function, significant changes in regional volumes may reveal underlying microstructural changes of functional relevance (Regeur, 2000). We report that the hypothalamus volume increases by about 30% after 8 weeks of HFD treatment (Table 15.3 and Figure 15.1). There are few data on volume changes of one or two nuclei in the hypothalamus, although some studies indicate that increase in BMI and obesity may be associated with changing in gray and white matter volume (Young, 1982; Pistell et al., 2010). A few studies have reported that high-fat feeding induces the expression of several proinflammatory cytokines and inflammatory responsive proteins in the brain and hypothalamus (De Souza et al., 2005; Moraes et al., 2009; Pistell et al., 2010; Langdon et al., 2011). Treatment with HFD reduces levels of brain-derived neurotrophic factor (BDNF), a molecule with direct anti-inflammatory effects in the brain (Granholm et al., 2008). Deletion of BDNF in hypothalamus of adult mice also resulted in hyperphagic behavior and obesity (Unger, 2007; Wang et al., 2010). These findings suggest that the volume increases in the hypothalamus reported here may result from inflammation caused by HFD. Although extracellular space was not quantified in this study, a qualitative increase was apparent (see Figure 15.4). Although short- and long-term HFD treatments decreased the numerical density of hypothalamic neurons by about 10% and 20%, respectively, this decrease was only significant for the long-term HFD group (Table 15.3 and Figure 15.2). However, this reduction in neuron density after long-term HFD may be explained by the fact that neuron density reflects the number of neuron per unit of volume (N_V). Because the total volume of hypothalamus increased after long-term HFD (Figure 15.1), the reduction in neuron density reflects this volume increase, rather than a reduction in neuron number *per se*. This conclusion is further supported by the calculation of total neuron number (Table 15.3 and Figure 15.3), which shows no changes in the hypothalamus for either short- or long-term treatment with HFD, that is, the so-called reference trap (for review, see Abusaad et al., 1999). The significant increase in hypothalamic volume may indicate that HFD increases intercellular space by induction of inflammation or gliosis (Pistell et al., 2010).

In summary, we conclude that long-term consumption of HFD may increase the volume of the hypothalamus, possibly due to inflammation and gliosis, but does not change the total number of neurons in the hypothalamus. Studies are needed to specifically address the effects of HFD on inflammation and gliosis in the hypothalamus. This study also illustrates the pitfall, the so-called reference trap, which may arise when relying on changes in neuronal density, rather than total neuron number.

Acknowledgments

We thank Biotechnology Research Center of Shiraz University for using their cryostat and the Histomorphometry and Stereology Research Center, SUMS, Shiraz, Iran. We also wish to thank Dr. Noura Al Menhali from the University of United Arabic Emirates for her kind assistance in this project. The present article was extracted from thesis written by Samira Raminfard and financially supported by Shiraz University of Medical Sciences Grant No. 89-5129.

References

Abusaad, I., MacKay, D., Zhao, J., Stanford, P., Collier, D. A., Everall, I. P. 1999. Stereological estimation of the total number of neurons in the murine hippocampus using the optical disector. *J Comp Neurol* **408** (4): 560–566.

Amin, K. A., Kamel, H. H., Abd Eltawab, M. A. 2011. The relation of high fat diet, metabolic disturbances and brain oxidative dysfunction: modulation by hydroxy citric acid. *Lipids Health Dis* **10**: 74–85.

Benes, F. M., Vincent, S. L., Todtenkopf, M. 2001. The density of pyramidal and nonpyramidal neurons in anterior cingulated cortex of schizophrenic and bipolar subjects. *Biol Psychiatry* **50**: 395–406.

Buettner, R., Parhofer, K. G., Woenckhaus, M., Wrede, C. E., Kunz-Schughart, L. A., Schölmerich, J., Bollheimer, L. C. 2006. Defining high-fat-diet rat models: metabolic and molecular effects of different fat types. *J Mol Endocrinol* **36** (3): 485–501.

Cammisotto, P., Bendayan, M. 2012. A review on gastric leptin: the exocrine secretion of a gastric hormone. *Anat Cell Biol* **45**: 1–16.

De Souza, C. T., Araujo, E. P., Bordin, S., Ashimine, R., Zollner, R. L., Boschero, A. C., Saad, M. J., Velloso, L. A. 2005. Consumption of a fat-rich diet activates a proinflammatory response and induces insulin resistance in the hypothalamus. *Endocrinology* **146** (10): 4192–4199.

De Souza, C. T., Pereira-da-Silva, M., Araujo, E. P., Morari, J., Alvarez-Rojas, F., Bordin, S., Moreira-Filho, D. C., Carvalheira, J. B., Saad, M. J., Velloso, L. A. 2008. Distinct subsets of hypothalamic genes are modulated by two different thermogenesis-inducing stimuli. *Obesity* **16** (6): 1239–1247.

Formiguera, X., Cantón, A. 2004. Obesity: epidemiology and clinical aspects. *Best Pract Res Clin Gastroenterol* **18** (6): 1125–1146.

Granholm, A. C., Bimonte-Nelson, H. A., Moore, A. B., Nelson, M. E., Freeman, L. R., Sambamurti, K. 2008. Effects of a saturated fat and high cholesterol diet on memory and hippocampal morphology in the middle-aged rat. *J Alzheimers Dis* **14** (2): 133–145.

Gundersen, H. J., Jensen, E. B., Kiêu, K., Nielsen, J. 1999. The efficiency of systematic sampling in stereology—reconsidered. *J Microsc* **193**: 199–211.

Howard, C. V., Reed, M. G. 1998. *Unbiased Stereology Three Dimensional Measurement in Microscopy*, 1st ed. Oxford: Bios Scientific Publisher.

Hsuchou, H., He, Y., Kastin, A. J., Tu, H., Markadakis, E. N., Rogers, R. C., Fossier, P. B., Pan, W. 2009. Obesity induces functional astrocytic leptin receptors in hypothalamus. *Brain* **132**: 889–902.

Korbo, L., Amrein, I., Lipp, H. P., Wolfer, D., Regeur, L., Oster, S., Pakkenberg, B. 2003. No evidence for loss of hippocampal neurons in non-Alzheimer dementia patients. *Acta Neurol Scand* **10**: 1–8.

Langdon, K. D., Clarke, J., Corbett, D. 2011. Long-term exposure to high fat diet is bad for your brain: exacerbation of focal ischemic brain injury. *Neuroscience* **182**: 82–87.

Moraes, J. C., Coope, A., Morari, J., Cintra, D. E., Roman, E. A., Pauli, J. R., Romanatto, T., Carvalheira, J. B., Oliveira, A. L., Saad, M. J., Velloso, L. A. 2009. High-fat diet induces apoptosis of hypothalamic neurons. *PLoS ONE* **4** (4): e5045.

Mouton, P. R. 2011. *Unbiased Stereology: A Concise Guide*. Baltimore, MD: The Johns Hopkins University Press.

Park, E. S., Yi, S. J., Kim, J. S., Lee, H. S., Lee, I. S., Seong, J. K., Jin, H. K., Yoon, Y. S. 2004. Changes in orexin-A and neuropeptide Y expression in the hypothalamus of the fasted and high-fat diet fed rats. *J Vet Sci* **5** (4): 295–302.

Paxinos, G., Franklin, K. R. 2001. *The Mouse Brain in Stereotaxic Coordinates*, 2nd ed. San Diego, CA: Academic Press.

Pirnik, Z., Bundzikova, J., Mikkelsen, J. D., Zelezna, B., Maletinska, L., Kiss, A. 2008. Fos expression in hypocretinergic neurons in C57B1/6 male and female mice after long-term consumption of high fat diet. *Endocr Regul* **42** (4): 137–146.

Pistell, P. J., Morrison, C. D., Gupta, S., Knight, A. G., Keller, J. N., Ingram, D. K., Bruce-Keller, A. J. 2010. Cognitive impairment following high fat diet consumption is associated with brain inflammation. *J Neuroimmunol* **219** (2): 25–32.

Rada, P., Bocarsly, M. E., Barson, J. R., Hoebel, B. G., Leibowitzm, S. F. 2010. Reduced accumbens dopamine in Sprague-Dawley rats prone to overeating a fat-rich diet. *Physiol Behav* **101** (3): 394–400.

Regeur, L. 2000. Increasing loss of the brain tissue with increasing dementia: a stereological study of post-mortem brains from elderly females. *Eur J Neurol* **7**: 47–54.

Sahu, A. 2003. Leptin signaling in the hypothalamus: emphasis on energy homeostasis and leptin resistance. *Front Neuroendocrinol* **24** (4): 225–253.

Townsend, K. L. 2008. Mechanisms of high fat induced-obesity in mice and premigration/prehibernation fattening in rats. Thesis in Graduate School of Arts and Sciences, Boston University, Boston, MA, pp. 170–172.

Townsend, K. L., Lorenzi, M. M., Widmaier, E. P. 2008. High-fat diet-induced changes in body mass and hypothalamic gene expression in wild-type and leptin-deficient mice. *Endocrine* **33** (2): 176–188.

Unger, T. 2007. *Examination of Deficits in Energy Balance and Affective Behavior Following Central or Hypothalamic Depletion of Brain-Derived Neurotrophic Factor*, Sackler School of Graduate Biomedical Sciences, p. 194. Medford, MA: Tufts University.

Valladolid-Acebes, I., Stucchi, P., Cano, V., Fernández-Alfonso, M. S., Merino, B., Gil-Ortega, M., Fole, A., Morales, L., Ruiz-Gayo, M., Del Olmo, N. 2011. High-fat diets impair spatial learning in the radial-arm maze in mice. *Neurobiol Learn Mem* **95** (1): 80–85.

Wang, C. F., Godar, R. J., Billington, C. J., Kotz, C. M. 2010. Chronic administration of brain-derived neurotrophic factor in the hypothalamic paraventricular nucleus reverses obesity induced by high-fat diet. *Am J Physiol Regul Integr Comp Physiol* **298** (5): R1320–R1332.

Yi, C. O., Jeon, B. T., Shin, H. J., Jeong, E. A., Chang, K. C., Lee, J. E., Lee, D. H., Kim, H. J., Kang, S. S., Cho, G. J., Choi, W. S., Roh, G. S. 2011. Resveratrol activates AMPK and suppresses LPS-induced NF-kB-dependent COZ-2 activation in RAW $26_{4.7}$ macrophage cells. *Anat Cell Biol* **44** (3): 194–203.

Young, J. K. 1982. A comparison of hypothalami of rats and mice: lack of gross sexual dimorphism in the mouse. *Brain Res* **239** (1): 233–239.

16   2D and 3D Morphometric Analyses Comparing Three Rodent Models

JiHyuk Park[1] and S. Omar Ahmad[2]

[1] *Yonsei University, Seoul, South Korea*
[2] *St. Louis University, St. Louis, MO, USA*

Background

Numerous theoretical papers have discussed the strengths and weaknesses of model-based morphometry (2D) and design-based stereology (3D), with the majority finding that the merits of design-based (unbiased) stereology exceed those of model-based image analysis (Gundersen, 1977, 1978, 1986; West, 1993; Saper, 1996; Guillery and Herrup, 1997; Benes and Lange, 2001; von Bartheld, 2001; Selemon and Rajkowska, 2002; Mandarim-de-Lacerda, 2003; Schmitz and Hof, 2005; Mouton, 2011). The purpose of the present study is to directly compare assumption- and model-based 2D approaches versus unbiased stereology for counts of tyrosine hydroxylase (TH)-positive neurons in three brain regions (substantia nigra pars compacta [SNpc], the ventral tegmental area [VTA], and the nucleus accumbens [NAc]) using brain sections from three different rodent models. Specifically, we compared results from unbiased stereology against results from a profile count/fractionator scheme (2D profile method) to estimate total number of profiles, an approach in which the Abercrombie correction factor is applied to the results of the profile count/ fractionator estimate of total profile number (model-based approach). We also obtained results using optical densitometry. The findings suggest 2D analyses may be adequate for rough screening but lacks accuracy and reliability for the estimation of total neuronal number and size. Since 3D unbiased stereology avoids all known sources of bias (systematic error), the accuracy and reliability of unbiased stereology far outweighs model-based methods for morphometric analysis of brain changes.

Materials and Methods

We analyzed brain tissue sections from three different rodent models. The chronic MPTP/ probenecid PD (MPD) model in C57BL/6 mice has relatively severe neuron loss compared with the alcohol-preferring (AP) model in the Wistar rat and the enriched environment (EE) model in Sprague-Dawley rats. Control groups were sedentary control (SC) in MPD mouse model, standard housing environment (SE) in the EE rat model, and alcohol nonpreferring (ANP) in the AP rat model.

Neurostereology: Unbiased Stereology of Neural Systems, First Edition. Edited by Peter R. Mouton.
© 2014 John Wiley & Sons, Inc. Published 2014 by John Wiley & Sons, Inc.

Animals and Tissue Samples

For the MPD model, 10 mice ($n = 5$ chronic MPD, $n = 5$ controls) were injected with a total of 10 doses of MPTP hydrochloride together with an adjuvant, probenecid, on a 5-week schedule and an interval of 3.5 days between consecutive doses (Lau et al., 1990; Ahmad et al., 2009b). Mice were anesthetized, transcardially perfused, and brain samples embedded with the Multi-Brain™ technology, sectioned coronally at 50 μm and immunostained with TH (NeuroScience Associates, Knoxville, TN). This preparation yielded about 12% shrinkage, with sections cut at an initial instrument setting of 50 μm reduced to about 31 μm. Second, 16 brains from adult female Wistar rats were obtained from AP ($n = 8$) and ANP ($n = 8$) rats (Indiana University School of Medicine). None of the rats were exposed to alcohol prior to sacrifice (Ahmad et al., 2009a). Finally, 16 Sprague-Dawley rats (8 males, 8 females) from the EE rat model were used, with 8 rats each exposed to EE and the SE for about 2 months (Almli et al., 2008). For the EE group, a variety of toys such as objects of wood, metal, plastic, leather, and cardboard were available in the cage at all times, with rotation of toys alternated every 3 days for novelty, along with meshed wire ladders for climbing and plastic pipes (polyvinyl chloride [PVC]) for tunneling and nesting. The SE had no toys in a transparent plastic laboratory cage lined with wood shavings. The same tissue preparation methods were used for both AP rat model and EE rat model (Almli et al., 2008; Ahmad et al., 2009a). All rats were anesthetized and then perfused through the left ventricle and then postfixed and sectioned coronally at 60 μm by NeuroScience Associates (Knoxville, TN) using MultiBrain™ Technology. Free-floating sections were stained for TH and mounted on gelatinized glass slides for viewing.

A computerized stereology system consisting of a Nikon Eclipse 80i microscope equipped to an ASI MS-2000 motorized stage, a Sony 3CCD Color Digital Video Camera, integrated to a Dell Precision 650 Server with high-resolution plasma monitor was used. The system software estimated total number of TH-positive neurons, mean neuron volume (MNV), and volume of reference space using the principles of design-based (unbiased) stereology. For the model-based approach, the system captured 2D images of sections through the reference space, which were then exported to the NIH *ImageJ* software (National Institutes of Health, Bethesda, MD) for quantification of TH-positive profiles, MVN, and reference space volumes.

Data Collection

Each reference space (area of interest) in the right hemisphere was analyzed using different approaches in the same sections from the same animals from each model. For the chronic MPD mouse model and EE rat model, the number and volume of TH-positive neurons in the SNpc was quantified by design-based stereology and profile counts. For TH-positive neuronal number and volume, every 8th section was sampled from the SNpc with a random start. For the AP rat model, these same parameters were quantified in the VTA. In AP rat model, the region volume of the NAc was quantified by design-based stereology, 2D profile counts, and the model-based approach. Every 4th section containing the NAc was sampled from a random initial start.

Neuron Number

For design-based stereology, the 3D optical disector approach was used to estimate the total number of TH-positive neurons. Briefly, at low magnification (4×), the area of interest was outlined using stereotaxic atlases of mouse and rat brains (Paxinos and Watson, 2007; Franklin and Paxinos, 2008). After the software placed the unbiased counting frames (disectors, Figure 16.1) across the reference area at systematic-random locations, TH-positive neurons were counted at high

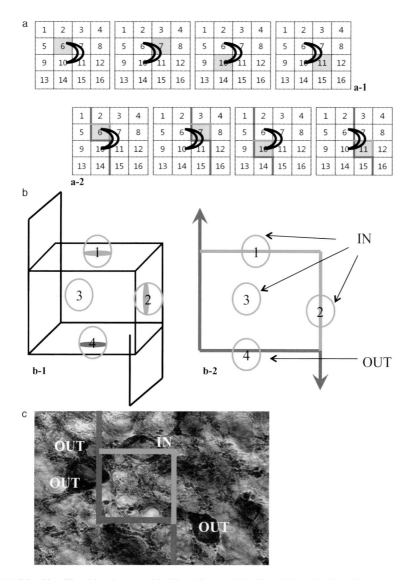

Figure 16.1 (a) Edge bias. The object is counted in biased frames 6, 7, 10, and 11 (a-1). The object, however, is counted in unbiased frame 10 only (a-2). (b) 3D unbiased probe. Unbiased disector counting frames showing inclusion (green) and exclusion (red) line (2D) and inclusion and exclusion (red) planes (3D) as shown in 3D (b-1) and 2D (b-2). (c) Optical disector principle. Neurons must be counted only appears for the first time within the unbiased count frame while the investigator optically sections from top to the bottom in the z-axis.

resolution using a 100×/NA1.4 immersion lens (3600× magnification). The guard height was 3 μm, and the thickness of each section was determined by the mean thickness of count frames using the 100×/1.4 aperture oil immersion lens.

For the 2D profile counts and model-based approaches, images of each section were captured at low power (20× lens) using the computerized stereology system and profiles of TH-positive neurons manually counted on each set of images in the reference space using ImageJ (NIH). For the 2D profile counts, profiles of TH-positive nuclei were counted for each animal and then the fractionator scheme was used to calculate the total number of neurons as the product of the sum of profiles counted and the reciprocal of the section sampling fraction (1/8). For the model-based approach, the Abercrombie correction (Abercrombie and Johnson, 1946) was applied to correct for split neurons: Nt = Na(T/D + T), where Nt = total number of neurons, Na = total number of neurons from the hybrid method, D = average diameter of neurons, and T = section thickness. For the Abercrombie correction, the 3D sphere diameter (D) of neurons was calculated from the average neuronal diameter (d) using the formula $D = 4d/\pi$ (Weibel, 1979; Rinne et al., 2008). The diameter (d) of neurons was estimated from the formula $d = \sqrt{4A/\pi}$ (Rinne et al., 2008). The profile areas of neurons (A) were measured by the ImageJ program with areas of $n = 10$ neurons measured for the calculation of the mean neuron diameter. The section thickness (T) was taken as the cut section thicknesses, that is, 50 μm for the chronic MPTP mice and 60 μm for AP and EE rats.

Optical Densitometry

Optical densitometry was used to quantify TH-positive neurons. For each image, the reference space was outlined precisely according to the stereotaxic atlas of Paxinos and Watson (2007) and optical density assessed using ImageJ. The optical density for the reference space in the reference volume for each animal was the sum of optical densities for all sample sections.

Mean Neuron Volume (MNV)

The number-weighted nucleator method (Gundersen and Jensen, 1985), a method of design-based stereology, was used to estimate the MNV of TH-positive neurons in the SNpc and the VTA (Figure 16.2). For the model-based approach to MNV estimation, the volume of neurons (V) was estimated from the formula $V = (4\pi/3)r^3$ where the radius of neurons (r) was back-calculated from the profile area using the formula $A = \pi r^2$. In the second method based on profile measure, the largest diameter of the neuron was measured by ImageJ and then divided by 2. For both of these 2D approaches, neuronal volume was estimated from the average of 10 neurons in each section.

Region Volume

For the unbiased stereology method, the Cavalieri-point counting approach in the computerized system was used to estimate the total volume from a systematic-random sample of sections through

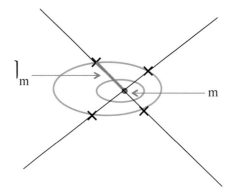

Figure 16.2 The nucleator method. m; the center of the cell, l_m; the line length between the center and the border of the cell.

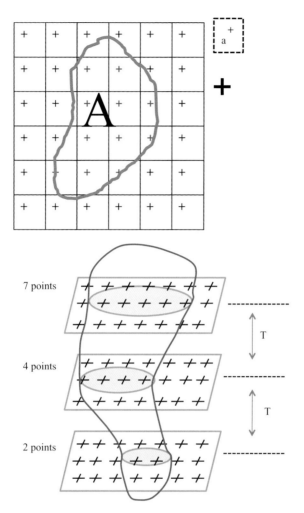

Figure 16.3 The Cavalieri-point counting method to estimate volume. The upper panel (2D) shows dimensionless points (arrow) spaced apart by area, a, and placed at random over profiles leads to unbiased estimates of the expected profile area, A. The lower panel shows point-counting and Cavalieri method in 3D object.

the NAc. The NAc on each section was outlined with low magnification (4×) and then point-grids were automatically overlaid in a random manner across the NAc (Figure 16.3). Points falling within the NAc were automatically counted and the thickness of each section measured with a 100×/1.4 aperture oil immersion lens. The volume of NAc was calculated as the product of the sum of outlined areas and the distance between each section.

For the model-based approach, images of each section were captured with 4× lenses, the area of the NAc in each section measured using ImageJ software. The volume of the NAc was estimated as the product of the sum of the NAc areas and the spacing distance (SD) between the sampled sections. The two estimates of the NAc volume were generated with section pre-stained cut thickness (60 µm) and actual section thickness after all tissue processing. All section thickness measurements were made at high magnification (100× oil).

Table 16.1 Quantification of TH+ neuronal number

Models	Group	Design-based stereology	Model-based stereology	Fractionator method	Densitometry
MPD	Control (SC)	5,272.28 ± 489.38 (100 ± 9.45)	3,034.50 ± 257.06** (100 ± 8.47)	4,046.00 ± 342.74 (100 ± 8.47)	100 ± 6.45
	Experimental (MPD)	2,393.86 ± 242.46* (45.40 ± 4.59*)	2,097.60 ± 184.20* (65.31 ± 3.87*, **)	2,796.80 ± 245.60* (65.31 ± 3.87*, **)	76.03 ± 3.90*, **
EE	Control (SE)	4,144.84 ± 244.31 (100 ± 5.89)	3,855.40 ± 160.43 (100 ± 4.16)	5,210.00 ± 246.80** (100 ± 4.16)	100 ± 5.56
	Experimental (EE)	4,853.59 ± 198.15* (117.09 ± 4.78*)	3,974.54 ± 111.79** (103.09 ± 2.89**)	5,371.00 ± 151.07 (103.09 ± 2.89**)	95.62 ± 3.23**
AP	Control (ANP)	8,683.95 ± 488.63 (100 ± 5.62)	4,037.88 ± 378.66** (100 ± 9.37)	5,244.00 ± 491.77** (100 ± 9.37)	100 ± 5.50
	Experimental (AP)	10,457.25 ± 494.16* (120.42 ± 5.69*)	4,375.80 ± 490.58** (108.36 ± 12.14)	5,610.11 ± 628.94** (106 ± 11.99)	110 ± 5.12

Indicated as percentage of control (mean ± SEM); *$p < 0.05$ versus control, **$p < 0.05$ versus design-based stereology.

Table 16.2 Quantification of TH+ neuronal volume (μ^3)

Models	Group	Design-based stereology	Model-based stereology	Profile measure
MPD	Control (SC)	1129 ± 76.33 (100 ± 6.76)	3995.04 ± 219.45** (100 ± 5.49)	3888.91 ± 123.05** (100 ± 3.16)
	Experimental (MPD)	1157 ± 33.93 (102 ± 3.00)	4012.35 ± 162.70** (100.43 ± 4.07)	3496.31 ± 148.87** (89.90 ± 3.82**)
EE	Control (SE)	1381.36 ± 54.90 (100 ± 3.97)	5011.96 ± 184.82** (100 ± 3.68)	3645.55 ± 118.89** (100 ± 3.26)
	Experimental (EE)	1403.73 ± 109.51 (101.61 ± 7.92)	5074 ± 314.40** (101.25 ± 6.27)	3323.05 ± 191.26** (91.15 ± 5.24)
AP	Control (ANP)	546.58 ± 37.01 (100 ± 6.77)	3028.71 ± 169.05** (100 ± 5.58)	1487.31 ± 219.73** (100 ± 7.37)
	Experimental (AP)	558.23 ± 40.05 (102.13 ± 7.32)	2758.47 ± 162.44** (91.07 ± 5.36)	1734.33 ± 67.23** (116 ± 4.52)

Indicated as percentage of control (mean ± SEM); *$p < 0.05$ versus control, **$p < 0.05$ versus design-based stereology.

Data Analysis

Data are presented as the mean (standard error of the mean [SEM]) actual estimates and percent (Table 16.1, Table 16.2, and Table 16.3), and normalized as a percentage of the mean value for the control group in each model. Student's t-test (two-tailed) was used to compare quantitative data of each analysis between control and experimental groups in each model. Student's t-test (two-tailed) was also used to compare quantitative data between design-based stereology and 2D analyses. Differences between groups were considered significant at $p < 0.05$.

Results

For the chronic MPD model, all quantitative analyses found significant differences in number of TH+ neurons between SC and MPD both for actual neuron number and normalized value

Table 16.3 Quantification of NAc volume (mm³)

Models	Group	Design-based stereology	Model-based stereology I	Model-based stereology II	Profile measure (mm²)
AP	Control (ANP)	2.13 ± 0.10 (100 ± 6.10)	2.94 ± 0.05** (100 ± 1.71)	1.96 ± 0.03 (100 ± 1.71)	12.27 ± 0.21 (100 ± 1.71)
	Experimental (AP)	1.76 ± 0.11* (82.89 ± 5.22*)	2.46 ± 0.10*· ** (83.52 ± 3.63*)	1.64 ± 0.07* (83.52 ± 3.63*)	10.25 ± 0.44 (83.52 ± 3.63*)

Indicated as percentage of control (mean ± SEM); *$p < 0.05$ versus control, **$p < 0.05$ versus design-based stereology.

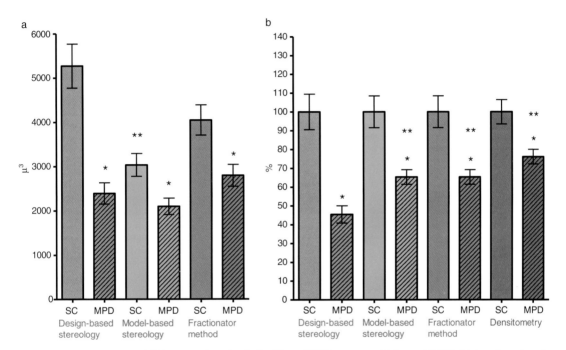

Figure 16.4 Quantification of TH+ neuronal number in the SNpc of MPD mouse model (mean ± SEM). (a) Actual number of neurons was estimated by three quantification methods: design-based stereology, model-based stereology, and the fractionator method. All three found significant DA neuronal loss in the SNpc of MPD. Both model-based stereology and the fractionator method estimate fewer neuronal number than design-based stereology. Only neuronal number of SC in model-based stereology was significantly different from the number of SC in design-based stereology. *$p < 0.05$ versus SC, **$p < 0.05$ versus design-based stereology. (b) Neuronal number was normalized in a percentage as respects the mean of the SC. All four found significant differences of neuronal number of DA neurons in the SNpc. However, three 2D methods, model-based stereology, the fractionator method, and densitometry, demonstrated fewer neuronal loss of DA neurons than design-based stereology. *$p < 0.05$ versus SC, **$p < 0.05$ versus design-based stereology. SC, sedentary control; MPD, chronic MPTP/probenecid PD.

(Figure 16.4). For actual number, the model-based approach, that is, fractionator profile counts with Abercrombie correction for split cells, showed a significant difference in SC from design-based stereology. After normalizing the results to controls, this approach found a significantly larger percentage of TH-positive neurons than design-based stereology.

For the EE rat model, design-based stereology revealed a significant difference between SE and EE for numbers of TH-positive neurons, while the profile counts either with or without Abercrombie correction showed no significant differences (Figure 16.5).

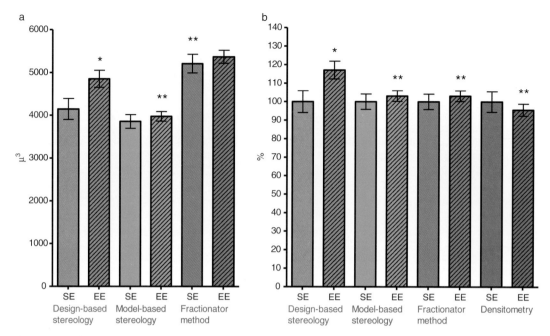

Figure 16.5 Quantification of TH+ neuronal number in the SNpc of EE rat model (mean ± SEM). (a) Actual number of neurons was estimated by three quantification methods: design-based stereology, model-based stereology, and the fractionator method. Only design-based stereology found a significant difference of DA neuronal number between SE and EE. 2D analyses, including model-based stereology and the fractionator method, did not find significant differences between SE and EE. DA neuronal number in EE of model-based stereology and SE of the fractionator method were significantly different from DA neuronal number in design-based stereology. *$p < 0.05$ versus SE, **$p < 0.05$ versus design-based stereology. (b) Neuronal number was normalized in a percentage as respects the mean of the SE. Only design-based stereology found a significant difference of DA neuronal number between SE and EE. All 2D analyses, including model-based stereology, the fractionator method, and densitometry, were significantly different from design-based stereology in EE. *$p < 0.05$ versus SE, **$p < 0.05$ versus design-based stereology. SE, standard environment; EE, enriched environment.

The model-based approach demonstrated a smaller actual number than design-based stereology, while the profile counts without model-based correction approach showed a larger number than design-based stereology. For normalized data, design-based stereology revealed a significant difference between SE and EE while the profile counts with or without model-based correction did not. The result from design-based stereology was significantly different from the two profile counting approaches and densitometry.

In the AP rat model, design-based stereology demonstrated a significant difference for TH-positive number between ANP and AP while neither of the profile counting method, that is, with or without Abercrombie correction, did for either actual number estimation nor normalized values (Figure 16.6). For actual number, the profile counts with and without correction estimated significantly smaller numbers of TH-positive neurons than design-based stereology. For normalized data, there were no significant differences between design-based stereology and the other methods.

For the chronic MPD model there was no significant difference in MNV of TH-positive neurons between SC and MPD (Figure 16.7) using unbiased stereology, the model-based correction, or the profile measure.

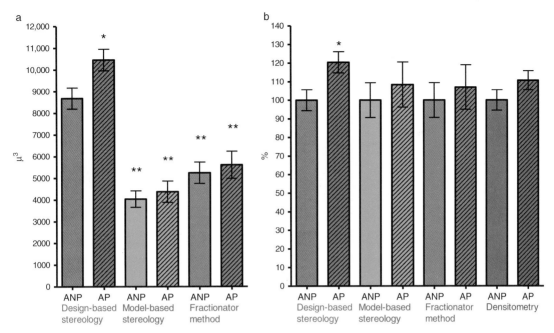

Figure 16.6 Quantification of TH+ neuronal number in the VTA of AP rat model (mean ± SEM). (a) Actual number of DA neurons was estimated by design-based stereology, model-based stereology, and the fractionator method. Only design-based stereology found a significant difference of DA neuronal number between ANP and AP. 2D analyses, including model-based, and the fractionator method, did not find a significant difference between ANP and AP. All 2D analyses demonstrated less neuronal number than design-based stereology. All neuronal numbers estimated by 2D analyses were significantly different from neuronal numbers estimated by design-based stereology. $*p < 0.05$ versus ANP, $**p < 0.05$ versus design-based stereology. (b) Neuronal number was normalized in a percentage as respects the mean of ANP. Only design-based stereology found a significant difference in DA neuronal number between ANP and AP. There is no significant difference between design-based stereology and 2D analyses. $*p < 0.05$ versus ANP, $**p < 0.05$ versus design-based stereology. ANP, alcohol nonpreferring; AP, alcohol preferring.

In actual volume estimation, the model-based approach and profile measurement showed significantly larger MNV than design-based stereology. For normalized data, the MPD estimate by profile measure was significantly smaller than that by design-based stereology. In EE rat model, there was no significant difference in MNV between SE and EE (Figure 16.8).

For the actual MNV results, both model-based and profile measure demonstrated significantly larger MNV than design-based stereology for both SE and EE, while for normalized data, there was no significant difference between design-based stereology and model-based methods and profile measure. In AP rat model, there was no significant difference between ANP and AP (Figure 16.9). In actual volume estimation, both model-based and profile measure demonstrated significantly larger MCV than design-based stereology for both ANP and AP. For normalized data, there was no significant difference between design-based stereology and 2D model-based methods and profile measure.

For the regional volume of the NAc, all approaches found a significant group difference between ANP and AP (Figure 16.10). As expected, the actual volume estimation based on pre-stained section thickness was significantly larger volume for both ANP and AP. The volume estimation using postprocessing section thickness was not significantly different from that obtained by design-based stereology.

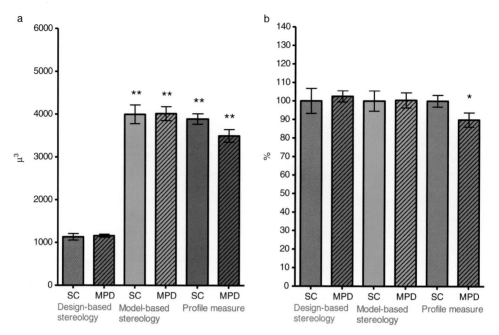

Figure 16.7   Quantification of TH+ neuronal volume in the SNpc of MPD mouse model (mean ± SEM). (a) Actual neuronal volume was estimated by design-based stereology, model-based stereology, and profile measure. All three analyses did not find a significant difference of neuronal volume between SC and MPD. 2D analyses, including model-based stereology and profile measure, estimated significantly different from design-based stereology in both SC and MPD. *$p < 0.05$ versus SC, **$p < 0.05$ versus design-based stereology. (b) Neuronal volume was normalized in a percentage as respects the mean of the SC. All three analyses did not find significant differences of neuronal volume between SC and MPD. MPD of profile measure was significantly different from MPD of design-based stereology. *$p < 0.05$ versus SC, **$p < 0.05$ versus design-based stereology. SC, sedentary control; MPD, chronic MPTP/probenecid PD.

Discussion

The purpose of this study is to directly compare 2D methods of model-based image analysis with 3D design-based stereology to quantify morphological differences between groups using the same sections from three different rodent models. Design-based stereology is the accepted gold standard for quantifying morphological and anatomical features in light microscopy (West and Gundersen, 1990; Saper, 1996; Mouton, 2011). Here we compared results from unbiased stereology with a 2D method based on profile counting and fractionator scheme to estimate total number of profiles, and a model-based approach that applies a correction factor for split cells to the results from the profile counting and fractionator method.

Estimates of total number of TH-positive using design-based stereology were not significantly different from the estimation of 3D reconstruction of serial sections in dopaminergic neurons of SNpc in the C57B/6J mouse (Baquet et al., 2009). This 3D reconstruction of serial sections provides a gold standard of sorts, an accurate determination of neuronal number obtained by counting all neurons in the reference volume (Coggeshall and Lekan, 1996; Guillery and Herrup, 1997). The advantage of design-based stereology is that the range of variations in cell size, cell shape, and section thickness that influence 2D profile counts and correction factors do not influence the estimate of total neuronal number (West, 1999; Selemon and Rajkowska, 2002; Mouton, 2011). These theoretical disadvantages of 2D analyses have led to the development of design-based

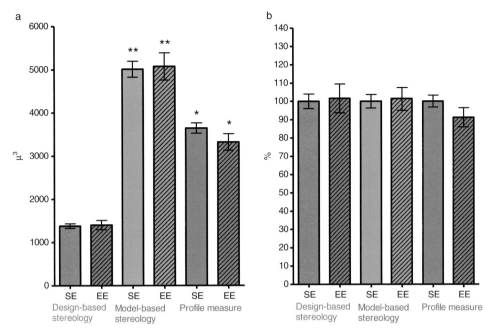

Figure 16.8 Quantification of TH+ neuronal volume in the SNpc of EE rat model (mean ± SEM). (a) Actual neuronal volume was estimated by design-based stereology, model-based stereology, and profile measure. All three methods did not find significant differences between SE and EE. 2D analyses, including model-based stereology and profile measure, demonstrated less neuronal volume significantly than design-based stereology in both SE and EE. *$p < 0.05$ versus SE, **$p < 0.05$ versus design-based stereology. (b) Neuronal volume was normalized in a percentage as respects the mean of the SE. All three methods did not find a significant difference between SE and EE. There is no significant difference between design-based stereology and 2D analyses. *$p < 0.05$ versus SE, **$p < 0.05$ versus design-based stereology. SE, standard environment; EE, enriched environment.

stereology; however, 2D analyses are still commonly used for comparisons of morphological and anatomical features.

The results of this study indicate that 2D analyses may be adequate for rough screening but inaccurate and unreliable for the estimation of total neuronal number. The fractionator method applied to profile counts underestimated the number of TH-positive neurons in both chronic MPD mouse model and AP rat model, and overestimated the number of TH-positive neurons in EE rat model. Comparing the difference between control and experimental groups, 2D analyses found a significant difference in chronic MPD mouse model with severe neuron loss but did not reveal less severe neuron loss in the EE rat model and AP rat model. In contrast, design-based stereology found significant differences in all three models. Thus, this study suggests that while profile-counting methods may detect relatively large differences between groups, these approaches lack reliability to estimate total neuronal number.

For quantification of neuronal volume, the result of the present study indicates that 2D analyses may be reliable in normalized data, but inaccurate for estimation of actual volume. Model-based approaches and profile measurement showed consistent overestimation of neuronal volume in all three approaches based on 2D measurements. Even though 2D analyses produced inaccurate estimates of MNV, normalized data from model-based stereology seemed to be reliable for a rough comparison or for large effects.

There are several possible explanations for the difference of estimations in total neuronal number between design-based stereology and 2D analyses. Many theoretical papers have argued

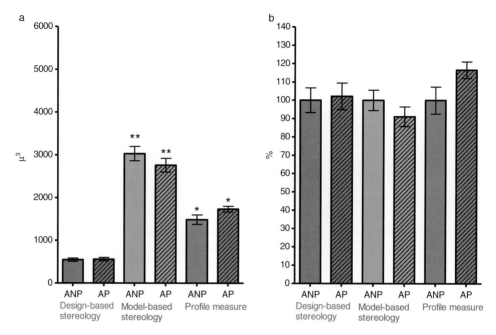

Figure 16.9 Quantification of TH+ neuronal volume in the VTA of AP rat model (mean ± SEM). (a) Actual neuronal volume was estimated by design-based stereology, model-based stereology, and profile measure. All three methods did not find a significant difference between SE and EE. 2D analyses, including model-based stereology and profile measure, demonstrated larger neuronal volume significantly than design-based stereology in both ANP and AP. *p < 0.05 versus ANP, **p < 0.05 versus design-based stereology. (b) Neuronal volume was normalized in a percentage as respects the mean of the SE. All three methods did not find a significant difference between SE and EE. There is no difference between design-based stereology and 2D analyses. *p < 0.05 versus ANP, **p < 0.05 versus design-based stereology. ANP, alcohol nonpreferring; AP, alcohol preferring.

that the major error in the use of profile counting arises from split-cells (Abercrombie and Johnson, 1946; West and Gundersen, 1990; Selemon and Rajkowska, 2002; Baquet et al., 2009). The fractionator method of profile counting overestimates total number of DA neurons by approximately 70% in samples with 10μ sections as compared to design-based stereology in the SNpc of the C57BL/6J mouse (Baquet et al., 2009). This bias from split-cells leads to overestimation of total neuronal number with the fractionator method, with the degree of bias a function of section thickness. The bias in profile counting is more severe for thin sections that generate more split-cells than thicker sections (Cooper and Sofroniew, 1996; Meredith et al., 1999). However, the present study demonstrated that the fractionator method would not always overestimate neuronal number because cross-sectional images of a sample section may not represent whole neurons of sample tissue in thick section. In the present study, thickness of sample tissue was 50μ (mouse) or 60μ (rat), and the diameter of neurons were about 10μ. The thickness of section was five or six times greater than the diameter of neurons. Thick sections of sample tissue may cause underestimation of neuronal number and attenuate overestimation due to split-cells because some neurons may overlap and become unfocused in the z-axis perspective. The effect of this bias depends on neuronal size. Smaller neurons have less probability to be split and may be more unfocused neurons in thick section, which could explain why 2D profile counting demonstrated significant underestimation of neuronal number in AP rat model. In this model, neuronal volume was about two times smaller than neuronal volume of the other models.

The model-based approach applies the Abercrombie correction factor to compensate for overestimation due to split-cells from the fractionator method (Abercrombie and Johnson, 1946;

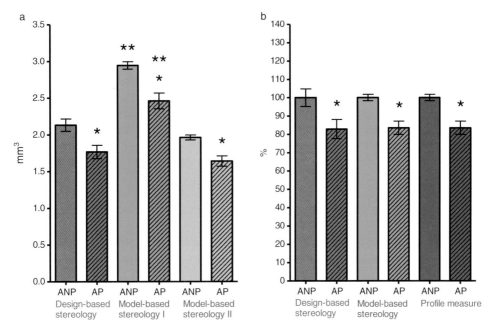

Figure 16.10 Quantification of NAc volume in the VTA of AP rat model (mean ± SEM). (a) Regional volume of the NAc was estimated by design-based stereology and model-based stereology. For design-based stereology, pre-stained cut thickness (60μ) was used, and model-based stereology used actual section thickness (40μ) for estimation. All three estimation demonstrated significant differences between ANP and AP. Model-based stereology showed significantly larger regional volume of the NAc than design-based stereology. $*p < 0.05$ versus ANP, $**p < 0.05$ versus design-based stereology (b) The volume of the NAc was normalized in a percentage as respects the mean of the ANP. All three methods found significant differences between ANP and AP. There is no significant difference between design-based stereology and 2D analyses. $*p < 0.05$ versus ANP, $**p < 0.05$ versus design-based stereology. NAc, nucleus accumbens; ANP, alcohol nonpreferring; AP, alcohol preferring.

Guillery and Herrup, 1997). However, the present study demonstrated the Abercrombie correction was not reliable for the estimation of neuronal number. Larger sampling intervals may cause a loss of precision in estimation of 2D neuronal counting method with the Abercrombie correction. Sample intervals larger than 150μ cause inaccuracy in estimating numbers of TH-positive neurons in the SNpc of the C57BL/6J mouse (Baquet et al., 2009). Thus, sampling intervals for profile count with Abercrombie correction should be less than $100\mu m$. In the present study, the sampling interval was $400\mu m$ for chronic MPD mouse model and $480\mu m$ for both EE rat model and AP rat model. This larger sampling interval may underestimate total neuronal number in the present study. Thus, the Abercrombie correction cannot compensate for biases causing underestimation of neuronal number in the fractionator method and model-based stereology. In addition, the Abercrombie correction demonstrated an unreliable adjustment for overestimation (Meredith et al., 1999; Baquet et al., 2009). These sources of systematic error affect not only estimation of total number but also normalized data for comparison in the ratio of the experimental group to the control group.

Normalized data of 2D analyses failed to accurately estimate differences between comparison groups in neuronal number. Model-based correction and the profile counting method estimated about 35% neuronal loss, while design-based stereology estimated 55% loss in chronic MPD mice. Densitometry also underestimated the extent of neuronal loss with more bias in the estimation of neuronal number by percentage since densitometry quantified not only TH-positive neurons, but also nonneuronal structures stained, such as dendrites. Normalization by percentage did not compensate for biases due to section thickness and section interval in model-based approach and the profile counting method. Previous studies indicate that the Abercrombie correction factor did not affect the ratio between comparison populations if neuronal size was not changed (Guillery and Herrup, 1997; Selemon and Rajkowska, 2002). Normalization to control values did not compensate for the bias of neuronal counting in 2D analyses, such as model-based correct and the profile counting method. Previous studies demonstrated similar differences in estimation between design-based stereology and 2D analyses on chronic MPD mice model with the same breed and induced Parkinsonism protocol. Profile counting estimated about 30% neuronal loss, but design-based stereology estimated about 50% neuronal loss (Petroske et al., 2001; Schintu et al., 2009). This difference may be caused not only by quantification methods but also other factors, such as tissue preparation, SD, and section thickness.

The present study supports the view that 2D analyses are inaccurate for both total number estimation and values normalized to controls. The inaccuracy due to 2D profile counts affects sensitivity for finding differences between groups, which conflicts with arguments by some researchers that model-based profile counting estimates accurately for the comparison of experimental groups to controls, provided neurons do not change in size, shape, or orientation between groups. This study shows that profile counting with and without correction factors generates inaccurate estimate of neuronal number even where there is no difference of neuronal volume between groups. The likely reason for this finding is that the profile ratio was not accurate and the Abercrombie correction did not compensate profile ratio. Neither profile counts nor profile ratios for comparison provide accurate estimates of neuronal number as suggested by some authors (Coggeshall and Lekan, 1996). In general, 2D analyses based on profile counts lack accuracy for total neuronal number or results normalized to controls.

The present findings indicate that 2D analyses do not have enough sensitivity to detect relatively small differences in neuronal number. 2D analyses did not identify the relatively small differences in neuronal number of the SNpc. Using unbiased stereology, the severe model (MPD) demonstrated more than 50% difference between control and experimental groups, while models with less severe neuron loss (EE, AP) showed less than 20% difference. Profile counting methods and densitometry showed a significant difference between control and experimental groups in the chronic MPD model but not in the other two models with less severe neuron loss.

Several previous studies have quantified TH+ neurons in the SNpc to investigate the effect of EE in different rodent species, including C57B1/6 mice, SAMP8 mice, Wistar rats, and Sprague-Dawley rats (Bezard et al., 2003; Faherty et al., 2005; Steiner et al., 2006; Yuan et al., 2009). Most of these 2D analyses of profile counts reported no significant differences in neuron number between control and EE groups in the SNpc; however, significant differences were revealed using design-based stereology (Bezard et al., 2003; Faherty et al., 2005). Also, counts of TH-positive profiles in ANP and AP rats did not find significant differences that were found using design-based stereology (Zhou et al., 1995; Ahmad et al., 2009a). The present study demonstrates how the low sensitivity of 2D profile counts could easily produce different results as compared to design-based stereology.

The 2D analyses overestimated the actual MNV of TH-positive neurons but generated comparable value to design-based stereology when normalized as a percentage of control. The explanation for these observations lies in the different approaches used to measure radius for the MNV calculations for design-based stereology versus the two profile-based approaches. For the volume, V, formula [$V = (4\pi/3)r^3$], one model-based approach measures the profile area and then back-calculates the radius from the Euclidean formula, area = πr^2. The second method based on 2D profile measurement allows ImageJ to find the longest diameter and then divides by 2 to calculate the radius. Both of these approaches for the volume calculation led to overestimation in MNV relative to the nucleator approach of unbiased stereology (Gundersen and Jensen, 1985). The nucleator uses the same equation $[V = (4\pi/3)r^3]$ to estimate MNV but quantifies the radius for this equation using stochastic geometry, rather than model-based Euclidean geometry. The nucleator method measures radius as the average of four random angles across the neuron. Since the radius is cubed in the formula for volume estimation $[V = (4\pi/3)r^3]$, relatively small overestimations of the radius using the model-based 2D approaches leads to correspondingly large overestimation of the MNV. Note that normalized MNV values for the 2D approach based on radius calculation from the profile area were not markedly different from the nucleator estimates, while the normalized MNV values with radius calculated as the longest diameter were different from the nucleator estimates. Thus, 2D model-based approaches have the potential to estimate MNV with the same accuracy as design-based stereology, depending on how the radius is calculated.

In summary, we find that 2D analyses may be a useful screening tool to identify large group difference in number and size of TH-positive neurons in rodent models. Caution must be used when interpreting future and previous reports of significant differences in numbers of TH-positive neurons based on 2D analyses of profile counts and Euclidean-based models. For studies of brains from humans and experimental animals, inaccurate determination of group differences may lead to incorrect conclusions about neuropathological severity or intervention effects.

References

Abercrombie, M., Johnson, M. L. 1946. Quantitative histology of Wallerian degeneration: I. Nuclear population in rabbit sciatic nerve. *J Anat* **80** (Pt 1): 37–50.

Ahmad, S. O., Park, J.-H., Penick, E., Manzardo, A. (2009a). Stereological examination of the mesocortical dopamine system in alcohol preferring and non preferring Wistar rats. 2009 Meeting Planner. Chicago, IL: Neuroscience Society for Neuroscience.

Ahmad, S. O., Park, J. H., Stenho-Bittel, L., Lau, Y. S. 2009b. Effects of endurance exercise on ventral tegmental area neurons in the chronic 1-methyl-4-phenyl-1,2,3,6-tetrahydropyridine and probenecid-treated mice. *Neurosci Lett* **450** (2): 102–105.

Almli, C., Abel, R., Levy, T., Switzer, R., Park, J., Ahmad, S. O. (2008). Effects of complex-enriched versus standard laboratory rearing environments on brain and behavioral development of rats. 2008 Meeting Planner. Washington, DC: Neuroscience Society for Neuroscience.

Baquet, Z. C., Williams, D., Brody, J., Smeyne, R. J. 2009. A comparison of model-based (2-D) and design-based (3-D) stereological methods for estimating cell number in the substantia nigra pars compacta (SNpc) of the C57BL/6J mouse. *Neuroscience* **161** (4): 1082–1090.

Benes, F. M., Lange, N. 2001. Two-dimensional versus three-dimensional cell counting: a practical perspective. *Trends Neurosci* **24** (1): 11–17.

Bezard, E., Dovero, S., Belin, D., Duconger, S., Jackson-Lewis, V., Przedborski, S. et al. 2003. Enriched environment confers resistance to 1-methyl-4-phenyl-1,2,3,6-tetrahydropyridine and cocaine: involvement of dopamine transporter and trophic factors. *J Neurosci* **23** (35): 10999–11007.

Coggeshall, R. E., Lekan, H. A. 1996. Methods for determining numbers of cells and synapses: a case for more uniform standards of review. *J Comp Neurol* **364** (1): 6–15.

Cooper, J. D., Sofroniew, M. V. 1996. Increased vulnerability of septal cholinergic neurons to partial loss of target neurons in aged rats. *Neuroscience* **75** (1): 29–35.

Faherty, C. J., Raviie Shepherd, K., Herasimtschuk, A., Smeyne, R. J. 2005. Environmental enrichment in adulthood eliminates neuronal death in experimental Parkinsonism. *Brain Res Mol Brain Res* **134** (1): 170–179.

Franklin, K. B. J., Paxinos, G. 2008. *The Mouse Brain in Stereotaxic Coordinates*, 3rd ed. New York: Academic Press.

Guillery, R. W., Herrup, K. 1997. Quantification without pontification: choosing a method for counting objects in sectioned tissues. *J Comp Neurol* **386** (1): 2–7.

Gundersen, H. J. 1978. Estimators of the number of objects per area unbiased by edge effects. *Microsc Acta* **81** (2): 107–117.

Gundersen, H. J. 1986. Stereology of arbitrary particles. A review of unbiased number and size estimators and the presentation of some new ones, in memory of William R. Thompson. *J Microsc* **143** (Pt 1): 3–45.

Gundersen, H. J. G. 1977. Notes on the estimation of the numerical density of arbitrary profiles: the edge effect. *J Microsc* **117** (143): 3–45.

Gundersen, H. J., Jensen, E. B. 1985. Stereological estimation of the volume-weighted mean volume of arbitrary particles observed on random sections. *J. Microsc* **138** (Pt 2): 127–142.

Lau, Y. S., Trobough, K. L., Crampton, J. M., Wilson, J. A. 1990. Effects of probenecid on striatal dopamine depletion in acute and long-term 1-methyl-4-phenyl-1,2,3,6-tetrahydropyridine (MPTP)-treated mice. *Gen Pharmacol* **21** (2): 181–187.

Mandarim-de-Lacerda, C. A. 2003. Stereological tools in biomedical research. *An Acad Bras Cienc* **75** (4): 469–486.

Meredith, S., Dudenhoeffer, G., Jackson, K. 1999. Single-section counting error when distinguishing between primordial and early primary follicles in sections of rat ovary of different thickness. *J Reprod Fertil* **117** (2): 339–343.

Mouton, P. R. 2011. *Unbiased Stereology: A Concise Guide*. Baltimore, MD: The Johns Hopkins Press.

Paxinos, G., Watson, C. 2007. *The Rat Brain in Stereotaxic Coordinates*, 6th ed. Amsterdam. Boston: Elsevier.

Petroske, E., Meredith, G. E., Callen, S., Totterdell, S., Lau, Y. S. 2001. Mouse model of Parkinsonism: a comparison between subacute MPTP and chronic MPTP/probenecid treatment. *Neuroscience* **106** (3): 589–601.

Rinne, J. O., Ma, S. Y., Lee, M. S., Collan, Y., Roytta, M. 2008. Loss of cholinergic neurons in the pedunculopontine nucleus in Parkinson's disease is related to disability of the patients. *Parkinsonism Relat Disord* **14** (7): 553–557.

Saper, C. B. 1996. Any way you cut it: a new journal policy for the use of unbiased counting methods. *J Comp Neurol* **364** (1).

Schintu, N., Frau, L., Ibba, M., Garau, A., Carboni, E., Carta, A. R. 2009. Progressive dopaminergic degeneration in the chronic MPTPp mouse model of Parkinson's disease. *Neurotox Res* **16** (2): 127–139.

Schmitz, C., Hof, P. R. 2005. Design-based stereology in neuroscience. *Neuroscience* **130** (4): 813–831.

Selemon, L. D., Rajkowska, G. 2002. Two-dimensional versus three-dimensional cell counting. *Biol Psychiatry* **51** (10): 838–840; author reply, 842–836.

Steiner, B., Winter, C., Hosman, K., Siebert, E., Kempermann, G., Petrus, D. S. et al. 2006. Enriched environment induces cellular plasticity in the adult substantia nigra and improves motor behavior function in the 6-OHDA rat model of Parkinson's disease. *Exp Neurol* **199** (2): 291–300.

von Bartheld, C. S. 2001. Comparison of 2-D and 3-D counting: the need for calibration and common sense. *Trends Neurosci* **24** (9): 504–506.

Weibel, E. R. 1979. *Stereological Methods: Practical Methods for Biological Morphometry*, Vol. 1. London: Academic Press.

West, M. J. 1993. New stereological methods for counting neurons. *Neurobiol Aging* **14** (4): 275–285.

West, M. J. 1999. Stereological methods for estimating the total number of neurons and synapses: issues of precision and bias. *Trends Neurosci* **22** (2): 51–61.

West, M. J., Gundersen, H. J. 1990. Unbiased stereological estimation of the number of neurons in the human hippocampus. *J Comp Neurol* **296** (1): 1–22.

Yuan, Z. Y., Gu, P., Liu, L., Wang, Y. Y., Liu, J., Cui, D. S. et al. 2009. Neuroprotective effects of enriched environment in MPTP-treated SAMP8 mice. *Neurosci Lett* **454** (1): 6–10.

Zhou, F. C., Zhang, J. K., Lumeng, L., Li, T. K. 1995. Mesolimbic dopamine system in alcohol-preferring rats. *Alcohol* **12** (5): 403–412.

17   A Stereologic Perspective on Autism Neuropathology

Neha Uppal and Patrick R. Hof

Fishberg Department of Neuroscience, Seaver Autism Center, Mount Sinai School of Medicine, New York, NY, USA
Friedman Brain Institute, New York, NY, USA

Background

Autism spectrum disorders are symptomatically defined conditions affecting 1 in 88 children in the United States, with an almost fivefold greater effect in boys (Center for Disease Control, 2012). Children throughout the spectrum have varying degrees of impairment in social communication and interactions, in addition to restricted interests and repetitive behaviors (American Psychiatric Association, 2000). Genetic studies to understand the cause of autism have revealed no single cause. Several potential candidate genes have been implicated (Aldinger et al., 2011), which explain approximately 25% of cases. The diversity of causes suggests that distinct genetic disruptions converge on similar pathways in the brain regions of affected patients, resulting in the characteristic phenotype of autism.

Abnormalities in minicolumns and microstructural defects have been qualitatively reported throughout ages and sexes in specific cortical areas (Weidenheim et al., 2001; Casanova and Trippe, 2009; Casanova et al., 2010; Wegiel et al., 2010), and many studies have even observed localized changes in neuron density (Bauman and Kemper, 2005). Since these changes appear restricted to a particular area or cortical layer, further studies require tools that are precise and accurate enough to detect subtle pathologic alterations in the brain. Unbiased stereology meets this potential using assumption- and model-free approaches to sample anatomically defined brain regions and make accurate estimates of total cell number (Schmitz and Hof, 2005).

Cortical Areas

Behavioral symptoms of autism patients combined with qualitative studies of brain sections indicate that pathology will be strongly represented in cerebral cortex (outlined in Figure 17.1). Casanova and colleagues determined that minicolumns, the structural cortical domains in which afferent, efferent, and local connections of pyramidal neurons come together, are smaller and more numerous throughout the cortex in autism (Casanova and Trippe, 2009; Casanova et al., 2010). Wegiel et al. (2010) explored the microarchitecture of cortical areas to determine patterns of developmental disparities between patients with autism and controls. Through a full spectrum of ages, an overall disorganization of gray and white matter along with more region- and patient-specific alterations was observed in many regions in patients with autism.

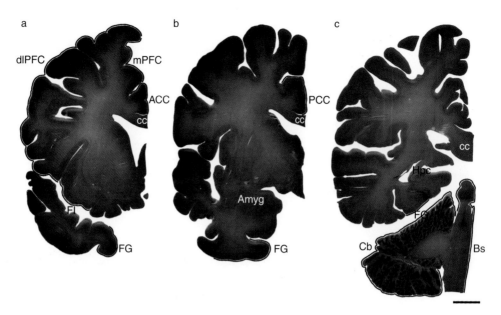

Figure 17.1 Nissl-stained left hemispheres depict areas in which neuropathology has been studied in autism. (a) Dorsolateral prefrontal cortex (dlPFC), medial prefrontal cortex (mPFC), anterior cingulate cortex (ACC), frontoinsular cortex (FI), and fusiform gyrus (FG); (b) posterior cingulate cortex (PCC), amygdala (Amyg), and fusiform gyrus (FG); (c) hippocampus (Hpc), fusiform gyrus (FG), cerebellum (Cb), and brainstem (Bs). Corpus callosum, cc; scale bar = 1 cm.

In addition to pathologic changes throughout the cerebral cortex, several studies have high-lighted the presence of lobe- and area-specific or even layer-specific cortical changes in patients affected by this disorder. For example, Bauman and Kemper (2005) have carried out many studies showing differences in neuron size and density in the hippocampal formation, anterior cingulate cortex (ACC), septum, and mammillary bodies. These analyses, coupled with knowledge from behavioral symptoms and results from imaging studies, have stimulated many researchers to investigate these areas in autism using unbiased stereology.

Prefrontal Cortex

The role for the prefrontal cortex (PFC), usually categorized as "executive functions," is thought to regulate planning, decision making and, most importantly, social behavior (Fuster, 2001; Miller and Cohen, 2001). To explore whether behavioral abnormalities in autism specific to PFC functions might begin early in life, Courchesne and colleagues assessed the medial and dorsolateral PFC in 7 boys with autism and 6 typically developing boys, ranging from age 2 to 16 (Courchesne et al., 2011; Table 17.1). The postmortem tissue was stained for Nissl substance to visualize cell bodies of neurons and glial cells. The materials available for this study varied from 50 to 200 μm in cut thickness and allowed for series of 8–12 sections per case for analysis. The materials were optimal for stereological quantification of total numbers of neuron and glia using the optical fractionator (West et al., 1991). The study design accounted for sampling about 100 sites per case to ensure precise estimates. The neurons and glia were counted through 10 μm of tissue with an 8-μm guard zone to avoid cutting bias. The authors also used the nucleator probe to measure neuronal volume in both regions (for review, see Mouton, 2011). Although no differences were found in glia number or neuron size between groups, boys with autism had a 67% higher mean numbers

Table 17.1 Summary of stereologic parameters in the prefrontal cortex

Study	Courchesne et al. (2011)	Jacot-Descombes et al. (2012)
Area, layers	DL-PFC and M-PFC, layers not specified	Areas 44 and 45, layers III, V, and VI
Number of autism, controls	7, 6	8, 6
Age range of autism, controls	2–16, 2–16	4–66, 4–52
Sex	M	M and F
Stain	Nissl—thionine, cresyl violet; PEG	Nissl—gallocyanin
Section thickness	Ranges from 50 to 200 µm	200 and 500 µm
Number of sections (average)	8–12	5
Objective	40–100× oil	40× air
Probes used	Optical fractionator, nucleator	Optical fractionator, nucleator, Cavalieri
Disector height	10 µm	20 µm
Guard zone	>8 µm	2 µm
Counting frame	n/a	50 × 50 µm
Grid size	n/a	500 × 500 µm
Coefficient of error	≤0.10	≤0.11
Results	↑79% in DL-PFC ↑29% in M-PFC	↓18% neuron volume in layer III ↓18.5% neuron volume in layer V ↓22% neuron volume in layer VI

Sources: Courchesne, E., Mouton, P. R., Calhoun, M. E., Semendeferi, K., Ahrens-Barbeau, C., Hallet, M. J., Barnes, C. C., Pierce, K. 2011. Neuron number and size in prefrontal cortex of children with autism. *J Am Med Assoc* **306** (18): 2001–2010. Jacot-Descombes, S., Uppal, N., Wicinski, B., Santos, M., Schmeidler, J., Giannakopoulos, P., Heinsen, H., Schmitz, C., Hof, P. R. 2012. Decreased pyramidal neuron size in Brodmann areas 44 and 45 in patients with autism. *Acta Neuropathol (Berl)* **124** (1): 67–79.

of neurons in two subregions of PFC as compared with typically developing boys (illustrated in Figure 17.2). There was a 79% increase in neuron number in boys with autism in the dorsolateral PFC (1.57 billion in autism, 0.88 billion in controls) and a 29% increase in the medial PFC (0.36 billion in autism, 0.28 billion in controls), complementing a parallel volume increase in these areas found by imaging studies of children with autism (Carper and Courchesne, 2005).

Cortical neurons are generated in excess early in gestation (Gohlke et al., 2007), and this over-abundance may be even larger in children with autism. Since neurons do not develop postnatally in the PFC (Samuelsen et al., 2003; Uylings et al., 2005; Bhardwaj et al., 2006; Larsen et al., 2006), the authors suggested that the pathology found in this study could result from a prenatal overabundance of neurons or reflect impairment in apoptotic mechanisms postnatally (Courchesne et al., 2011). The increase in brain weight and size typically reported in autism may reflect the abnormal increase in neuron number reported in this study, as shown in animals (Chenn and Walsh, 2002). Impairment in apoptosis during early postnatal life, which typically removes subplate neurons, may also contribute to the excess amount of cortical neurons in autism.

While this study revealed striking autism-related neuropathology of the PFC, the authors stressed that the study was preliminary in several ways. Like all of the neuropathology studies discussed in this chapter, it would have greatly benefited from a larger number of cases and controls; unfortunately, the amount of available tissue is limited. With regard to the evaluation of the PFC, the authors analyzed two large, generic cortical domains but did not assess separate Brodmann areas or layers. Because many subregions of the PFC contribute differently to cognitive functioning and each layer has a distinct role in information processing, future studies to analyze these components separately could help to shed light on the specific neuropathology in autism.

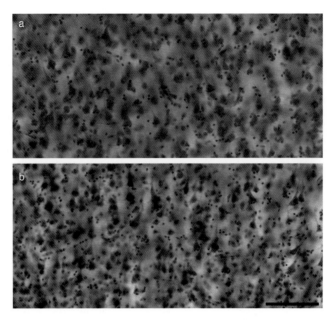

Figure 17.2　Illustration of the reported increase in neuron number in children with autism in layer III of the prefrontal cortex. Note the qualitative increase in neurons in the patient with autism (b) when compared to the typically developing control (a). Scale bar = 100 μm.

Hof and colleagues have begun delineating the PFC by focusing on areas 44 and 45, which are involved in language processing, imitation, and sociality (Bookheimer, 2002; Williams, 2008; Tyler et al., 2011; Senju, 2012). The study included patients and controls 4–66 years old with both sexes and hemispheres represented (Jacot-Descombes et al., 2012; Table 17.1). Layers III, V, and VI were compared in eight patients with autism and six age-comparable controls, assessing the layer volume with the Cavalieri principle, neuron number with the optical fractionator probe, and neuron size with the nucleator probe. These analyses were completed on Nissl-stained tissue, on sets of 4–12 sections per case. The neurons were counted and measured through 20 μm of tissue with a 2-μm guard zone in a 50-μm square grid.

No differences in neuron number and layer volume in autism were found, but a significant decrease in the size of neurons was reported in patients with autism throughout the age range. In layer III, patients with autism had an 18% reduction in neuron size compared to controls (2034 μm^3 in autism, 2482 μm^3 in controls), 18.5% reduction in layer V (2148 μm^3 in autism, 2637 μm^3 in controls), and 22% reduction in layer VI (1947 μm^3 in autism, 2499 μm^3 in controls). When separated into subgroups, the trajectory of neuronal volume was distinct between groups and ages; controls showed a reduction in size of neurons with increasing age (29% reduction in layer III, 11% in layer V, and 13% in layer VI), but the neuronal size in autism was consistently reduced (16% difference between children and adults with autism in layer III, 2% in layer V, and 1.5% in layer VI). Typically developing controls had an average neuron size of 3026 μm^3 as children and 2156 μm^3 as adults in layer III, whereas children with autism had an average neuron size of 2264 μm^3 and adults with autism had an average size of 1897 μm^3. In layer V, typically developing children averaged 2828 μm^3 large neurons, and adults had neurons 2523 μm^3 in size. Children with autism had neuronal size of 2120 μm^3 and adults had an average of 2166 μm^3. In layer VI, typically developing children had an average of 2714 μm^3, where adults had an average of 2369 μm^3. Children with autism averaged 1965 μm^3 neuronal size, and adults were similarly sized at 1937 μm^3.

Importantly, reduced perikaryal size may have an impact on connectivity within this region's network. This may be substantiated by the reduced neuron size in the fusiform gyrus (FG), which is connected functionally with areas 44 and 45 (van Kooten et al., 2008; see later discussion).

A previous nonstereologic study similarly found no difference in pyramidal neuron density, other neurons, or glia between patients with autism and controls (Coleman et al., 1985). Results from the present study do not, however, substantiate the drastic changes seen in the PFC as a whole (Courchesne et al., 2011). The discovery of the subtle changes in areas 44 and 45 may be attributed to the specificity of the area and layers assessed in this study. The differences in results between these two studies highlight the importance of having both detailed analysis of individual areas and broad analysis of regions, as they both give distinct views on the effect of autism on brain pathology.

Fusiform Gyrus

van Kooten et al. (2008) carried out one of the first rigorous stereologic studies in the brains of autistic individuals (Table 17.2). The authors focused on the fusiform gyrus (FG), a cortical region important for facial processing and, therefore, social behaviors, as well as the primary visual cortex (area 17) and the whole cortical gray matter as comparison and internal control regions. The study evaluated postmortem tissue from 7 patients with autism and 10 controls of both sexes, aged 4–65 years. The tissue was Nissl-stained and was processed at either 200 or 500 μm; 20 μm of the tissue thickness were analyzed with a 10-μm guard zone. Layers II, III, IV, V, and VI were assessed separately in the FG to determine neuron number, layer volume, and neuron volume with the optical fractionator, Cavalieri principle, and nucleator probe, respectively. The results showed significant and specific neuropathology in layers III, V, and VI in the FG in patients with autism that was not found in the control areas. Layer III neurons were less numerous and less dense, and layer V and VI neurons were less numerous and smaller in size in the FG compared to the cortex as a whole and to area 17. All three layers had smaller volumes in autism compared to controls. These results suggest that patients with autism either have a reduced number of neurons in this area when they are born, or that a potential overabundance of abnormal synapses at a young age leads to pruning of neurons that are nonfunctional. Regardless of the cause, the effect of having smaller perikaryal volume is a parallel reduction in dendritic length, which implies that these neurons are not sending information to their intended target. This, as well as a reduced number of neurons, may cause a defect in connectivity between the FG and the areas that it receives input and sends output to, suggesting problems in cortical circuitry. This hypothesis is corroborated by a similar effect seen in areas connected to the FG, such as the amygdala (Schumann and Amaral, 2006) and areas 44 and 45 (Jacot-Descombes et al., 2012).

The lack of pathology in the control areas (area 17 and whole cortex), provide evidence that these neuropathological alterations are region-specific and do not occur in a widespread manner or randomly through the brain. However, the evidence would have been more convincing had the layers in the control areas been individually analyzed as the FG was; as illustrated by the results in the FG, there were layer-specific changes that may have been overlooked as the layers in the internal control regions were grouped together.

This study was followed a few years later with a more focused analysis of different neuronal types in the FG in autism (Oblak et al., 2011; Table 17.2). Blatt and colleagues looked at the parvalbumin- and calbindin-expressing GABAergic interneurons as well as the thionine-stained cell bodies with the optical fractionator to determine their densities in this area. The FG was analyzed in two laminar domains, the superficial (I–IV) and deep (V–VI) layers, with a 63× oil objective. For the Nissl-stained materials, a guard zone of 5 μm and disector of 20 μm was used

Table 17.2 Summary of stereologic parameters in the fusiform gyrus

Study	van Kooten et al. (2008)	Oblak et al. (2011)
Area, layers	Fusiform gyrus (FG), layers II–VI, VI; Area 17, cortical gray matter (CGM)	Fusiform gyrus (Area 37), superficial (I–IV) and deep (V–VI) layers
Number of autism, controls	7, 10	9, 7
Age range of autism, controls	4–23, 4–65	14–32, 16–36
Sex	M and F	M and F
Stain	Nissl—gallocyanin	Nissl—thionin, parvalbumin, calbindin
Section thickness	200 and 500 µm	40–80 µm
Number of sections (average)	FG: 10.8 Area 17, CGM: 20.2	n/a
Objective	20× oil	63× oil
Probes used	Optical fractionator, nucleator, Cavalieri	Optical fractionator
Disector	20 µm	Thionin: 20 µm Parvalbumin and calbindin: 10 µm
Guard zone	10 µm	Thionin: 5 µm Parvalbumin and calbindin: 4 µm
Counting frame	FG: 70×70 µm (I–V) and 80×80 µm (VI) Area 17: 6241 µm^2 CGM: 80×80 µm	Thionin: 1600 µm^2 (area) Parvalbumin and calbindin 4800 µm^2 (area)
Grid size	FG: 650×650–900×900 µm CGM: 6500×6500 µm Area 17: 1100×1100 µm	950×950 µm
Coefficient of error	≤0.05	≤0.09
Results	↓ volume of layers III, V, VI ↓ neuron density in layer III ↓ mean neuron number in layers III, V, VI ↓ neuron volume in layers V, VI	No significant differences found

Sources: van Kooten, I. A., Palmen, S. J., von Cappeln, P., Steinbusch, H. W., Korr, H., Heinsen, H., Hof, P. R., van Engeland, H., Schmitz, C. 2008. Neurons in the fusiform gyrus are fewer and smaller in autism. *Brain* **131** (Pt 4): 987–999.
Oblak, A. L., Rosene, D. L., Kemper, T. L., Bauman, M. L., Blatt, G. J. 2011. Altered posterior cingulate cortical cyctoarchitecture, but normal density of neurons and interneurons in the posterior cingulate cortex and fusiform gyrus in autism. *Autism Res* **4** (3): 200–211.

with a counting frame area of 1600 µm^2. The parvalbumin- and calbindin-immunoreactive inter-neurons were analyzed with a guard zone of 4 µm, a disector of 10 µm, and a counting frame area of 4800 µm^2. Unlike the previous FG study, the authors reported no difference in cytoarchitecture, Nissl-stained cell body density, parvalbumin- or calbindin-immunoreactive interneuron density, or relative density of either interneuron population with Nissl-stained cell bodies in autism.

The discrepancy between these two studies provides an interesting situation to explore the effects of the methods used. As both groups measured neuron density in Nissl-stained materials in the same area, the overall amounts of neurons should have been comparable. Four major differences (applicable to Nissl-stained material only) were tissue thickness, magnification, grid size, and layer grouping, with the first three differences alleviated by using stereological procedures. The collective analysis of layers may have restricted the ability to find the more delicate changes in the brain. However, there was a clear diagnostic difference in layers V and VI in the van Kooten study, which was not seen in the Oblak study even though layers V and VI were analyzed together.

This may be due to an age effect, as the van Kooten study included typically developing controls at a much older age. In addition the boundaries of the FG were cytoarchitecturally defined in the Oblak study, which was not done in the van Kooten study. The cytoarchitecture of the FG does vary along its rostrocaudal axis, so the area assessed in the Oblak study may have been a more restricted area of cortex. This suggests the interesting possibility that the changes seen the FG in the van Kooten study may reflect the location of the fusiform face area and the changes found through imaging studies (Kanwisher et al., 1999; Pierce et al., 2001, 2004; Piggot et al., 2004; Bolte et al., 2006; Kleinhans et al., 2008).

Frontoinsular Cortex

The frontoinsular cortex (FI) is located in the anterior inferior portion of the insular cortex. It is involved in our understanding of our body's sensations, which contributes to our emotional self-awareness and social interactions (Craig, 2002, 2003, 2009; Critchley et al., 2004). This area is also home to particular neurons, the von Economo neurons (VENs), which are large, slender, bipolar cells found in layer V of the FI and ACC (Figure 17.3c; see comparison of morphology with pyramidal cells in Figure 17.3a,b). Because of their location and morphology as well as being a specific target in neuropsychiatric disorders (Seeley et al., 2006, 2007; Kaufman et al., 2008; Brüne et al., 2010; Seeley, 2010; Kim et al., 2012; for review see Butti et al., 2011), VENs are speculated to be involved in our ability to process information quickly in complex social situations (Allman et al., 2005, 2010). Since representation of emotions and bodily sensation is potentially altered in autism given its social symptoms, Courchesne and colleagues evaluated the FI in four males with autism and five male controls (Kennedy et al., 2007; Table 17.3). The patients with autism were aged 3, 15, 34, and 41 years, while the controls were 2, 16.5, 21, 44, and 75 years. These Nissl-stained materials were analyzed with a 63× oil objective using the optical fractionator probe to determine VEN number across ages and diagnosis. The guard zone spanned 4 μm above the disector and 2 μm below, with a disector between 6 and 10 μm. The grid size was a square of 200 μm, containing a counting frame of 125 by 100 μm.

The authors reported no difference in the number of VENs in the FI between groups after stereological analysis, though there was a slight nonsignificant increase in VEN number in autism (mean number of VENs in autism was 35,329 whereas controls had 29,125). However, this

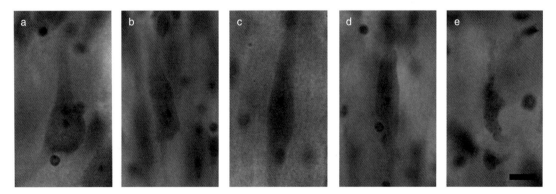

Figure 17.3 Morphology of pyramidal neurons and abnormal morphology of von Economo neurons (VENs) in the frontoinsular cortex. (a) Typical pyramidal neuron in a control subject; (b) typical pyramidal neuron in a patient with autism; (c) typical VEN in a control subject; (d) abnormal morphology of a VEN in a patient with autism—note the abnormal placement of a glial cell; (e) abnormal morphology of a VEN in a patient with autism—note the corkscrew shape of the dendrite. Scale bar = 10 μm.

Table 17.3 Summary of stereologic parameters in the frontoinsular cortex

Study	Kennedy et al. (2007)	Santos et al. (2011)
Area, layers	FI, layer V	FI, layer V
Number of autism, controls	4, 5	4, 3
Age range of autism, controls	3–41, 2–75	4–11, 4–14
Sex	M	M and F
Stain	Nissl—thionin, Gallyas silver stain	Nissl—gallocyanin
Section thickness	20–100 μm	200 and 500 μm
Number of sections (average)	Range of 9–25	11
Objective	60× oil	40× air
Probes used	Optical fractionator	Optical fractionator, Cavalieri
Disector	6–10 μm	20 μm
Guard zone	4 μm top, 2 μm bottom	2 μm
Counting frame	125 × 100 μm	VENs: 220 × 180 μm Pyramidal neurons: 50 × 50 μm
Grid size	200 × 200 μm	VENs: 220 × 180 μm Pyramidal neurons: 650 × 400 μm
Coefficient of error	≤0.09	≤0.1
Results	No significant difference in VEN number	↑53% in ratio of VENs to pyramids No significant difference in VEN number (though trend toward significant ↑ in autism) No difference in pyramidal neuron number between autism and controls No difference in layer V volume

Sources: Kennedy, D. P., Semendeferi, K., Courchesne, E. 2007. No reduction of spindle neuron number in frontoinsular cortex in autism. *Brain Cogn* **64** (2): 124–129.
Santos, M., Uppal, N., Butti, C., Wicinski, B., Schmeidler, J., Giannakopoulos, P., Heinsen, H., Schmitz, C., Hof, P. R. 2011. von Economo neurons in autism: a stereologic study of the frontoinsular cortex in children. *Brain Res* **1380**: 206–217.

increase was due to an outlier in the autism group, and when removed from the average, VEN number in the FI in autism reduced to 29,557. The authors also measured neuron size using four rays in the vertical nucleator probe, and found no difference in VEN size between autism and controls.

This area was explored once more by Hof and colleagues, but with a more specific age focus (Santos et al., 2011; Table 17.3). The study assessed four patients with autism 4–11 years of age and three controls 4–14 years of age. The tissue sections were either 200- or 500-μm thick, and Nissl-stained to allow for identification of VEN and pyramidal cell bodies (Figure 17.3a,b). Each case had an average of 11 sections analyzed for VEN and pyramidal neuron number as well as layer volume in layer V of the FI. The counting frame and grid size for VEN population estimation in the optical fractionator probe were equivalent at 220 μm by 180 μm—as VENs are not evenly distributed throughout layer V in autism, the authors counted exhaustively throughout the layer to ensure an unbiased estimate of the VEN population. Pyramidal neurons were counted with a square counting frame of 50 μm in a 650- by 400-μm grid. The authors used the ratio of VENs to pyramidal neurons as their output for this study so results across ages, sexes, and hemispheres would be more comparable. The main result of the analysis was a 53% increase in the ratio of VENs to pyramidal neurons in children with autism as well as qualitative observation of alterations in VEN morphology (Figure 17.3d,e). There was no difference in VEN number (though there was a trend toward significantly higher numbers in autism, with a mean of 28,995 VENs in autism, and 18,889 in controls), pyramidal number, VEN density, or layer volume. The striking increase in ratio of VENs to pyramidal neurons in children with autism may reflect the higher level of interoception some children experience, as the pathology is specific to the neuron that may modulate this emotion.

As commonly found in neuropathologic studies of this size, the two studies on the FI found seemingly conflicting results. However, the studies are not easily comparable, as many of their methods differ. The Kennedy study used both a Nissl and silver stains on their cases, whereas the Santos study only used Nissl staining. More importantly the Kennedy study's age range was much broader than that of Santos and colleagues, which is likely the cause of the distinct results. The Santos study also counted exhaustively through the x and y planes to ensure an accurate count of VENs, whereas the Kennedy study estimated the population in all planes. However, at the ages that the two studies overlapped, the estimated number of VENs found was very similar, suggesting that age was likely the largest factor in the difference of results.

Anterior Cingulate Cortex

Blatt and colleagues published a study on the possible involvement of VENs in the anterior cingulate cortex (ACC) in autism (Simms et al., 2009; Table 17.4). The ACC is involved in autonomic functions, and more pertinent to autism, cognitive functions such as empathy, reward anticipation, decision making, and emotion (Devinsky et al., 1995; Allman et al., 2001; Schmitz and Rezaie, 2008; Schmitz et al., 2008). The study included nine males with autism (15–54 years old) and four male controls (20–55 years old). The study was limited to area 24, and separated into area

Table 17.4   Summary of stereologic parameters in the anterior cingulate cortex

Study	Simms et al. (2009)
Area, layers	Area 24, layer I–III, V–VI (pyramidal neurons); layer V (VENs)
Number of autism, controls	9, 4
Age range of autism, controls	15–54, 20–55
Sex	M
Stain	Nissl—thionin
Section thickness	80 μm
Number of sections (average)	7
Objective	n/a
Probes used	Optical fractionator, nucleator
Disector	7 μm
Guard zone	1 μm
Counting frame	Pyramidal neurons: 50×50 μm
Grid size	Pyramidal neurons: 290×290 μm
Coefficient of error	≤0.1
Results	No difference in overall VEN density ↑pyramidal neuron density in layers I–III in left hemisphere versus right of 24a ↓neuron size in 24b ↓neuron packing density in layers V–VI of 24c

Source: Simms, M. L., Kemper, T. L., Timbie, C. M., Bauman, M. L., Blatt, G. J. 2009. The anterior cingulate cortex in autism: heterogeneity of qualitative and quantitative cytoarchitectonic features suggests possible subgroups. *Acta Neuropathol (Berl)* **118** (5): 673–684.

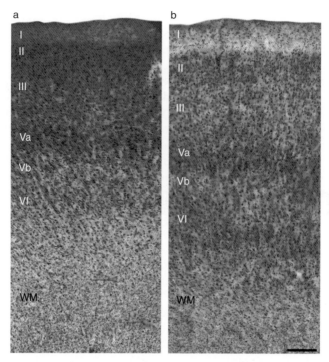

Figure 17.4   Cortical layers I–IV of the anterior cingulate cortex. Note that the cortical lamination is similar in both the control (a) and patient with autism (b), highlighting the need for further stereologic study to determine whether there are changes at the cellular level. Scale bar = 200 μm.

24a, b, and c as defined by Vogt et al. (1995). The tissue was 80 μm thick and Nissl-stained. Seven sections were analyzed per case with the optical fractionator probe to determine whether there were differences in VEN or pyramidal neuron number. Layers I–III were analyzed together, as were layers V and VI. The pyramidal neurons were counted through these layers in a square counting frame of 50 μm within a square grid of 290 μm. VENs were counted with no exclusionary parameters in two randomly selected sections per case throughout layer V. Neuron volume was also measured with the vertical nucleator using four rays. The results demonstrated no difference in lamination in the majority of autism cases (Figure 17.4) or in overall VEN density, although more specific changes were observed. There was a laterality difference in area 24a in autism, with significantly higher pyramidal neuron densities in layers I–III in the left hemisphere as compared to the right. There was also a significant reduction in pyramidal neuron size in autism through all layers analyzed in area 24b, which substantiated qualitative findings of reduced neuron size by Kemper and Bauman (1993; 1998). Neuronal packing density was significantly reduced in layers V–VI in area 24c as well, which is consistent with previously reported reductions in neuronal density in the FG and amygdala (Schumann and Amaral, 2006; van Kooten et al., 2008), though not consistent with the above-mentioned qualitative studies, which reported increased neuronal density. As each subarea in area 24 presented a unique pathology, the authors speculated that areas in which neuronal size and density are altered may be those in which neuronal development or circuitry have been selectively affected in autism.

Although there was no overall effect on VEN density in the autism group as a whole, there were distinct subgroups present with differences in VEN density in comparison to controls. Three patients with autism, all with abnormal cytoarchitecture, had significantly higher VEN density when compared to controls in areas 24a and 24b. Of the remaining six patients, two had cytoar-chitecture irregularities and all had significantly lower density of VENs than controls in 24a, b, and c. The authors suggested that the reduction in VENs may cause a disruption in information processing in the ACC, and may result in a reduction in the ability of patients with autism to modulate social interaction. The presence of subgroups points to the potential reflection of the "spectrum" of autism spectrum disorders—the interindividual variability is quite large, and it would be advantageous to be able to separate postmortem tissue into subgroups based on their place on the spectrum. It is also possible that these subgroups were formed because of the method used to estimate VEN population in these cases. VEN density changes throughout the expanse of the ACC, and as VENs were only counted in two random sections in each case, it is possible that estimates of VEN number were not accurate because all sections of the ACC were not included.

Posterior Cingulate Cortex

Blatt and colleagues also assessed the posterior cingulate cortex (PCC, area 23) because of its role in processing the significance of faces and events (Oblak et al., 2011; Table 17.5). The study used thionine-stained materials for neuronal density and parvalbumin- and calbindin-immunoreactive sections for GABAergic interneuron densities. There were eight patients with autism (19–54 years old) and eight controls (20–63 years old) from both sexes. Using the optical fractionator, the authors examined the superficial (layers I–IV) and deep (layers V–VI) layers. Thionine-stained

Table 17.5   Summary of stereologic parameters in the posterior cingulate cortex

Study	Oblak et al. (2011)
Area, layers	Area 23, superficial (I–IV) and deep (V–VI) layers
Number of autism, controls	8, 8
Age range of autism, controls	19–54, 20–63
Sex	M and F
Stain	Nissl—thionin, parvalbumin, calbindin
Section thickness	Thionin: 80 μm Parvalbumin and calbindin: 40 μm
Number of sections (average)	n/a
Objective	63× oil
Probes used	Optical fractionator
Disector	Thionin: 20 μm Parvalbumin and calbindin: 10 μm
Guard zone	Thionin: 5 μm Parvalbumin and calbindin: 4 μm
Counting frame	Thionin: 1600 μm^2 (area) Parvalbumin and calbindin: 4800 μm^2 (area)
Grid size	Thionin: 1050 × 1050 μm (layers I–IV), 830 × 830 μm (layers V–VI) Parvalbumin and calbindin: 330 × 330 μm
Coefficient of error	≤0.09
Results	No significant differences found

Source: Oblak, A. L., Rosene, D. L., Kemper, T. L., Bauman, M. L., Blatt, G. J. 2011. Altered posterior cingulate cortical cyctoarchitecture, but normal density of neurons and interneurons in the posterior cingulate cortex and fusiform gyrus in autism. *Autism Res* **4** (3): 200–211.

neurons were counted in an area of $1600\,\mu m^2$ through $20\,\mu m$ of tissue in a square grid of $1050\,\mu m$ in superficial layers and $830\,\mu m$ in deep layers. Parvalbumin- and calbindin-immunolabeled interneurons were counted through $10\,\mu m$ of tissue in a $4800\,\mu m^2$ area of a $330\,\mu m$ square grid. Their stereologic results showed no significant differences in neuron and interneuron density, nor a difference in relative density and percentage of parvalbumin- or calbindin-immunoreactive interneurons, although the calbindin-expressing interneurons showed a trend toward a reduced density in autism. The authors did observe abnormal cytoarchitecture in all patients with autism, though the layers in which alterations were present were not consistent. Some cases also presented with an uncharacteristic increase in white matter neurons in the PCC. Because of the abnormal neuronal distribution and density of white matter neurons in autism, the authors suggested that this reflects a failure of proper cortical development during cortical plate migration. The reduced amount of calbindin-expressing interneurons may support this hypothesis, as these interneurons are critical for minicolumn organization (Mountcastle, 1997). This pathology could affect the social and emotional processing that occurs in the PCC, which may then affect areas the PCC interacts with, such as the FG.

Hippocampus

The hippocampus is a broadly studied area in regard to the mechanisms of memory formation and storage. It is also known as a structure of the "limbic system," a group of midline cortical areas that have consistently been implicated in autism. Blatt and colleagues assessed the hippocampal and subiculum areas in 5 males with autism and 5 male controls, aged 13–54 and 14–63, respectively (Lawrence et al., 2010; Table 17.6). The tissue was stained for calbindin, parvalbumin, and

Table 17.6 Summary of stereologic parameters in the hippocampus

Study	Lawrence et al. (2010)
Area, layers	Hippocampal and subicular subfields
Number of autism, controls	5, 5
Age range of autism, controls	13–54, 14–63
Sex	M
Stain	Calbindin, parvalbumin, calretinin
Section thickness	$50\,\mu m$
Number of sections (average)	≥7
Objective	63× oil
Probes used	Optical fractionator, Cavalieri
Disector	n/a
Guard zone	$2\,\mu m$
Counting frame	$50 \times 50\,\mu m$
Grid size	$100 \times 100\,\mu m$
Coefficient of error	≤0.1
Results	↑ density of parvalbumin interneurons in CA1, CA3, anterior body of the hippocampal formation ↑density of calbindin interneurons in dentate gyrus ↑ density of calretinin interneurons in CA1

Source: Lawrence, Y. A., Kemper, T. L., Bauman, M. L., Blatt, G. J. 2010. Parvalbumin-, calbindin-, and calretinin-immunoreactive hippocampal interneuron density in autism. *Acta Neurol Scand* **121** (2): 99–108.

calretinin immunoreactivity, which are all proteins that bind to calcium to prevent an overabundance of intracellular calcium. The study aimed to determine potential differences in the density of interneurons and their relative densities between areas and diagnoses. A disruption in regulation by these interneurons may be a cause of autism, and a difference in their densities may provide support for the excitation/inhibition imbalance hypothesis of autism (e.g., see Gogolla et al., 2009; Yizhar et al., 2011; Dinstein et al., 2012). For this study, the authors analyzed at least seven 50-μm-thick sections per case using the optical fractionator probe. The interneuron population was estimated with a counting frame of $50 \times 50\,\mu m$ in a grid of $100 \times 100\,\mu m$ with a guard zone of $2\,\mu m$. The authors used the Cavalieri principle to determine area volume as well. The results of this study showed differences throughout the interneuron populations between autism and controls. There was an increase in density of parvalbumin-immunoreactive interneurons in the CA1 and CA3 subfields and the anterior body of the hippocampal formation in patients with autism. Patients with autism also had an increased density of calbindin-expressing interneurons in the dentate gyrus and an increased density of calretinin-expressing interneurons in the CA1. A qualitative analysis of densities across ages showed no major difference in these calcium-binding proteins in controls, though they seemed to be smaller and denser in autism, particularly in the subiculum subfields. The potential implication of these results is an impact on information interchanged in the hippocampus, and could even stem beyond the hippocampus to areas such as the PFC, which receives input from the CA1. On the other hand, it is also possible that pathology in the PFC (as described above) may be causing the abnormalities in the hippocampus.

Previous nonstereologic reports have also found increased cell packing density in autism (Bauman and Kemper, 1985, 2005) and a reduction in GABAergic receptors in autism (Blatt et al., 2001; Guptill et al., 2007). In addition, morphological abnormalities have been observed in the neurons and cytoarchitecture in the hippocampus in autism (Weidenheim et al., 2001; Wegiel et al., 2010).

Noncortical Areas

There are several studies analyzing noncortical structures in autism, chiefly the amygdala and cerebellum (outlined in Figure 17.1). These regions communicate with the cortex and provide important feedback to many areas that have been investigated for neuropathologic changes. These cortical alterations may be caused by or be reflections of changes in these ventral portions of the brain, and researchers are beginning to investigate what these differences might be.

Amygdala

Another area closely tied in the neural circuitry thought to modulate social behavior is the amygdala, most well known for its role in emotional learning (Cahill et al., 1995; Phelps and LeDoux, 2005; LeDoux, 2007). Bauman and Kemper (1985) and Kemper and Bauman (1993) qualitatively assessed the amygdala of seven patients with autism, reporting a decreased size and increased neuron density in the medial, central, and cortical nuclei. More recently, this area was studied with stereologic techniques to determine whether differences in neuron number were present in male controls, aged 11–44 years of age (Schumann and Amaral, 2005), and males with autism, aged 10 to 44 years of age (Schumann and Amaral, 2006; Table 17.7). The study was first carried out in controls in 2005 and was compared with patients with autism a year later. The 100 μm-thick tissue was Nissl-stained, and neuron number in each individual nucleus in the amygdala was determined using the optical fractionator probe. The authors counted through 9 μm of tissue using a 3-μm guard zone in a square counting frame of 60 μm. Neuron size was estimated using six rays in the

Table 17.7   Summary of stereologic parameters in the amygdala

Study	Schumann and Amaral (2006)
Area, layers	Amygdalar nuclei
Number of autism, controls	9, 10
Age range of autism, controls	10–44, 11–44
Sex	M
Stain	Nissl—thionin
Section thickness	100 μm
Number of sections (average)	25
Objective	100× oil
Probes used	Optical fractionator, nucleator, Cavalieri
Disector	9 μm
Guard zone	3 μm
Counting frame	60 × 60 μm
Grid size	Lateral nucleus: 6250 μm^2 Basal nucleus: 4000 μm^2 Accessory basal nucleus: 2250 μm^2 Central nucleus: 1000 μm^2 Remaining nuclei: 4000 μm^2
Coefficient of error	≤0.1
Results	↓ neuron number in amygdala and in lateral nucleus and in amygdala as a whole

Source: Schumann, C. M., Amaral, D. G. 2006. Stereological analysis of amygdala neuron number in autism. *J Neurosci* **26** (29): 7674–7679.

nucleator probe, and amygdala nuclei volumes were assessed with the Cavalieri probe. The results of this study showed no difference in the volume of the amygdala or its nuclei, nor any difference in neuron size. However, there was a significant reduction in neuron number in autism in the amygdala as a whole, with controls having a mean of 12.21×10^6 compared to a mean of 10.74×10^6 neurons in patients with autism. Several individual nuclei had a trend toward a decrease in neurons, but the lateral nucleus showed a significant reduction in patients with autism (3.47×10^6) compared to controls (4.00×10^6). The authors speculated that the reduction in neuron number in the amygdala is due to the generation of a reduced amount of neurons during development or to abnormal degeneration that may occur after a typical early development. As the age range of the cases spanned from 10 to 44 years, a closer look at younger developmental ages may provide insight toward the cause of this neuropathology. The differences between the results of these two studies may be accounted for by the presence of epileptic comorbidity in many of the cases in Bauman and Kemper's study, as well as by the differences in quantification methodologies.

Cerebellum

Initially thought to be primarily involved in the coordination of motor actions, the role of the cerebellum in the regulation of affect has progressively come to light. The study of clinical cases revealed that lesions, usually involving the vermis and fastigial nucleus, consistently resulted in newly diagnosed neuropsychiatric impairments such as a lack of impulse-control, tactile defensiveness, ritualistic behaviors, and the inability to appreciate social boundaries (Schmahmann et al., 2007). In this context, the presence of cerebellar alterations in autism became an area of interest and, even though results are still controversial, the cerebellum is certainly one of the most extensively explored brain regions in the field of autism neuropathology. From 1980 to 2002, 8 studies have assessed the effect on Purkinje cells in patients with autism, 20 out of 27 cases having showed a reduction in Purkinje cell number or density. Fatemi and colleagues determined that the mean size of Purkinje cells in patients with autism was 24% smaller compared to controls (Fatemi et al., 2002). Despite these rather convincing results, a weakness of these studies is the presence, in the autism cases, of comorbidities such as epilepsy that can themselves cause a reduction in neuron number and thus bias the results (Haut et al., 2004; Schmitz and Rezaie, 2008).

To more accurately determine the potential involvement of Purkinje cell loss in autism, Whitney et al. (2008) reevaluated the area using stereology to quantify cell populations (Table 17.8). Unlike previous analyses of this area that used a Nissl stain, the authors used immunohistochemistry with an anti-calbindin antibody, which labels the vast majority of Purkinje cells. Six patients with autism aged 13–54 and four controls aged 17–53 were assessed for Purkinje cell number in Crus II. Both sexes were included in this study, and ten 30μm-thick sections were analyzed using the optical fractionator. The Purkinje cells were counted exhaustively through 7.5–8.5 μm of the tissue, excluding the Purkinje cells found at the top or bottom of the plane. The authors found no significant difference in density of Purkinje cells between the two groups. However, as several studies in other areas have observed, there were two subgroups of patients with autism. Three patients had similar densities to the control group, but the other three patients had a reduction in Purkinje cell number. By using precise stereologic methods, this study pointed out possible inconsistencies in the previous findings that had reported a reduction of Purkinje cell number in autism. More

Table 17.8 Summary of stereologic parameters in the cerebellum

Study	Whitney et al. (2008)	Whitney et al. (2009)
Area, layers	Cerebellar hemisphere lobule crus II, Purkinje cell layer	Cerebellar hemisphere lobule crus II, molecular layer
Number of autism, controls	6, 4	6, 4
Age range of autism, controls	13–54, 17–53	13–54, 17–53
Sex	M and F	M and F
Stain	Calbindin	Parvalbumin
Section thickness	30μm	30μm
Number of sections (average)	10	10
Objective	40×	40×
Probes used	Optical fractionator	Optical fractionator
Disector	7.5–8.5μm	7.5–8.5μm
Guard zone	None—top and bottom cells excluded	None—top and bottom interneurons excluded
Counting frame	None—exhaustive counting	$100 \times 75\mu m$
Grid size	None—exhaustive counting	$600 \times 450\mu m$
Coefficient of error	≤0.09	n/a
Results	No significant differences found overall; two subgroups identified, one with ↓ Purkinje cells	No significant differences found

Sources: Whitney, E. R., Kemper, T. L., Bauman, M. L., Rosene, D. L., Blatt, G. J. 2008. Cerebellar Purkinje cells are reduced in a subpopulation of autistic brains: a stereological experiment using calbindin-D28k. *Cerebellum* 7 (3): 406–416.
Whitney, E. R., Kemper, T. L., Rosene, D. L., Bauman, M. L., Blatt, G. J. 2009. Density of cerebellar basket and stellate cells in autism: evidence for a late developmental loss of Purkinje cells. *J Neurosci Res* **87** (10): 2245–2254.

importantly, these results demonstrated the presence of significant interindividual differences and of possible distinct subgroups, highlighting the heterogeneous nature of the disorder.

A subsequent study by the same group used the same cases but immunostained for parvalbumin to quantify the inhibitory GABAergic basket and stellate interneurons that innervate the Purkinje cells (Whitney et al., 2009; Table 17.8). Once again, ten 30 μm-thick sections were analyzed with the optical fractionator to determine interneuron number in the molecular layer. The interneurons were counted in 7.5–8.5 μm of tissue in a counting frame of 100 by 75 μm in a grid of 600 by 450 μm. No guard zones were used, but all interneurons in the top and bottom of the plane were excluded. No significant difference was found between groups in packing density of either type of interneuron or in their ratio to Purkinje neurons. The loss of Purkinje cells in patients with autism, despite a normal amount of innervating interneurons, was interpreted with regard to neurodevelopment: Purkinje cells were initially present in normal numbers and distribution but later degenerated, probably between 32 weeks of gestation and early postnatal life (Blatt, 2005).

These stereologic data are complemented by other nonstereologic studies; a recent study on the molecular pathogenesis of Fragile X syndrome demonstrated a 40% decrease in the number of Purkinje cells in the cerebellum in all three patients, one of which was also diagnosed with autism (Greco et al., 2011). Other alterations were noted, namely incorrect orientation and abnormal clustering of Purkinje cells, undulations of the internal granular layer, abnormalities in axons, and the presence of astrocytes in the white matter. Atrophy in the anterior and posterior parts of the vermis was also quantitatively determined. Other groups confirmed these results, consistent with the hypothesis of compromised cerebellar development in patients with autism. Wegiel and collaborators (2010) reported the presence of flocculonodular dysplasia in the cerebellum of 6 out of 13 patients ranging from age 7 to 56 and in the vermis of a 13-year-old patient, as well as of cerebellar hypoplasia in a 60-year-old patient. In addition, Weidenheim et al. (2001) observed swollen axon terminals, called spheroids, in the cerebellum of one patient with autism. Even though we do not fully understand the mechanisms underlying the relationship between the neuropathologic alterations observed in the cerebellum in autism and the symptomatic manifestations of the disorder, the previously discussed studies clearly point to the implication of this region in its etiopathogeny.

Brainstem

Although no stereologic studies have been performed so far, many qualitative studies exist in the brainstem. Apart from the frequently cited social impairments characteristic of autism, a less well-known comorbidity is the presence of hearing deficits (Tomchek and Dunn, 2007). This led Kulesza and Mangunay (2008) to explore an auditory brainstem structure, the medial superior olive. Confirming their hypothesis, five patients with autism (aged 8–32) showed a significant disruption in cell morphology, particularly in cell body shape and orientation, compared to the two controls (aged 26 and 29). Another study focusing on the brainstem reported that in young patients with autism, deep cerebellar nuclei and inferior olivary neurons appeared enlarged, but in older patients these neurons become pale and reduced in size (Kemper and Bauman, 1993). In the same line, a case study by Rodier et al. (1996) reported the presence of marked alterations in the brainstem of a 21-year-old patient with autism. They found an almost complete lack of facial nucleus and superior olive as well as a global shortening of the brainstem between the trapezoid body and inferior olive. Similarly, Bailey et al. (1998) described the presence of olivary dysplasia in three out of five cases of autism and, in two cases, abnormally placed neurons, relatively to the olivary complex, were observed. Taking a closer look at cellular morphology in several areas of the brainstem, Weidenheim et al. (2001) observed the presence of spheroids (also described in other brain regions in autism, see earlier discussion) in the periaqueductal gray matter and reticular formation of the midbrain, the dorsal raphe, locus coeruleus and interpeduncular nucleus of the pons, and the sensory nuclei of the medulla. Although not conclusive given the low number of cases and the lack of precise quantitative data, these findings provide a strong case for further exploration of the brainstem and its possible implication in autism.

Conclusions

Stereology provides researchers with a set of tools to explore neuropathology and anatomy quantitatively and may allow us to uncover a plethora of alterations among diagnoses within the spectrum. While qualitative assessments and nonstereologic design are at risk of yielding incorrect data when determining parameters such as cell density, the studies summarized above are invaluable in the detail and precision of their outcome, in spite of the low number of cases available.

The available stereologic studies point to consistent, yet in some studies, subtle neuronal alterations in autism. To understand what causes one person to develop autistic symptoms requires delving deeper into the delicate differences in the patterning, type, and number of cells that populate the human brain. Brain regions involved in functions such as social cognition may be affected, especially in layers that process high-order information, while areas delegated for functions unaffected in autism are spared. One such network is the face processing circuit, involving the FG, amygdala, orbital PFC, ACC, and superior temporal gyrus. Each of these areas has been studied in autism and has either been implicated neuropathologically or through functional imaging (Saitovitch et al., 2012).

Pathways are not exclusive, however, and similar brain regions are involved in many different processes. An effect in neuron size in an output layer will affect outputs to each area that receives its projections. An alteration in the FG may not only affect face processing but also the social-affective brain circuits, and in turn the areas that send and receive their information, such as the amygdala, PFC, ACC, FI, and ventral striatum. Once again, this theory is validated by both neuropathologic and imaging studies (Davidson and Irwin, 1999) and lends support to the importance of assessing not only individual areas, but also the layers and cells within them.

Despite the advances made since the advent of stereology, there are still several factors limiting the impact and interpretation of most neuropathologic studies of autism. The need for studies with a higher number of subjects and the use of precise quantitative methodologies are essential, considering the inconsistent results of different studies focusing on each brain region. Several studies have also emphasized the importance of investigating autism as a heterogeneous condition, and of acknowledging its developmental and highly individual characteristics. We can no longer simply compare a group of patients with autism to controls; we must consider their age, severity of autism, intelligence, and comorbidities. An increase in donations to brain banks and more centralized collections will ideally allow for more specific distinctions between groups, separating by age, sex, hemisphere, and even autism severity. As shown through the comparison of studies investigating one area using cases with distinct demographics, these details can lead to very different results. Stereology does allow the freedom for investigators to compare overall results between cases with different tissue staining, thicknesses, and stereologic parameters, which is a vital resource in a field in which tissue is sparse.

The quantitative and reliable definition of cell-type specific alterations and determination of phenotypes of vulnerability along the course of the disease are avenues we are beginning to explore through neuropathologic studies in autism. One day these findings may shed light on the pathogenic mechanisms in autism and possibly point toward therapeutic avenues for prevention and/or cure.

References

Aldinger, K. A., Plummer, J. T., Qiu, S., Levitt, P. 2011. SnapShot: genetics of autism. *Neuron* **72** (2): 418–8 e1.

Allman, J. M., Hakeem, A., Erwin, J. M., Nimchinsky, E., Hof, P. 2001. The anterior cingulate cortex: the evolution of an interface between emotion and cognition. *Ann N Y Acad Sci* **935**: 107–117.

Allman, J. M., Watson, K. K., Tetreault, N. A., Hakeem, A. Y. 2005. Intuition and autism: a possible role for Von Economo neurons. *Trends Cogn Sci* **9** (8): 367–373.

Allman, J. M., Tetreault, N. A., Hakeem, A. Y., Manaye, K. F., Semendeferi, K., Erwin, J. M., Goubert, V., Hof, P. R. 2010. The von Economo neurons in frontoinsular and anterior cingulate cortex of great apes and humans. *Brain Structure and Function* **214**: 495–517.

American Psychiatric Association. 2000. *Diagnostic and Statistical Manual of Mental Disorders*. Washington, DC: American Psychiatric Association.

Bailey, A., Luthert, P., Dean, A., Harding, B., Janota, I., Montgomery, M., Rutter, M., Lantos, P. 1998. A clinicopathological study of autism. *Brain* **121** (Pt 5): 889–905.

Bauman, M., Kemper, T. L. 1985. Histoanatomic observations of the brain in early infantile autism. *Neurology* **35** (6): 866–874.

Bauman, M. L., Kemper, T. L. 2005. Neuroanatomic observations of the brain in autism: a review and future directions. *Int J Dev Neurosci* **23** (2–3): 183–187.

Bhardwaj, R. D., Curtis, M. A., Spalding, K. L., Buchholz, B. A., Fink, D., Bjork-Eriksson, T., Nordborg, C., Gage, F. H., Druid, H., Eriksson, P. S., Frisen, J. 2006. Neocortical neurogenesis in humans is restricted to development. *Proc Natl Acad Sci U S A* **103** (33): 12564–12568.

Blatt, G. J. 2005. GABAergic cerebellar system in autism: a neuropathological and developmental perspective. *Int Rev Neurobiol* **71**: 167–178.

Blatt, G. J., Fitzgerald, C. M., Guptill, J. T., Booker, A. B., Kemper, T. L., Bauman, M. L. 2001. Density and distribution of hippocampal neurotransmitter receptors in autism: an autoradiographic study. *J Autism Dev Disord* **31** (6): 537–543.

Bolte, S., Hubl, D., Feineis-Matthews, S., Prvulovic, D., Dierks, T., Poustka, F. 2006. Facial affect recognition training in autism: can we animate the fusiform gyrus? *Behav Neurosci* **120** (1): 211–216.

Bookheimer, S. 2002. Functional MRI of language: new approaches to understanding the cortical organization of semantic processing. *Annu Rev Neurosci* **25**: 151–188.

Brüne, M., Schobel, A., Karau, R., Benali, A., Faustmann, P. M., Juckel, G., Petrasch-Parwez, E. 2010. Von Economo neuron density in the anterior cingulate cortex is reduced in early onset schizophrenia. *Acta Neuropathol (Berl)* **119** (6): 771–778.

Butti, C., Santos, M., Uppal, N., Hof, P. R. 2011. Von Economo neurons: clinical and evolutionary perspectives. *Cortex* **49**: 312–316.

Cahill, L., Babinsky, R., Markowitsch, H. J., McGaugh, J. L. 1995. The amygdala and emotional memory. *Nature* **377** (6547): 295–296.

Carper, R. A., Courchesne, E. 2005. Localized enlargement of the frontal cortex in early autism. *Biol Psychiatry* **57** (2): 126–133.

Casanova, M., Trippe, J. 2009. Radial cytoarchitecture and patterns of cortical connectivity in autism. *Philos Trans R Soc Lond B Biol Sci* **364** (1522): 1433–1436.

Casanova, M. F., El-Baz, A., Vanbogaert, E., Narahari, P., Switala, A. 2010. A topographic study of minicolumnar core width by lamina comparison between autistic subjects and controls: possible minicolumnar disruption due to an anatomical element in-common to multiple laminae. *Brain Pathol* **20** (2): 451–458.

Center for Disease Control. 2012. Prevalence of autism spectrum disorders—Autism and Developmental Disabilities Monitoring Network, 14 sites, United States, 2008. *MMWR Morb Mortal Wkly Rep* **61** (SS03): 1–19.

Chenn, A., Walsh, C. A. 2002. Regulation of cerebral cortical size by control of cell cycle exit in neural precursors. *Science* **297** (5580): 365–369.

Coleman, P. D., Romano, J., Lapham, L., Simon, W. 1985. Cell counts in cerebral cortex of an autistic patient. *J Autism Dev Disord* **15** (3): 245–255.

Courchesne, E., Mouton, P. R., Calhoun, M. E., Semendeferi, K., Ahrens-Barbeau, C., Hallet, M. J., Barnes, C. C., Pierce, K. 2011. Neuron number and size in prefrontal cortex of children with autism. *J Am Med Assoc* **306** (18): 2001–2010.

Craig, A. D. 2002. How do you feel? Interoception: the sense of the physiological condition of the body. *Nat Rev Neurosci* **3** (8): 655–666.

Craig, A. D. 2003. Interoception: the sense of the physiological condition of the body. *Curr Opin Neurobiol* **13** (4): 500–505.

Craig, A. D. 2009. How do you feel-now? The anterior insula and human awareness. *Nat Rev Neurosci* **10** (1): 59–70.

Critchley, H. D., Wiens, S., Rotshtein, P., Ohman, A., Dolan, R. J. 2004. Neural systems supporting interoceptive awareness. *Nat Neurosci* **7** (2): 189–195.

Davidson, R. J., Irwin, W. 1999. The functional neuroanatomy of emotion and affective style. *Trends Cogn Sci* **3** (1): 11–21.

Devinsky, O., Morrell, M. J., Vogt, B. A. 1995. Contributions of anterior cingulate cortex to behaviour. *Brain* **118** (Pt 1): 279–306.

Dinstein, I., Heeger, D. J., Lorenzi, L., Minshew, N. J., Malach, R., Behrmann, M. 2012. Unreliable evoked responses in autism. *Neuron* **75** (6): 981–991.

Fatemi, S. H., Halt, A. R., Realmuto, G., Earle, J., Kist, D. A., Thuras, P., Merz, A. 2002. Purkinje cell size is reduced in cerebellum of patients with autism. *Cell Mol Neurobiol* **22** (2): 171–175.

Fuster, J. M. 2001. The prefrontal cortex—an update: time is of the essence. *Neuron* **30** (2): 319–333.

Gogolla, N., Leblanc, J. J., Quast, K. B., Sudhof, T. C., Fagiolini, M., Hensch, T. K. 2009. Common circuit defect of excitatory-inhibitory balance in mouse models of autism. *J Neurodev Disord* **1** (2): 172–181.

Gohlke, J. M., Griffith, W. C., Faustman, E. M. 2007. Computational models of neocortical neuronogenesis and programmed cell death in the developing mouse, monkey, and human. *Cereb Cortex* **17** (10): 2433–2442.

Greco, C. M., Navarro, C. S., Hunsaker, M. R., Maezawa, I., Shuler, J. F., Tassone, F., Delany, M., Au, J. W., Berman, R. F., Jin, L.-W., Schumann, C., Hagerman, P. J., Hagerman, R. J. 2011. Neuropathologic features in the hippocampus and cerebellum of three older men with fragile X syndrome. *Mol Autism* **2** (1): 2.

Guptill, J. T., Booker, A. B., Gibbs, T. T., Kemper, T. L., Bauman, M. L., Blatt, G. J. 2007. [3H]-flunitrazepam-labeled benzodiazepine binding sites in the hippocampal formation in autism: a multiple concentration autoradiographic study. *J Autism Dev Disord* **37** (5): 911–920.

Haut, S. R., Veliskova, J., Moshe, S. L. 2004. Susceptibility of immature and adult brains to seizure effects. *Lancet Neurol* **3** (10): 608–617.

Jacot-Descombes, S., Uppal, N., Wicinski, B., Santos, M., Schmeidler, J., Giannakopoulos, P., Heinsen, H., Schmitz, C., Hof, P. R. 2012. Decreased pyramidal neuron size in Brodmann areas 44 and 45 in patients with autism. *Acta Neuropathol (Berl)* **124** (1): 67–79.

Kanwisher, N., Stanley, D., Harris, A. 1999. The fusiform face area is selective for faces not animals. *Neuroreport* **10** (1): 183–187.

Kaufman, J. A., Paul, L. K., Manaye, K. F., Granstedt, A. E., Hof, P. R., Hakeem, A. Y., Allman, J. M. 2008. Selective reduction of Von Economo neuron number in agenesis of the corpus callosum. *Acta Neuropathol (Berl)* **116** (5): 479–489.

Kemper, T. L., Bauman, M. 1998. Neuropathology of infantile autism. *J Neuropathol Exp Neurol* **57** (7): 645–652.

Kemper, T. L., Bauman, M. L. 1993. The contribution of neuropathologic studies to the understanding of autism. *Neurol Clin* **11** (1): 175–187.

Kennedy, D. P., Semendeferi, K., Courchesne, E. 2007. No reduction of spindle neuron number in frontoinsular cortex in autism. *Brain Cogn* **64** (2): 124–129.

Kim, E.-J., Sidhu, M., Gaus, S. E., Huang, E. J., Hof, P. R., Miller, B. J., DeArmond, S. J., Seeley, W. W. 2012. Selective frontoinsular von Economo neuron and fork cell loss in early behavioral variant frontotemporal dementia. *Cereb Cortex* **22** (2): 251–259.

Kleinhans, N. M., Richards, T., Sterling, L., Stegbauer, K. C., Mahurin, R., Johnson, L. C., Greenson, J., Dawson, G., Aylward, E. 2008. Abnormal functional connectivity in autism spectrum disorders during face processing. *Brain* **131** (Pt 4): 1000–1012.

Kulesza, R. J., Mangunay, K. 2008. Morphological features of the medial superior olive in autism. *Brain Res* **1200**: 132–137.

Larsen, C. C., Bonde Larsen, K., Bogdanovic, N., Laursen, H., Graem, N., Samuelsen, G. B., Pakkenberg, B. 2006. Total number of cells in the human newborn telencephalic wall. *Neuroscience* **139** (3): 999–1003.

Lawrence, Y. A., Kemper, T. L., Bauman, M. L., Blatt, G. J. 2010. Parvalbumin-, calbindin-, and calretinin-immunoreactive hippocampal interneuron density in autism. *Acta Neurol Scand* **121** (2): 99–108.

LeDoux, J. 2007. The amygdala. *Curr Biol* **17** (20): R868–R874.

Miller, E. K., Cohen, J. D. 2001. An integrative theory of prefrontal cortex function. *Annu Rev Neurosci* **24**: 167–202.

Mountcastle, V. B. 1997. The columnar organization of the neocortex. *Brain* **120** (Pt 4): 701–722.

Mouton, P. R. 2011. *Unbiased Stereology: A Concise Guide*, Baltimore, MD: The Johns Hopkins University Press.

Oblak, A. L., Rosene, D. L., Kemper, T. L., Bauman, M. L., Blatt, G. J. 2011. Altered posterior cingulate cortical cyctoarchitecture, but normal density of neurons and interneurons in the posterior cingulate cortex and fusiform gyrus in autism. *Autism Res* **4** (3): 200–211.

Phelps, E. A., LeDoux, J. E. 2005. Contributions of the amygdala to emotion processing: from animal models to human behavior. *Neuron* **48** (2): 175–187.

Pierce, K., Muller, R. A., Ambrose, J., Allen, G., Courchesne, E. 2001. Face processing occurs outside the fusiform "face area" in autism: evidence from functional MRI. *Brain* **124** (Pt 10): 2059–2073.

Pierce, K., Haist, F., Sedaghat, F., Courchesne, E. 2004. The brain response to personally familiar faces in autism: findings of fusiform activity and beyond. *Brain* **127** (Pt 12): 2703–2716.

Piggot, J., Kwon, H., Mobbs, D., Blasey, C., Lotspeich, L., Menon, V., Bookheimer, S., Reiss, A. L. 2004. Emotional attribution in high-functioning individuals with autistic spectrum disorder: a functional imaging study. *J Am Acad Child Adolesc Psychiatry* **43** (4): 473–480.

Rodier, P. M., Ingram, J. L., Tisdale, B., Nelson, S., Romano, J. 1996. Embryological origin for autism: developmental anomalies of the cranial nerve motor nuclei. *J Comp Neurol* **370** (2): 247–261.

Saitovitch, A., Bargiacchi, A., Chabane, N., Brunelle, F., Samson, Y., Boddaert, N., Zilbovicius, M. 2012. Social cognition and the superior temporal sulcus: implications in autism. *Rev Neurol (Paris)* **168**: 762–770.

Samuelsen, G. B., Larsen, K. B., Bogdanovic, N., Laursen, H., Graem, N., Larsen, J. F., Pakkenberg, B. 2003. The changing number of cells in the human fetal forebrain and its subdivisions: a stereological analysis. *Cereb Cortex* **13** (2): 115–122.

Santos, M., Uppal, N., Butti, C., Wicinski, B., Schmeidler, J., Giannakopoulos, P., Heinsen, H., Schmitz, C., Hof, P. R. 2011. von Economo neurons in autism: a stereologic study of the frontoinsular cortex in children. *Brain Res* **1380**: 206–217.

Schmahmann, J. D., Weilburg, J. B., Sherman, J. C. 2007. The neuropsychiatry of the cerebellum—insights from the clinic. *Cerebellum* **6** (3): 254–267.

Schmitz, C., Hof, P. R. 2005. Design-based stereology in neuroscience. *Neuroscience* **130** (4): 813–831.

Schmitz, C., Rezaie, P. 2008. The neuropathology of autism: where do we stand? *Neuropathol Appl Neurobiol* **34** (1): 4–11.

Schmitz, N., Rubia, K., van Amelsvoort, T., Daly, E., Smith, A., Murphy, D. G. 2008. Neural correlates of reward in autism. *Br J Psychiatry* **192** (1): 19–24.

Schumann, C. M., Amaral, D. G. 2005. Stereological estimation of the number of neurons in the human amygdaloid complex. *J Comp Neurol* **491** (4): 320–329.

Schumann, C. M., Amaral, D. G. 2006. Stereological analysis of amygdala neuron number in autism. *J Neurosci* **26** (29): 7674–7679.

Seeley, W. W. 2010. Anterior insula degeneration in frontotemporal dementia. *Brain Struct Funct* **214** (5–6): 465–475.

Seeley, W. W., Carlin, D. A., Allman, J. M., Macedo, M. N., Bush, C., Miller, B. L., DeArmond, S. J. 2006. Early frontotemporal dementia targets neurons unique to apes and humans. *Ann Neurol* **60** (6): 660–667.

Seeley, W. W., Allman, J. M., Carlin, D. A., Crawford, R. K., Macedo, M. N., Greicius, M. D., DeArmond, S. J., Miller, B. L. 2007. Divergent social functioning in behavioral variant frontotemporal dementia and Alzheimer disease: reciprocal networks and neuronal evolution. *Alzheimer Dis Assoc Disord* **21** (4): S50–S57.

Senju, A. 2012. Spontaneous theory of mind and its absence in autism spectrum disorders. *Neuroscientist* **18** (2): 108–113.

Simms, M. L., Kemper, T. L., Timbie, C. M., Bauman, M. L., Blatt, G. J. 2009. The anterior cingulate cortex in autism: heterogeneity of qualitative and quantitative cytoarchitectonic features suggests possible subgroups. *Acta Neuropathol (Berl)* **118** (5): 673–684.

Tomchek, S. D., Dunn, W. 2007. Sensory processing in children with and without autism: a comparative study using the short sensory profile. *Am J Occup Ther* **61** (2): 190–200.

Tyler, L. K., Marslen-Wilson, W. D., Randall, B., Wright, P., Devereux, B. J., Zhuang, J., Papoutsi, M., Stamatakis, E. A. 2011. Left inferior frontal cortex and syntax: function, structure and behaviour in patients with left hemisphere damage. *Brain* **134** (Pt 2): 415–431.

Uylings, H. B., Malofeeva, L. I., Bogolepova, I. N., Jacobsen, A. M., Amunts, K., Zilles, K. 2005. No postnatal doubling of number of neurons in human Broca's areas (Brodmann areas 44 and 45)? A stereological study. *Neuroscience* **136** (3): 715–728.

van Kooten, I. A., Palmen, S. J., von Cappeln, P., Steinbusch, H. W., Korr, H., Heinsen, H., Hof, P. R., van Engeland, H., Schmitz, C. 2008. Neurons in the fusiform gyrus are fewer and smaller in autism. *Brain* **131** (Pt 4): 987–999.

Vogt, B. A., Nimchinsky, E. A., Vogt, L. J., Hof, P. R. 1995. Human cingulate cortex: surface features, flat maps, and cytoarchitecture. *J Comp Neurol* **359** (3): 490–506.

Wegiel, J., Kuchna, I., Nowicki, K., Imaki, H., Wegiel, J., Marchi, E., Ma, S. Y., Chauhan, A., Chauhan, V., Bobrowicz, T. W., de Leon, M., Louis, L. A., Cohen, I. L., London, E., Brown, W. T., Wisniewski, T. 2010. The neuropathology of autism: defects of neurogenesis and neuronal migration, and dysplastic changes. *Acta Neuropathol (Berl)* **119** (6): 755–770.

Weidenheim, K. M., Goodman, L., Dickson, D. W., Gillberg, C., Rastam, M., Rapin, I. 2001. Etiology and pathophysiology of autistic behavior: clues from two cases with an unusual variant of neuroaxonal dystrophy. *J Child Neurol* **16** (11): 809–819.

West, M. J., Slomianka, L., Gundersen, H. J. 1991. Unbiased stereological estimation of the total number of neurons in the subdivisions of the rat hippocampus using the optical fractionator. *Anat Rec* **231** (4): 482–497.

Whitney, E. R., Kemper, T. L., Bauman, M. L., Rosene, D. L., Blatt, G. J. 2008. Cerebellar Purkinje cells are reduced in a subpopulation of autistic brains: a stereological experiment using calbindin-D28k. *Cerebellum* **7** (3): 406–416.

Whitney, E. R., Kemper, T. L., Rosene, D. L., Bauman, M. L., Blatt, G. J. 2009. Density of cerebellar basket and stellate cells in autism: evidence for a late developmental loss of Purkinje cells. *J Neurosci Res* **87** (10): 2245–2254.

Williams, J. H. 2008. Self-other relations in social development and autism: multiple roles for mirror neurons and other brain bases. *Autism Res* **1** (2): 73–90.

Yizhar, O., Fenno, L. E., Prigge, M., Schneider, F., Davidson, T. J., O'Shea, D. J., Sohal, V. S., Goshen, I., Finkelstein, J., Paz, J. T., Stehfest, K., Fudim, R., Ramakrishnan, C., Huguenard, J. R., Hegemann, P., Deisseroth, K. 2011. Neocortical excitation/inhibition balance in information processing and social dysfunction. *Nature* **477** (7363): 171–178.

Index

Note: Entries followed by "f" denote figures; "t" denotes tables.

Neurostereology: Unbiased Stereology of Neural Systems, First Edition. Edited by Peter R. Mouton.
© 2014 John Wiley & Sons, Inc. Published 2014 by John Wiley & Sons, Inc.

Keep up with critical fields

Would you like to receive up-to-date information on our books, journals and databases in the areas that interest you, direct to your mailbox?

Join the **Wiley e-mail service** - a convenient way to receive updates and exclusive discount offers on products from us.

Simply visit **www.wiley.com/email** and register online

We won't bombard you with emails and we'll only email you with information that's relevant to you. We will ALWAYS respect your e-mail privacy and NEVER sell, rent, or exchange your e-mail address to any outside company. Full details on our privacy policy can be found online.

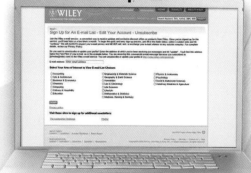

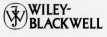 WILEY-BLACKWELL

www.wiley.com/email

17841